AF836005

PRINCIPLES OF PATHOBIOLOGY

PRINCIPLES OF

Edited by Mariano F. LaVia

New York · OXFORD UNIVERSITY PRESS

PATHOBIOLOGY

and Rolla B. Hill, Jr.

London · 1971 · Toronto

Copyright © 1971 by Oxford University Press, Inc.
Library of Congress Catalogue Card Number: 79-146041
Printed in the United States of America

FOREWORD

Classically, the pathologist has contributed to the study of human disease by describing advanced changes in cells and tissues, and it has often appeared that disease states differed fundamentally from the normal condition. More recently, because of tremendous advances in our knowledge of biochemistry, physiology, and microbiology as applied to medicine, we have been able to trace the pathogenesis of many disorders from their early onset. This new book presents the concept of disease as an abnormal biological process which differs quantitatively, rather than qualitatively, from normal biological mechanisms. This approach will illuminate for medical, dental, and biology students the study of disease and will fill a significant deficit in the textual material presently available.

The book consists of seven chapters covering the basic areas of pathology. The chapters on cellular changes, inflammation, and host-parasite relationships discuss several states in the reaction to injury, progressing from the molecular to the organismal level. These sections are written by active experimental pathologists who recognize that the compartmentalization of knowledge, a laudable and necessary goal in the research laboratory, cannot be the objective of students. Rather, students must integrate an infinite number of changes in ultrastructural organization and intermediary metabolism caused by multiple insults at the cellular level, and superimpose an awareness of the interactions and control processes of cells and tissue at the organ and organismal level.

Although growth is a response to injury as well as a normal phase of development, uncontrolled growth or neoplasia has assumed a unique role in pathology. Recent progress in understanding the implications of viruses, hormones, and immunological factors in carcinogenesis is of intense current interest to all biologists; in addition, the older work on physical and chemical carcinogens has taken on a new relevance. The chapter on neoplasia is one of the few available in the literature which makes a careful review of the entire field.

Immunological mechanisms play a dual role in injury and defense reactions. Antibody response to foreign moieties, such as bacteria and viruses, may protect an individual against clinical disease. Acute and delayed hypersensitivity, formerly associated with anaphylaxis, serum sickness, and tuberculosis, have now proven to be a serious problem in organ transplantation. "Self-injury" or autoimmunization has become of great importance in diseases affecting all organs, but particularly the kidney, thyroid, bowel, heart, and central nervous system.

In the final chapter, we are reminded that, in addition to well-documented biochemical inborn errors of metabolism, cytogenetic abnormalities, and teratologic defects in development, all disease states have a genetic basis which eventually determines the fate of the organism.

The editors have done a splendid job of identifying six basic areas of pathobiology or general pathology. They have presented their information in a succinct, integrated manner in a beautifully illustrated text, small enough to be used in core curricula, and large enough to provide an excellent review of the current state of the field.

DONALD WEST KING
Delafield Professor of Pathology
College of Physicians and Surgeons
Columbia University

PREFACE

It is a truism that several conflicting forces are making the design of curricula in the biological and medical sciences very difficult. The much touted information explosion of recent years must somehow be dealt with in these curricula. Disciplines are losing their discrete identities, and it is not always clear what is medical and what is biological. Disciplinary teaching time in required courses in medical schools is rapidly diminishing to allow for more electives and "integrated," interdisciplinary courses.

In its own field this textbook is an attempt to reconcile these conflicts and to fill a void that has existed for several years. The subject matter is that which has been known as General Pathology—the interface between biology and pathology, encompassing growth, metabolism, and biologic interaction as well as the effects of external and internal injuries on these general processes. It will be useful in those medical and dental schools where pressures have forced the adoption of a limited "core" curriculum in general pathology; it will be equally appropriate for biology or zoology departments that feel the need to expose their students to the principles governing some of the extremes of biological activity known as disease. The book is designed for easy use by busy students; it deals with current knowledge directly and intelligibly, avoiding the reconditeness and jargon of research papers.

In organizing this book it has been necessary to make some hard decisions. Some areas in general pathology that might be considered important have been either omitted or dealt with very briefly because of space limitations. Other relatively rare entities have been stressed because of fundamental concepts which they illuminate. We make no apologies for these decisions, which have been made consciously but which will obviously differ from the decisions that might have been made by others. Similar thought has gone into the bibliographies, which are thorough but in no sense exhaustive. It has been our abiding rule to consider the needs and capabilities of the student in the modern curriculum.

ROLLA B. HILL, JR.
MARIANO F. LA VIA

February 1971

ACKNOWLEDGMENTS

Chapter 2 Supported by USPHS grant AM-10698 from the National Institute of Arthritis and Metabolic Diseases. The authors wish to express their appreciation to the following colleagues who reviewed the manuscript and made many helpful suggestions:

Ruth Ellen Bulger, Charles A. Daniels, Fred L. Ginn, Peter J. Goldblatt, Hal K. Hawkins, Hugo O. Jauregui, Wolfgang J. Mergner, Bernard Poeschel, Norman B. Ratcliff, Somphong Sahaphong, and John D. Shelburne.

Chapter 3 Supported by grant AI-07291 from the Institute of Allergy and Infectious Diseases.

Chapter 4 The author wishes to express his appreciation to Miss Ala Jo Tester for secretarial work.

Chapter 5 Supported by USPHS grant AI-9294-01 and grant T-290D from the American Cancer Society. The author wishes to express his thanks to the following colleagues and students who reviewed the manuscript and made many helpful suggestions:

Council Dudley, Joseph Feldman, Richard Franson, and William Monteforti.

Chapter 6 Supported by USPHS grants CA-08856, CA-06927 and FR-05539 from the National Cancer Institute, grant IN-49 from the American Cancer Society, and by an appropriation from the Commonwealth of Pennsylvania.

Chapter 7 The author wishes to express his appreciation to C. Nash Herndon for reviewing the manuscript and making many useful suggestions.

A special note of gratitude goes to Mrs. Emily Cook for her untiring energy in typing and retyping the entire manuscript, to Mrs. Barbara De Weerd for her help in compiling the Subject Index, and to Mr. John Mc Intyre for proofreading.

CONTRIBUTORS

ANTTI U. ARSTILA, M.D.
Associate Professor of Pathology
Director, Electron Microscopy Laboratory
University of Turku
Turku, Finland

ROLLA B. HILL, JR., M.D.
Professor and Chairman
Department of Pathology
State University of New York
Upstate Medical Center
Syracuse, New York 13210

MARIANO F. LA VIA, M.D.
Professor
Department of Pathology
Emory University School of Medicine
Atlanta, Georgia 30322

CHARLES E. MCCALL, M.D.
Assistant Professor of Medicine
Associate in Pharmacology
The Bowman Gray School of Medicine
Winston-Salem, North Carolina 27103

RICHMOND T. PREHN, M.D.
Senior Member
The Institute for Cancer Research
Fox Chase
Philadelphia, Pennsylvania 19111

BENJAMIN F. TRUMP, M.D.
Professor and Chairman
Department of Pathology
University of Maryland
Baltimore, Maryland 21201

PETER A. WARD, M.D.
Chief, Immunobiology Branch
University of Connecticut
School of Medicine
Hartford, Connecticut 06105

ROBERT H. SHIKES
Assistant Professor
Department of Pathology
University of Colorado
Medical Center
Denver, Colorado 80220

CONTENTS

PRINCIPLES OF PATHOBIOLOGY

1

PATHOBIOLOGY AND THE MEDICAL SCIENCES

Rolla B. Hill, Jr., M.D.

> "Contemplations of nature and of bodies in their simple form break up and distract the understanding, while contemplations of nature and bodies in their composition and configuration overpower and dissolve the understanding . . . for that school is so busy with the particles that it hardly attends to the structure, while the others are so lost in admiration of the structure that they do not penetrate to the simplicity of nature."
>
> Francis Bacon

During its short life the discipline of cellular biology has grown with astonishing rapidity. Enormous and unenvisioned knowledge has been gained. The mechanism of transfer of genetic information is being steadily clarified; the mysteries of the control and expression of that genetic information are gradually yielding to experimentation; tools are being applied which allow the forbidding problems of morphogenesis, differentiation, and maturation to be approached.

Progress toward general understanding of disease at the molecular or cellular level has not kept pace with advances in normal biology, yet there are many isolated examples of brilliant work illuminating aspects of abnormal biology. For instance, our understanding of the nature of viral parasitism, of the specific enzymatic defects in the inborn errors of metabolism, of aspects of immunological deficiencies and diseases, and of the causes of hemoglobinopathies, has been greatly enriched by knowledge gained in the study of normal biology.

These new contributions to the study of disease have been achieved by close co-operation among scientists from disciplines previously devoted separately to normal or abnormal biology. From this fruitful union came pathobiology, a science integrating cell biology and classical pathology, encompassing normal processes of growth, metabolism, and biologic interaction, and the effects of external and internal injuries on these processes.

This science has not been with us long enough to have generated a strong philosophical basis, and we still grope at times to find applicability and meaning. Nevertheless, we must attempt a modern approach to what, in the heyday of descriptive morphologic pathology, was the unity of structure and function, when disease (dysfunction) was to be understood as a reflection of altered anatomy. Dyspnea and cyanosis in pneumonia were caused by the presence of inflammatory debris in the alveoli. Jaundice occurred because blockage of ducts prevented the excretion of bilirubin. Even this approach, which may seem grossly mechanistic to us, is little more than two hundred years old. For the long centuries prior to Morgagni, Bernard, Pasteur, and Virchow, the concept of a direct pathogenetic relation between altered structure and disease was foreign to medical thinking. The concept still has considerable utility, but the time is ripe for a refinement of thought not possible previously.

In 1943, W. D. Forbus, in his book *Reaction to Injury,* attempted to crystallize what was then a relatively new viewpoint in pathology: that disease did not exist except as a reaction to injury. A monumental two-volume tome classifying diseases according to types of injurious agents instead of topology set forth this view. Although the format was not widely adopted in teaching programs, the vision insinuated itself into pathology. A dialectical outgrowth of Forbus's contribution has been the concept that disease is *not the imposition of new, different structure and function, but simply the quantitative alteration–increase or decrease –of existing pathways.* The synthesis of these views is that to understand pathology we must understand the changes in structures and functions which occur in response to various injuries. The injurious agents themselves may determine the direction that a reaction will take, but they are bystanders to the disease itself. Once an injury has occurred, forces within the cell, tissue, or organism are brought into action; the interaction of these forces is what produces disease. Responses to injury can be isolated, dissected, and classified, and eventually the individual factors making up the total response can be identified. Although these individual responses are not infinite, they can occur in a bewildering number of combinations and strengths.

This is the subject of pathobiology–the alterations in normal biological mechanisms that occur in response to injury. Alterations in ribosome structure are as important as alterations in cardiac structure, and interference with oxidative phosphorylation is as crippling as interference with blood flow. Neoplasia and immunity are two parts of a general problem of control of cell division, cell growth, and cell differentiation. The proteins which are important in blood coagulation are synthesized by the same mechanisms and under the same general controls as intracellular enzymes.

The long list of etiological agents of disease does not reflect an equally long list of pathogenetic mechanisms. The dictum that all life processes depend on the cell leads inevitably to questions about these mechanisms. Which category of cellular processes determines the integrity of the cell in response to injury? Although gene action may be a primary directing force, the manifestations of disease must reflect disturbances of enzymatic activity.[1]

This is not to suggest that each injurious agent has a specific enzymatic target. Enzymatic anactivity, hypoactivity, and hyperactivity may result from a direct change in the number of enzyme molecules (through interference with genetic control or any of the steps leading to its expression), or from changes in the physical state of the molecule, or from effects on cofactors, pH, substrates, etc. Study of the purified enzyme *in vitro* may often not reveal these effects; since this highly artificial situation introduces vast changes in availability of cofactors and substrates, ionic strength and physical state, factors of architectural or spatial relationships (for example, enzyme complexes and membrane-bound enzymes) may be totally shattered. Evaluation of enzymes under these conditions may thus indicate an enzyme deficiency which is not in fact present, or it may fail to reveal the presence of an actual functional deficiency. In addition, injuries usually have more than a single target and produce much wider effects than a single enzymatic defect. The enormous discoveries of molecular biology have focused attention on the isolated cell and on isolated injury. The multicellular and the multi-organ organism have so many interlocking, mutually dependent, often mutually corrective mechanisms, that such isolation *in vivo* is indeed rare.

In analyzing injury one can distinguish injuries immediately affecting enzymatic activity from injuries which directly affect a mediating process that then deranges enzymatic activity. These mediators of injury may be chemical structures, e.g. DNA, from which activity of the enzymes originally springs, or physical structures such as a membrane or a polysome, or aggregations of cells whose functions interdependently rely on architectural relationships among them.

Variations in enzymatic activity occur frequently in tissue under normal physiological conditions; in fact, such variations are completely essential to survival. Hormones, differentiation and biological rhythms control enzymatic activities, and it may be difficult to distinguish between normal variation and variation due to injury, which can be identical quantitatively and qualitatively. Indeed,

[1] I am indebted to Dr. Renzo Rendi for making clear to me the central importance of this.

small, virtually undetectable injuries are constantly occurring and the slight corrective responses which approximate servo-mechanisms constitute homeostasis—the means by which an organism maintains its precarious identity in spite of the myriad internal and external injuries which beset living things.

It is the reaction to injury, not the injury itself, that produces the manifestations of disease. In the hereditary condition known as glucose-6-phosphate dehydrogenase deficiency, *in vitro* tests reveal a decrease in assayed enzyme activity of erythrocytes. This certainly reflects a genetic injury, but there are no symptoms, no overt responses, unless a second circumstance (the ingestion of fava beans, for instance, or doses of the drug primaquin) supervenes. The disease, characterized by hemolysis, does not occur without a secondary agent, but the genetic injury is demonstrably present throughout life.

It must be emphasized that pathology and pathobiology are not separate disciplines but simply subdisciplines of the over-all science of biology. There are no new metabolic pathways which occur in an injured cell, there is simply accentuation, diminution, or loss of existing pathways.[2] There are no new structures, there is simply an increase or decrease in structures which occur in so-called normal cells. Paul Weiss has said: "Even the grossest deformity is produced by the same rigorously lawful molecular and cellular interactions that govern normal development" (1960). Minor injuries occur constantly and cause small perturbations in homeostasis which are corrected as servo-mechanisms are thrown into play. All organisms float restlessly between the states of health and disease.

By now the reader is becoming aware of the difficulties surrounding the use of the word *injury*. It is almost axiomatic that traumatic damage, e.g. a knife wound in the skin, causes injury to tissues which elicits certain predictable homeostatic responses in the injured tissues. It is clear that sustained anoxia causes predictable damage and death to cells; a mild degree of hypoxia, however, causes qualitatively similar changes which result not in death, but in a reversibly altered, viable cell. Is this injury? When a recumbent person stands up, striking alterations in vascular physiology occur to accommodate for the alterations related to gravity and change of position—is this injury? Somebody bumps you slightly so that you lose your balance. If you happen to have your feet firmly planted, you can quickly recover your balance without falling. If not, you may fall and this may lead to a bruise or a broken bone, depending on where you are standing. The primary force is the same; the result may be anything from a reflexive rebalancing of muscular tension to severe damage or death.

[2] There are a very few exceptions. For instance, in cellular infection by some RNA viruses, the RNA acts as a repository of genetic information, and a template for the synthesis of messenger or DNA. These have not yet been identified as functions of RNA in normal animal cells.

Can one say, then, that injury occurs whenever the "steady state" is forcibly unbalanced? The agents of injury include anything that is capable of causing unbalance, whether the degree of unbalance is minute or severe, and whether it is correctable or not. Injuries may originate inside or outside the cell. Any minor variation in the external environment requires an adjustment by the cell, and major variations of course, require major adjustments. Injuries originating within the cell are mainly "genetic" mistakes, including those in transcription or translation. In general, external agents of injury fall into the following categories: drugs, parasites (viruses, bacteria, fungi, protozoa, metazoa, etc.), radiation, trauma, temperature, pH, nutrition, and immunologic phenomena.

The pattern formed by combinations of ultrastructural alterations in reaction to injury may occasionally be so characteristic that one can recognize the injury from the changes observed. The repertory of alterations is sharply limited, however, and usually a great many agents act through a common morphologic pathway. Specific diagnosis can rarely be made with the electron microscope.

At the light microscope level, tissues undergo a broader range of morphological alteration, and the permutations and combinations of these alterations are much more likely to give a characteristic diagnostic pattern. These alterations involve the relationships between cells, the cell types, the direction of differentiation of cells, and various degenerative alterations in cells and extracellular materials. Recognition of the patterns formed by these microscopic alterations is the essence of diagnostic pathology, which enables the pathologist to differentiate on morphologic grounds between pneumonia due to pneumococcus and pneumonia due to staphylococcus, between arthritis due to infection and degenerative arthritis, and to detect the precise kind of liver disease which is causing the patient to become jaundiced.

Inflammatory and immunological reactions, both accorded considerable attention in this book, are natural properties of vertebrates. Both are complex combinations of interacting humoral and cellular forces, which contribute considerably to survival in the evolutionary struggle and help in coping with a variety of foreign agents, both living and inanimate. Both are subject also to occasional errors which pervert the reactions, so that considerable damage to host tissue ensues.

Only rarely does an injury lead to disability. It is what happens after the injury that usually causes disease. Certainly the severing of the head with an ax is an injury which in itself causes observable damage and disability. However, the injection of several million *Staphylococcus aureus* under the skin by itself is quite harmless; it is the reaction of the body to the *Staph. aureus* that causes the development of inflammation, abscesses, and pus. In many diseases we do not even know what the injurious agent is. The vast group of diseases collectively called cancer, for instance, has been classified and subclassified and reclassified, but in only a very few cases do we have any clear understanding of the injurious agent. It is the hyperplastic-neoplastic responses to the injury that we see and that cause damage.

Most commonly, injuries are followed by homeostatic responses which restore normalcy. Sometimes a new steady state, differing from the normal but compatible with continued existence, is achieved. Sometimes the compensatory mechanisms which the cell or the body uses constantly to maintain the status quo are insufficient, and balance is not restored. The cell, organ, or body can utilize a great variety of compensatory mechanisms, but in the face of overwhelming or continued injury, these may not be enough. Failure may occur (1) because of a greatly increased load on the cell's adaptive mechanisms or (2) because of damage to the adaptive mechanisms. In the case of energy metabolism, for instance, a cell may under certain circumstances be required to produce an extraordinary amount of ATP. The adaptive mechanisms will allow a mild increase in ATP production from existing structures and pathways, but substantially to alter energy production requires new mitochondria. To make mitochondria, however, takes time and ATP. The cell then can be said to be failing prior to the time when new mitochondria are available. The demands for energy may be so great in fact, that the cell is unable to make enough mitochondria to provide this energy. On the other hand, even normal energy requirements cannot be met by the cell exposed to cyanide, which by poisoning cytochrome oxidase prevents normal energy metabolism.

The broad areas of biological injury dealt with in this book have been traditionally known as general pathology. We have attempted to relate them more closely to the science of general biology in order to provide an anchor in modern biology for the student of pathology and an anchor in pathology for the student of biology.

References

Forbus, W. D. (1943), Reaction to Injury; Pathology for Students of Disease, Williams and Wilkins Co., Baltimore.

Weiss, Paul (1960), Deformities as cues to understanding development of form, *in* Disease and the Advancement of Science, H. K. Beecher, Ed., Harvard University Press, Cambridge, Mass.

2

CELL INJURY AND CELL DEATH

Benjamin F. Trump, M.D., and Antti U. Arstila, M.D.

A. Introduction

The description of general morphologic and functional reactions of cells to injury is central to an understanding of pathologic processes. Although recent developments in cell biology have lead to the concept of molecular diseases, as in sickle cell anemia, and although it may soon be possible to describe and define diseases in terms of organelle reaction to injury, the cell remains the most useful unit for understanding and describing disease.

Traditional concepts regarding the effects of injury on cells have been based on a rather simple notion of the cell as composed of nucleus and cytoplasm. Until the electron microscope was developed the organization of the cytoplasm was also the subject of considerable debate because of the limited resolving power of the light microscope. The modern concept of the cell as composed of a series of organized membrane systems is much more complex, but consideration of cell injury in terms of changes within organelles simplifies the study of cell pathology.

This simplification is in large part due to the ultrastructural similarity of most cells even in widely differing species (Fig. 2-1). The human fibroblast is similar to the amoeba and at the same time to a human neuron. The modern analysis of disease thus has revealed a similarity at the ultrastructural level between such disparate disorders as multiple sclerosis and myocardial infarction (Trump and Ericsson, 1965). These similarities have at the same time afforded the opportunity to develop general hypotheses of cellular reactions to injury and have increased the efficiency of studying the pathogenesis and therapy of human disease.

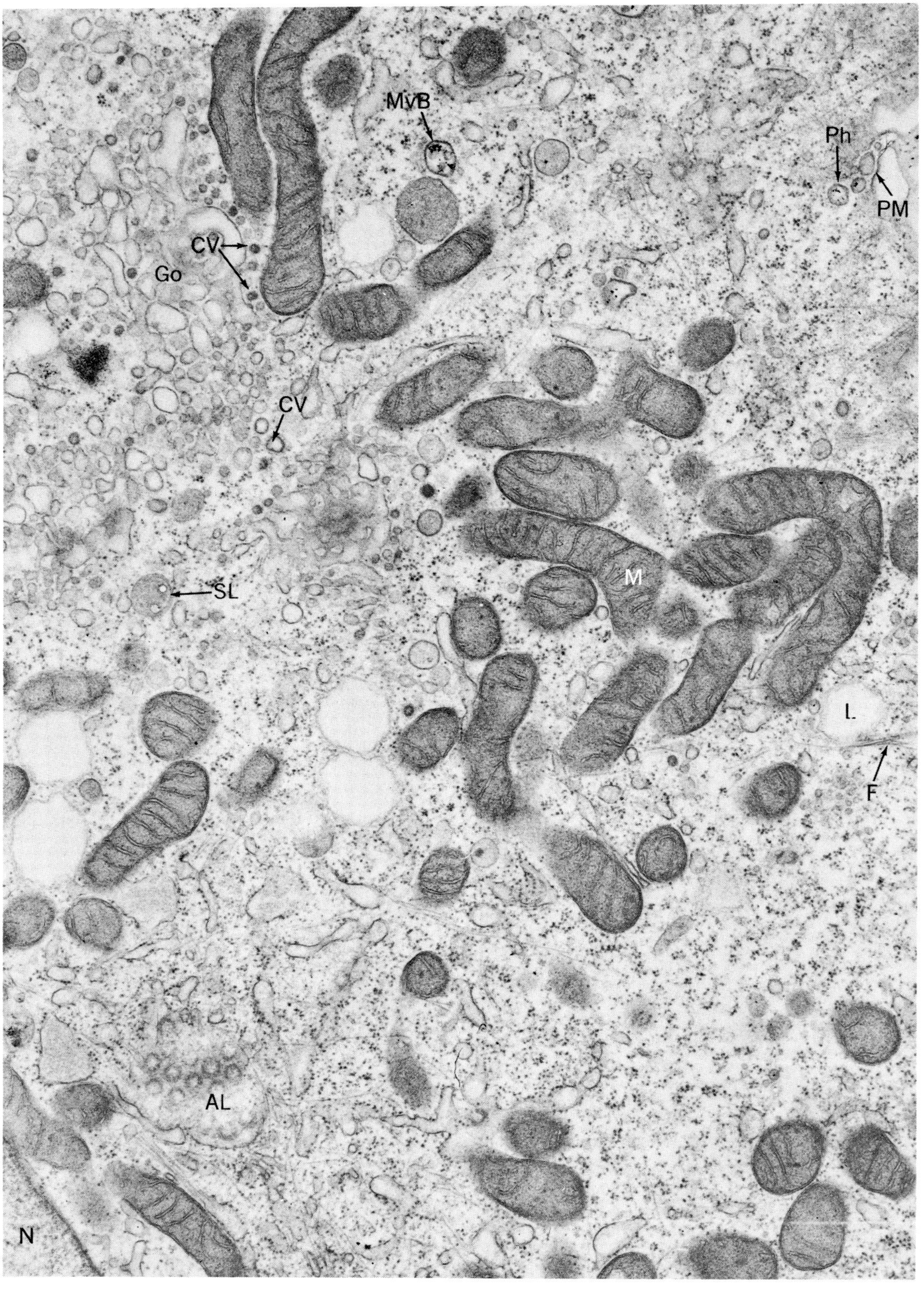

MvB
Ph
PM
CV
Go
CV
SL
M
L
F
AL
N

The study of disease processes in humans is limited by the nature of present techniques and by the difficulty of obtaining repeated data as a function of time and in producing controlled lesions in human subjects. Accordingly, most of our knowledge of disease in the human is derived from models of cell injury produced in other living forms (Trump and Ginn, 1969; Farber and Magee, 1965; de-Reuck and Knight, 1963).

B. Dynamics of Cell Injury

A useful conceptualization of the effects of injury on cells is shown in Fig. 2-2. When a cell in a normal state of homeostasis is injured, it is assumed that homeostasis is altered. Some injuries, even if prolonged, are sublethal; that is, the cell is able to adjust to the presence of continued abnormal stimuli by attaining some new or altered steady state, homeostatically maintained although at a different level. Such adaptations on the part of cells are of great importance in understanding human disease. Examples of new or altered steady states include fat deposition in cells, increased autophagic activity, increased storage of either exogenous or endogenous materials, hypertrophy, atrophy, cell swelling or loss of cell volume control, and even malignant transformation.

A lethal injury is defined as an injury that, if prolonged, results in the cell passing a point beyond which homeostatic mechanisms are unable to operate effectively to restore a steady state, even if the injurious stimulus is removed. This point, or "point of no return," might also be referred to as the point of cell death. It should be emphasized that this is a theoretical point and that conclusions regarding life or death of cells or whole organisms must, at the present state of knowledge, be based on essentially negative experiments (Majno *et al.,* 1960). Following the point of no return the cell can be considered to enter a degradative phase leading ultimately to debris or a state of physicochemical equilibrium (Trump and Ginn, 1969). This phase, from the point of no return to equilibrium, is the phase of necrosis. During this phase many of the reactions are essentially

Figure 2-1. Electron micrograph of a portion of a HeLa Cell illustrating characteristic features of the cytoplasm of mammalian cells. This cell was grown in a medium containing colloidal thorium dioxide, which was phagocytosed by the cells and is present within phagocytic vacuoles. Note the prominent Golgi apparatus (Go) and the appearance of the mitochondria (M), lipid droplets (L), annulate lamellae (AL), phagosomes (Ph), and a multivesicular body (MvB). Coated vesicles (CV) are present near the Golgi apparatus. Cytoplasmic filaments (F) course through the cytoplasm. A secondary lysosome (SL) can be seen, (PM) plasma membrane, and (N) nucleus.

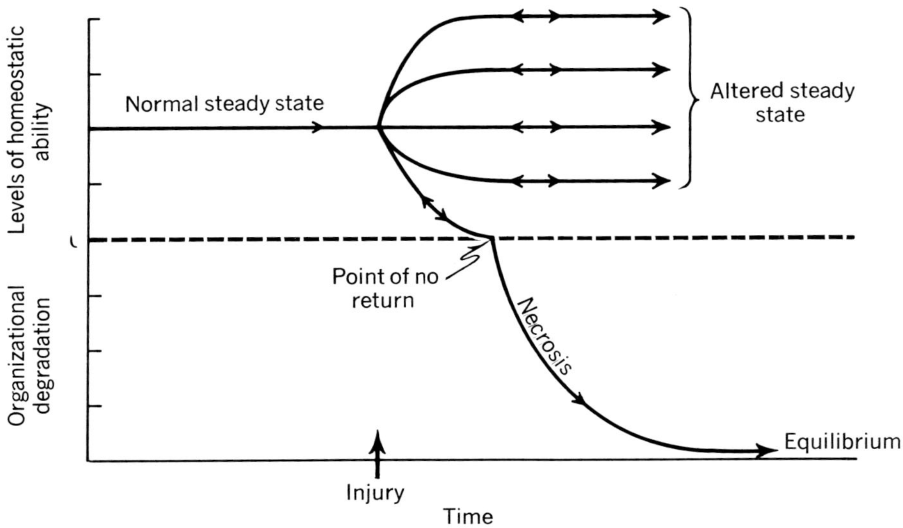

Figure 2-2. Conceptualization of cell injury. Following injury, a cell that is previously in a normal steady state can be considered to enter a phase where the homeostatic mechanisms are altered, resulting in new or altered steady states, such as fatty metamorphosis, hypertrophy, or atrophy. The cell may remain in this new steady state for long periods of time while the injury is continued. In the case of lethal injuries, on the other hand, the cell can eventually be assumed to pass a point, shown as zero level of homeostatic ability, beyond which it is unable to restore equilibrium even if the injury is eliminated. The zero level of homeostatic ability may be referred to as the **point of no return** or the **point of cell death.** Beyond this, the cell undergoes a series of degradative reactions leading to the production of cell debris or a state of physicochemical equilibrium (Trump and Ginn, 1969).

autolytic; they involve digestion of cell components by the cell's own hydrolytic enzymes.

Changes that occur in the necrotic phase are important determinants of the histologic patterns observed in many kinds of disease processes; these are considered in more detail below. Ultimately, necrotic cells may be reabsorbed by the animal or may undergo calcification or desiccation (mummification). In many instances organs are able to repair the defects resulting from necrosis by regenerating new cells from adjacent ones, resulting in reformation of the structures that have been destroyed.

C. Light Microscopy of Injured Cells (Figs. 2-3 and 2-4)

The light microscope remains an extremely useful instrument for the study of injured cells. In recent years the study of fixed tissue sections stained by empiric combinations of dyes such as hematoxylin and eosin (H & E) has been supplemented by a variety of specific staining methods, the use of which can localize many important cellular chemical constituents and enzymes. In addition, the development of other light optical methods such as fluorescence microscopy, phase contrast microscopy, interference microscopy, and polarization microscopy has permitted many observations to be made on unfixed or living cells, thus facilitating detailed analysis of the kinetics of cell injury responses.

1. Lethal reactions

In sectioned and stained preparations it is difficult, if not impossible, to observe changes before the point of no return is reached. The initial changes often involve accentuation of the chromatin clumps in the nucleus. Because of variations with fixation, which may induce chromatin clumping, this alteration is difficult to discern. The earliest cytoplasmic change often observed is increased eosinophilia, resulting partially from increased binding of eosin by cytoplasmic proteins. At the pH conventionally used in staining, eosin is negatively charged; the increased binding has been interpreted as representing the effects of greater exposure of positively charged reactive sites along polypeptide chains following denaturation. Another cause of the increased eosinophilia is the loss of cytoplasmic basophilia (loss of hematoxylin [a "basic" or cationic dye] binding in preparations stained with H & E). This usually reflects detachment and scattering of polysomes from the rough-surfaced endoplasmic cisternae. Another change that can be discerned in the cytoplasm in good preparations is swelling of mitochondria, visible as eosinophilic globules because of their high content of basic proteins. The cell margins may show irregularities and protrusions related to the blebbing phenomena described below (Fig. 2-3a). Late in the course of necrosis, granulation and irregular spaces in the cytoplasm represent the effects of denaturation and digestion of cytoplasmic organelles.

Later changes in the nucleus consist of coarsening and increased basophilia of the chromatin clumps (pyknosis) (Fig. 2-3d), fragmentation of chromatin clumps or nuclei (karyorrhexis), or disappearance of all stainable chromatin material (karyolysis) (Fig. 2-34d). The nuclear changes observed depend in part on the cell type. A common change in the necrotic phase is deposition of complex calcium phosphates within the cytoplasm, often related to mitochondrial damage as described below.

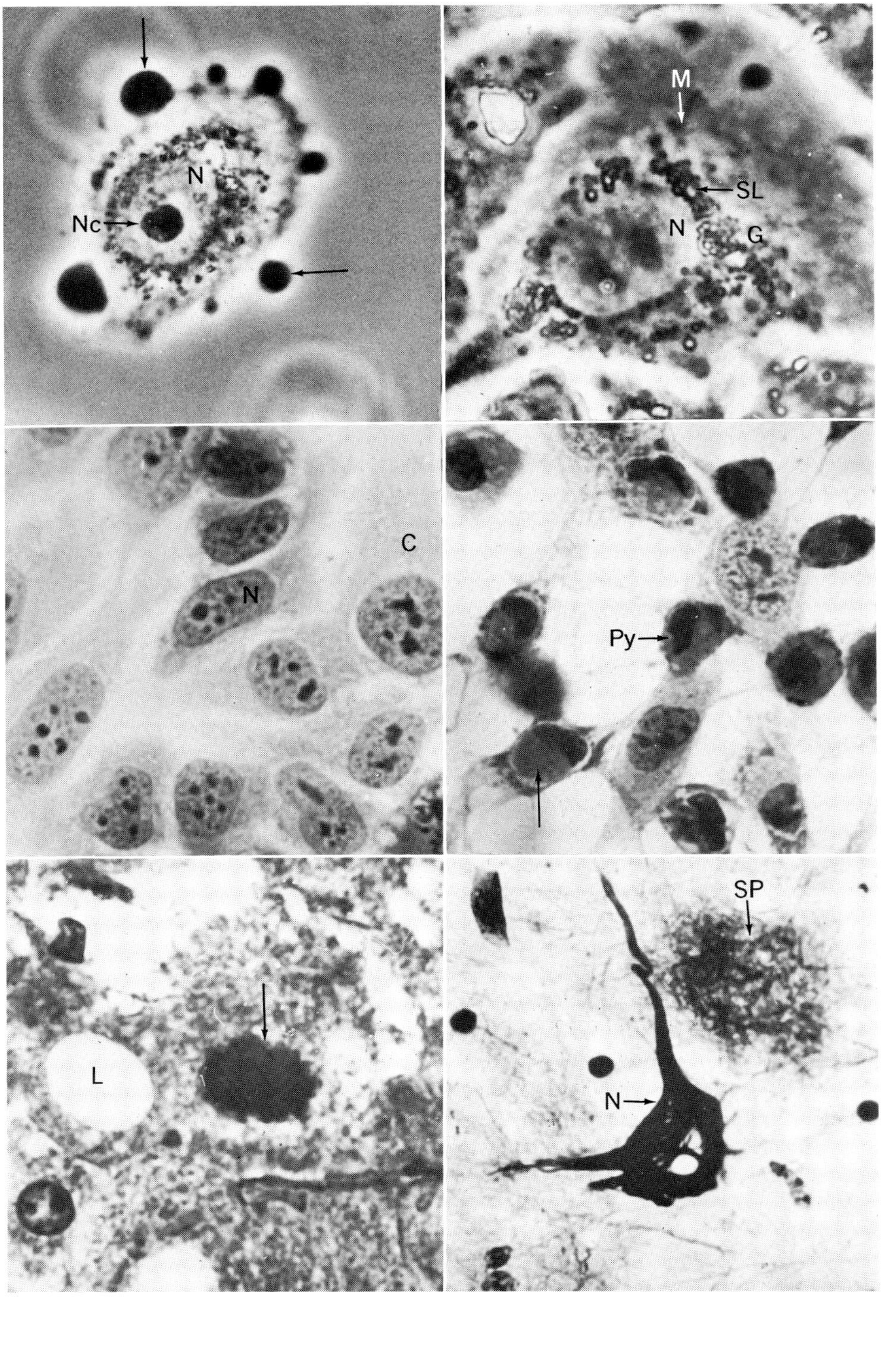
N
Nc
a
M
SL
N
G
b
C
N
c
Py
d
L
e
SP
N
f

2. Pre-lethal or sub-lethal reactions

Vacuoles. Clear "vacuoles," often seen in conventionally stained preparations of injured cells, may be diverse in origin and often difficult or impossible to distinguish or characterize with this technique alone. Accumulations of triglyceride within the cell commonly appear as vacuoles (fatty metamorphosis) (Fig. 2-4d) because of the solubility of such lipids in the materials used for preparing the section. In tissues prepared without lipid solvents, e.g. frozen sections, the lipid may be rather specifically stained by fat-soluble dyes such as Sudan IV or oil red 0. Acid mucopolysaccharides in storage diseases such as Hurler's disease may be removed by aqueous fixatives and also give rise to vacuoles. Other types of irregular clear areas in cells stained with hematoxylin and eosin may simply be due to accumulations of material such as glycogen which do not stain with this technique. In these cases, appropriate staining methods may be used. Glycogen, for example, can readily be stained with the periodic acid-Schiff (PAS) technique.

Many vacuoles, however, represent accumulations of fluid, usually isosmotic with plasma, in various intracellular compartments such as the endoplasmic cis-

Figure 2-3. **a.** HeLa cell 15 minutes after addition of potassium cyanide (10^{-3}M) and iodoacetic acid (10^{-4}M) to the medium. These compounds inhibit both glycolysis and respiration. Blebs (arrows) have appeared at the cell surface. The nucleus (N), the nucleolus (Nc), and the cytoplasmic organelles, visualized as granules in the perinuclear area, have a normal appearance. Phase contrast.

b. Untreated living HeLa cell photographed under phase contrast. Note the thin cytoplasm and cytoplasmic processes. N, nucleus; G, Golgi; SL, secondary lysosomes; M, mitochondrion.

c. Untreated HeLa cells photographed after fixation, sectioning, and staining. The nucleus (N), nucleoli, and cytoplasm (C) appear quite different from those of the unfixed cell in Figure 3b (Courtesy of Dr. C. A. Daniels).

d. HeLa cells 12 hours after infection with polio virus. Note the necrotic cell with shrunken pyknotic nucleus (Py) and eosinophilic cytoplasmic inclusion (arrow). Long cytoplasmic strands emerge from the cell surface. An adjacent nucleus is less altered. These are fixed cells viewed with conventional light microscopy (Courtesy of Dr. C. A. Daniels).

e. Liver cell from a patient with alcoholic cirrhosis. The arrow indicates a mass of alcoholic hyalin in the cytoplasm of a hepatic parenchymal cell. A lipid droplet (L) is also present.

f. Neuron (N) from brain of elderly person showing cytoplasmic staining characteristic of neurofibrillary tangles. A senile plaque (SP) is seen in the upper right.

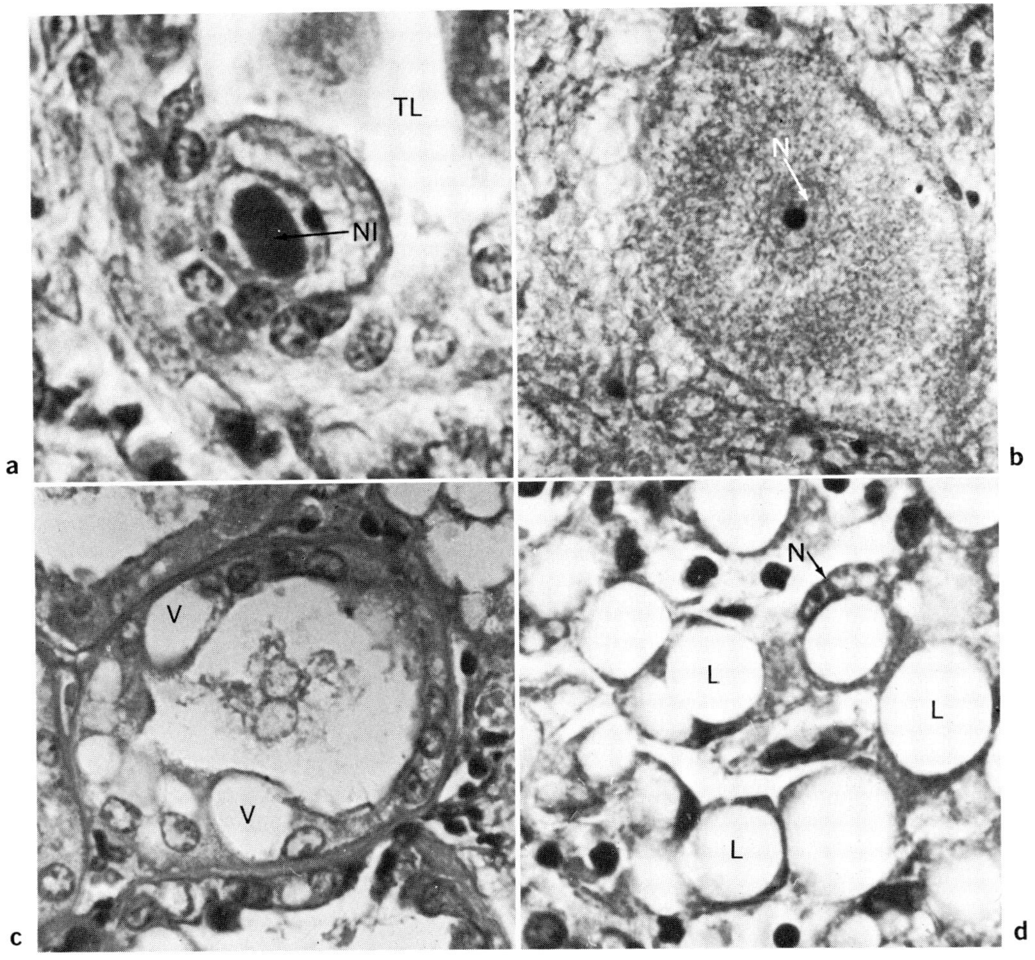

Figure 2-4. **a.** Kidney tubule cell from a patient with cytomegalic inclusion disease; the large nucleus contains an inclusion body (NI) which consists of virus particles. TL, tubular lumen. H & E stain.

b. Spinal neuron from a patient with Tay Sachs disease; the fine, scattered lipid inclusions are basophilic and consist principally of gangliosides. N, nucleus. H & E stain.

c. Kidney tubules from a patient with hypokalemic nephrosis; scattered large vacuoles (V) appear in the proximal tubular epithelium in such patients. H & E stain.

d. Liver cells from a patient with alcoholic cirrhosis. The hepatic parenchymal cells contain large triglyceride droplets (L). Nuclei (N) are indented by the lipid. H & E stain.

ternae, the mitochondria, the digestive vacuoles or lysosomes, the cell sap, or the nucleus. Their nature cannot be established unless specific histochemical or electron microscopic methods are used as detailed below. Such vacuoles are those occurring in renal proximal tubular cells in hypokalemic nephrosis (Fig. 2-4c), those resulting from massive enlargement of endoplasmic cisternae in the liver cell shortly after administration of hepatotoxins such as carbon tetrachloride, and the large intranuclear spaces seen after clumping of the nuclear chromatin.

Inclusions. This term is commonly used to refer to stainable accumulations of material within the nucleus or cytoplasm. Inclusions may be spherical or irregular, and homogeneous or granulofibrillar. Again, the precise identification of such inclusions depends on detailed analysis by cytochemistry and electron microscopy and may require their isolation by differential or density gradient centrifugation. Many inclusions represent accumulations of material within heterophagic or autophagic digestive vacuoles, such as the hyaline droplets of the renal proximal tubules associated with proteinuria. Masses of virus particles may be visible as inclusions (Fig. 2-4a). Mallory's alcoholic hyalin in the liver cells of alcoholics (Fig. 2-3e) (see p. 66) and the neurofibrillary change seen in neurons of the elderly (Fig. 2-3f) or in Alzheimer's disease are examples of inclusions consisting of filaments or microtubules.

Pigment. Many types of pigment may accumulate in cells. These may be endogenous such as lipofuscin or "aging" pigment, hemosiderin, and ferritin, or exogenous such as tattoo pigments or phagocytosed carbon particles. In most cases pigment accumulations are found in hetero- or auto-digestive vacuoles; melanin is an example of a pigment which may occur in exosecretory vacuoles of melanocytes. Accumulation of lipofuscin pigment commonly occurs in cells as a general manifestation of sublethal injury representing a residuum of autophagocytosis.

Inorganic deposits. Abnormal depositions of inorganic material such as calcium phosphate may occur in pathologically altered cells. In Wilson's disease, copper-containing deposits are often seen in digestive vacuoles of the liver and other organs. Crystalline masses are sometimes found in or about injured cells. These may be exogenous, as in the case of foreign bodies, but they may also originate from accumulation of abnormal amounts of metabolites such as oxalate or cystine. Analysis of such deposits often requires the use of polarization microscopy, the electron probe microanalyzer, or analysis by X-ray diffraction.

D. Plasma Membrane (Figs. 2-5 to 2-11)

The plasma membrane (or cell membrane) is in a strategic yet vulnerable position between the extracellular and intracellular compartments. Strategic, because

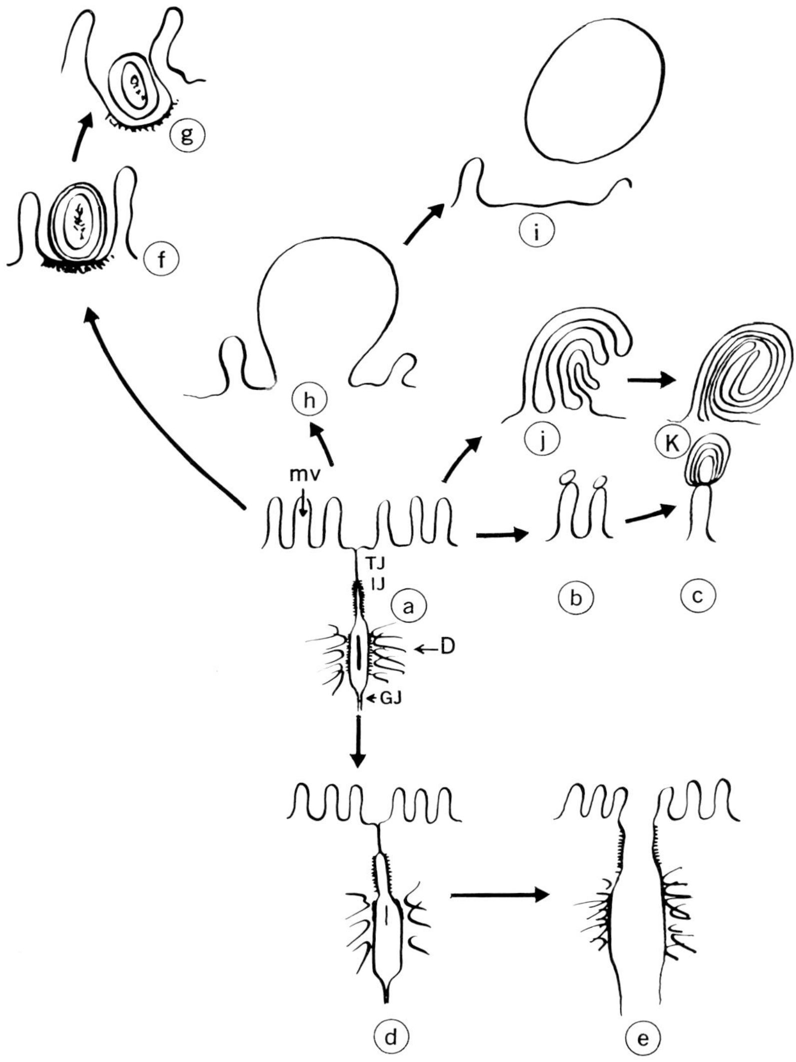

Figure 2-5. Diagrams illustrating configurational changes in the cell membrane after cell injury.

a. A typical normal membrane with microvilli (MV) and components of junctional complex, including tight junction (TJ), intermediate junction (IJ), desmosome (D), and gap junction (GJ).

b & c. Myelin forms involving elaboration of bimolecular leaflets representing extracted phospholipid.

its activities are of great importance in the regulation of homeostasis of the cell interior; vulnerable, because it is exposed to extracellular noxious agents and because it depends so heavily on energy metabolism for maintenance of its functional integrity. Modifications of the plasma membrane are therefore of vital importance in understanding cell injury. Some aspects of normal membrane structure are reviewed by Branton and Park (1968) and Dowben (1969).

1. Configurational changes

Changes in the configuration of plasma membrane structure can be related to changes in activity of membrane-associated enzymes, to changes in permeability, and to changes in electrical resistance. One example of such modification is the thickening of the plasma membrane that results when calcium levels are lowered in the extracellular fluid (Fig. 2-5). This results in increased permeability of the membrane as measured by decreased electrical resistance and is reflected at the cell level by increased uptake of water, sodium, and chloride in approximately isosmotic proportions. Depletion of membrane lipid by treatment of cells with fat solvents or enzymes such as phospholipase has been shown to increase membrane thickness reversibly and to reversibly inhibit membrane-associated enzyme activity (Trump *et al.*, 1970). Anesthetics, which are often lipid soluble, may exert effects on cells which are related to modifications of the physicochemical characteristics of the plasma membrane.

A dramatic example of lytic action on the structure of the membrane is provided by studies of complement-mediated hemolysis in human red cells (Dourmashkin and Rosse, 1966) (see Chapter 5). When such hemolysis occurs, large pores of the order of 90 Å in diameter appear in the membrane. Isosmotic swelling ensues, as described below, followed by stretching and finally bursting of the membrane.

Lipid peroxidation is another important way in which cell membrane structure and function can be modified (Barber and Bernheim, 1967). Peroxidation

d & e. Stages of separation of junctional complexes, occurring as a result of removal of calcium or treatment with chelating agents such as EDTA.

f & g. Stages in absorption of bacteria in small intestine, showing induced formation of spine-like coatings on cytoplasmic surface of membrane adjacent to the ingested organism.

h & i. Two stages in elaboration of an exotropic bleb from the membrane surface.

j & k. Elaboration of tubular forms with formation of concentric arrangements when these protrude into a constrained space such as a kidney tubule or a bile canaliculus.

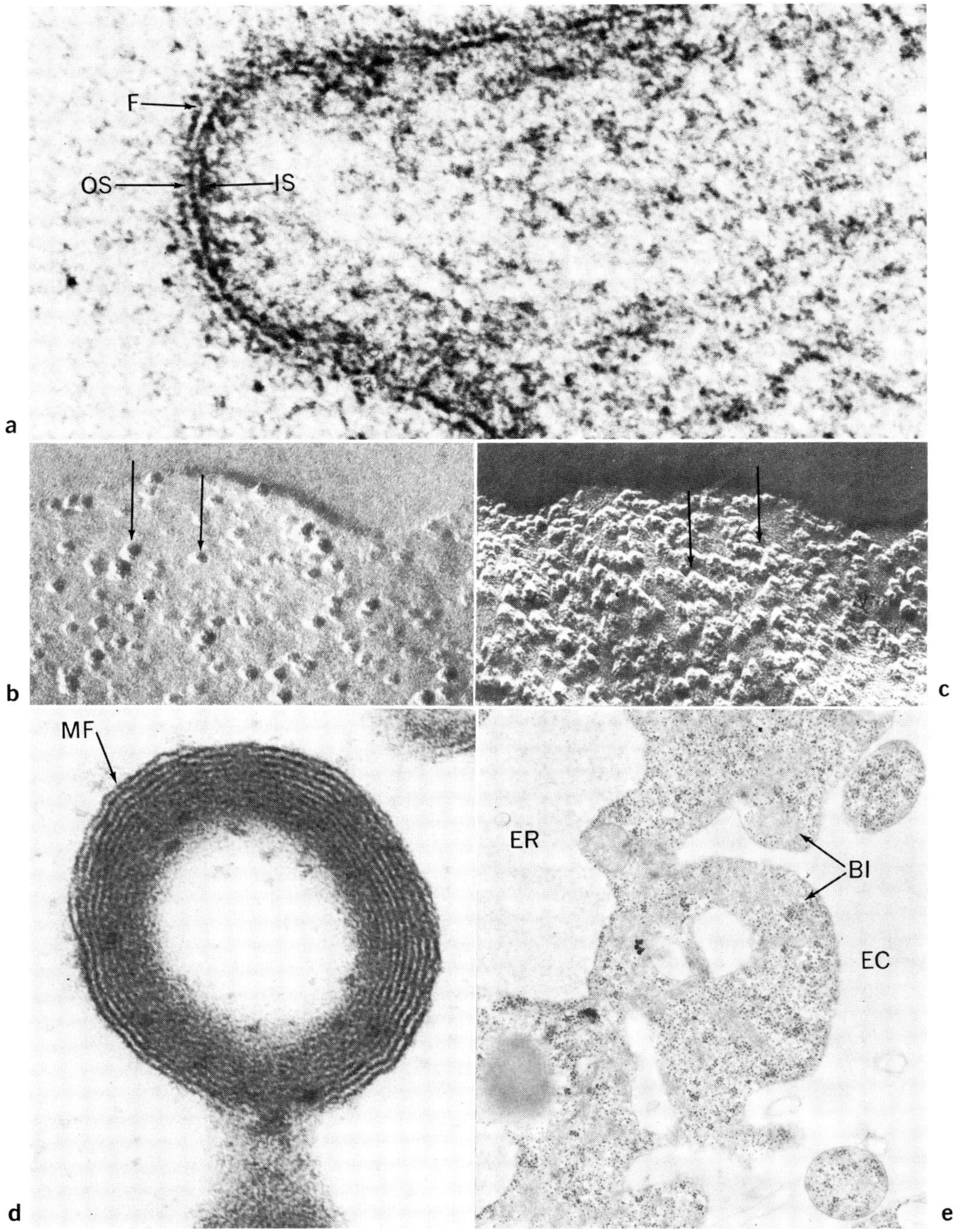
F
OS
IS
a
b
c
MF
ER
BI
EC
d
e

induced by free radical attack on unsaturated membrane lipids is often an important feature of injury to cells, for instance, in ionizing or in ultraviolet irradiation or in deficiency of antioxidants such as Vitamin E. Peroxidative damage to membranes is associated with changes in the architecture of the membrane leading to ultimate breakdown and liberation of phospholipids, which may form adjacent myelin figures.

2. Changes in cell membrane conformation

The plasma membrane is an extremely dynamic structure. In time-lapse movies of normal cells, ruffling movements, vacuole formation, and extrusion of blebs (Fig. 2-3a) are apparent. Changes of surface contour in injury are probably complex phenomena related to changes in electrical charge at the cell interface, compositional changes in the membrane, and/or changes in the surface pressure on the interior or exterior of the membrane itself. In their response to such abnormal environmental conditions, cells exhibit characteristic conformational changes.

Folds, microvilli, and invaginations (Figs. 2-7 and 2-8). The plasma membrane is essentially impermeable to hydrophilic particles much larger than 5Å in diameter; however, larger molecules including proteins, nucleic acids, and polysaccharides can exert effects on cells and apparently enter cells. An important means of entry of macromolecules to the cell is through the phenomenon known as *pinocytosis* or *phagocytosis* or collectively as *endocytosis*.

Figure 2-6. **a.** High magnification picture of a plasma membrane illustrating typical appearance of "unit membrane" in thin sections. OS, outer surface; IS, inner surface; F, "fuzz" coating on outer surface, also known as **glycocalyx.**

b. Human red blood cell membrane prepared by freeze etching. In this preparation the membrane has been cleaved. One is looking at the surface of the inner membrane. Frequent knob-like particles (arrows) are seen in the membrane. (Courtesy of Dr. Gary Kirk).

c. Human red blood cell membrane prepared by freeze etching. In this case one is looking at the inner surface of the outer portion of the membrane. Similar knobs to those seen in Figure 2-6b are present (arrows) (Courtesy of Dr. Gary Kirk).

d. Complex myelin figure at the surface of microvilli in a toad bladder treated with the detergent, cetyl pyridinium chloride. (Courtesy of Mr. Hal K. Hawkins).

e. Electron micrograph of an Ehrlich ascites cell showing a bleb (BL) at the cell surface following treatment with an antibody prepared against Ehrlich ascites cells in the presence of complement. Note dilated ER. EC, extracellular compartment. (Courtesy of Dr. James Hagadorn).

a

b

c

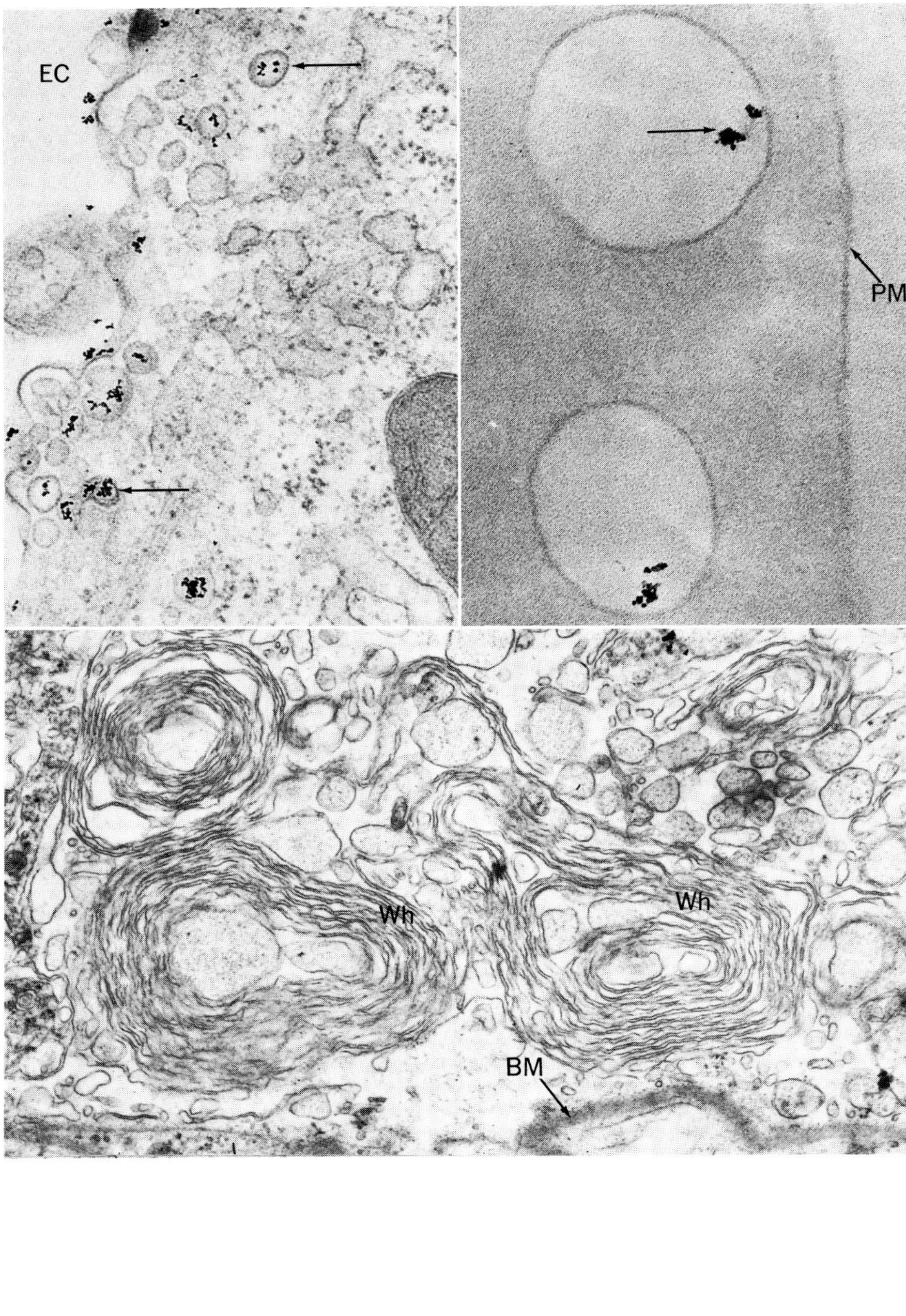

Endocytosis involves the invagination of plasma membranes forming caveolae and then vesicles in which solutes may be concentrated (Figs. 2-7a, 2-7b). This concentration may involve binding of solute particles to the cell surface, possibly to the glycocalyx or polysaccharide coat. Some caveolae, thought to be important in protein uptake, are coated also on the cytoplasmic side. It is probable that most, if not all, cells are capable of endocytosis, although general rules regarding the importance of this to the over-all economy of mammalian cells have not been formulated. It is evident, however, that in some unicellular forms, such as amoeba, virtually the entire nutrition of the cell is based on the uptake of food via endocytosis. It is also conceivable that such events as antigen processing, memory transfer, and interferon production are related to endocytic uptake of macromolecules by cells. Viruses are often taken up by this process (Fig. 2-8).

Endocytosis is also an important means of defense against microorganisms (Figs. 2-5 and 2-8), and certain cells such as the polymorphonuclear leukocyte are especially fit for such a digestive endocytic function. Other cells such as those of the reticuloendothelial system and those lining the proximal tubules of the kidney are very active in clearing particles, including antigens, bacteria, and cell debris, from the circulation via endocytosis. Further details of this process will be discussed in the section on the cytocavitary network.

In amoeba and in cultured mammalian cells endocytic vacuole formation can be induced by addition of suitable compounds to the extracellular fluid. Soluble proteins such as albumin are important inducers of pinocytosis. Increased membrane activity commonly occurs in endothelial cells in areas of inflammation, resulting in the formation of elaborate surface folds or cytofolds along the luminal surface of endothelial cells. Such situations can be observed in many human diseases. One example is the induction of pinocytosis in the proximal tubular cells which occurs in kidney disease when the glomerular filtrate contains large quantities of protein.

Blebs (Figs. 2-3a, 2-6e). Formation of blebs at the cell surface has long been

Figure 2-7. **a.** HeLa cell after a 30-minute pulse with colloidal thorium dioxide (Thorotrast) particles. Ingested particles are present in phagosomes (arrows) along the cell surface and attached to the exterior membrane surface. EC, extracellular compartment.

b. Human red cell treated with primaquine in the presence of glucose; the induced phagosomes contain ingested thorotrast (arrows). PM, plasma membrane. (Courtesy of Dr. Fred L. Ginn).

c. Base of kidney tubules 24 hours after administration of mercuric chloride showing characteristic whorls (Wh) derived from basilar cell membrane. BM, basement membrane.

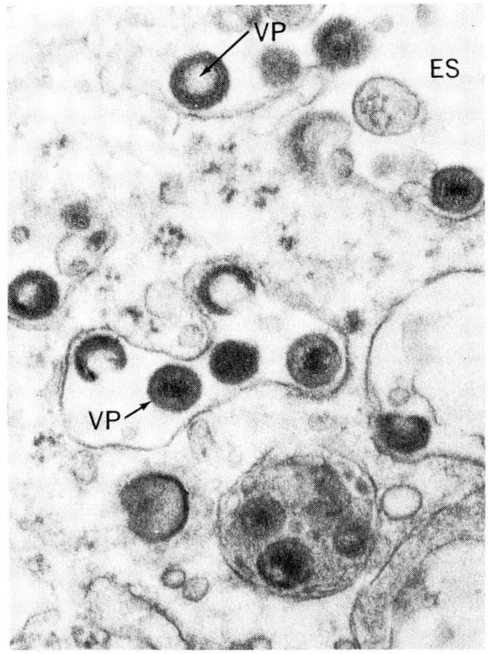

Figure 2-8. Surface of cultured fibroblast showing ingestion of herpes simplex virus particles (VP) in large phagosomes. ES, extracellular space. (Courtesy of Dr. William Bradford).

known to occur at the time of cell division. Time-lapse movies demonstrate that during telophase the cell surface becomes extremely active with a bubbling, effervescent appearance; numerous bleb-like processes are protruded and withdrawn in rapid sequence. Material within the blebs is of low viscosity as compared with the surrounding cytoplasm; this is shown by the increased Brownian movement of particles such as mitochondria found in these regions. Formation of blebs at the surface is also a very early reaction of many cells to a wide variety of injuries (anoxia, metabolic inhibitors, specific antibodies). The molecular basis of this phenomenon is not clear, but, it seems to occur when cell volume control has been lost; it is ordinarily accompanied by increased water uptake by the cells.

Tubular forms and membrane whorls (Fig. 7c). These are vermicular tubes which protrude from the surface of injured cells. They are visible by phase contrast microscopy in unfixed cells as long, undulating, thread-like extensions of the cell surface into the extracellular medium. With the electron microscope these are observed as membrane-bound projections, each limited by a trilaminar membrane resembling the original plasma membrane. When many of these projections exist in a confined space, for example, a kidney tubule lumen or a bile canaliculus, they coil around each other and result in multilaminated configurations (Ginn *et al.*,

a
b

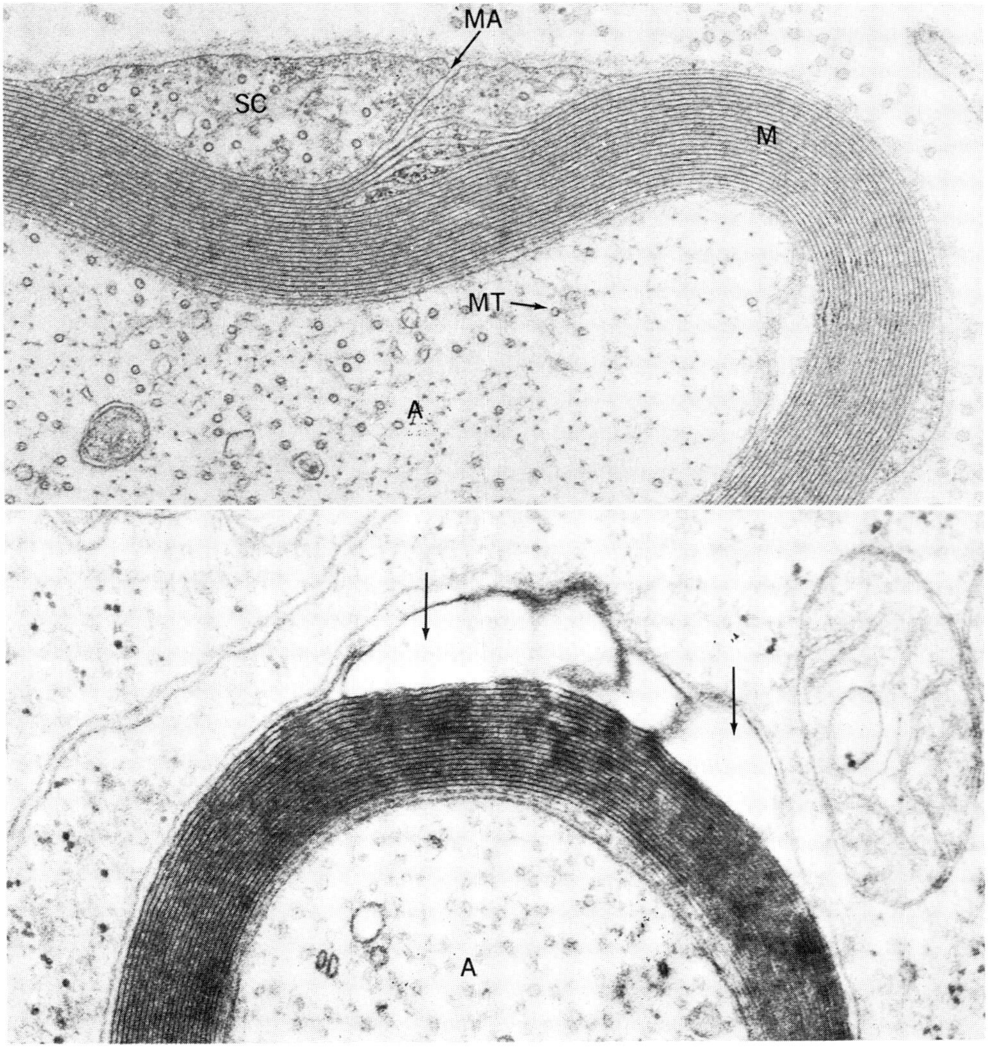

Figure 2-9. a. Normal peripheral nerve showing axon (A) with microtubules (MT), myelin (M), and Schwann cell (SC). MA, mesaxon. (Courtesy of Dr. Peter W. Lampert).

b. Peripheral nerve from an animal with experimental allergic neuritis. The central axon (A) is surrounded by myelin sheath consisting of regular, closely packed membranes. The arrows indicate blebs (bubbly degeneration) between myelin lamellae, an early sign of demyelination. (Courtesy of Dr. Peter W. Lampert).

1968). Multilaminated configurations often develop from complex parallel membrane infoldings such as those at the base of the kidney tubule. These are presumably different from the tubular forms although they appear somewhat similar in electron micrographs. It is evidently an energy-dependent function of the cell to maintain the normal complex parallel infoldings; following damage to the cell these structures revert to coiled or concentric spherical configurations.

Alterations in myelin (Fig. 2-9). Myelin sheaths are multilayered structures derived from plasma membranes of Schwann cells in peripheral nerves and from oligodendroglia in the central nervous system. Because of its repeating substructure, myelin can be studied by X-ray diffraction as well as by electron microscopy, and its molecular structure has been characterized better than that of any other membrane system. Changes in myelin, usually involving degeneration (so-called demyelination), are important in many diseases of the central and peripheral nervous system such as multiple sclerosis and allergic encephalomyelitis, and in the axonal reaction which appears after surgical or traumatic interruption of peripheral or central axons. Such changes also occur as part of the response to virtually any lesion in the nervous system which involves tissue destruction.

One type of change in myelin, consisting of separation of myelin lamellae with splitting of both minor and major dense lines, can occur in cases of cerebral edema due to vascular injury or the administration of certain chemical poisons. In these cases large amounts of fluid accumulate and form big vacuoles (spongy encephalopathy) easily visible with the light microscope. This is not the only cause of brain swelling, however, which may also result from swelling of astrocytic processes, from distended extracellular spaces, from vacuolated oligodendrocytes, or from swollen axons.

Demyelination occurring in allergic encephalomyelitis, multiple sclerosis, and many other central demyelinating diseases as well as in certain chemical toxicities of the peripheral nervous system such as lead poisoning, is presumably the result of primary injury to the oligodendrocyte or Schwann cell. The myelin lamellae are transformed into granular debris and many undergo vesiculation. In the case of allergic encephalomyelitis the primary injury may involve binding of antigen, antibody, and complement to the oligodendroglia and/or myelin sheath with release of lipases and other esterases, in a mechanism analogous to immune cytolysis of the red blood cell.

Intercellular attachments. An important determinant of the integrity of cell junctions is the concentration of calcium within the extracellular fluid. In the absence of calcium, these junctions dissociate and the cells separate. It is also possible to interfere with the integrity of cell junctions by proteolytic enzyme attack; trypsin or other proteolytic enzymes are used for dissociating multicellular tissues.

Dramatic changes in cell shape and internal organization occur after the junctional complexes have been dissociated by calcium depletion. The cell junctions thus seem to be important in the maintenance of cell shape; possibly they serve as sites of attachment for tonofilaments. Disruption of cell junctions, especially gap junctions, also affects electrical and therefore ionic communication between cells. In malignant hepatomas the electrical connections present between adjacent hepatic parenchymal cells are lost and the structure of the cell junctions is considerably modified. Improper development of junctional complexes in neoplastic cells may also have significance in the explanation of tumor cell invasion and metastasis.

3. **Abnormal cell volume regulation** (Figs. 2-10 and 2-11)

In mammalian cells the intracellular ionic composition differs markedly from that of the extracellular fluid. The intracellular fluid in addition to ions has a high concentration of negatively charged protein. Since the plasma membrane can be shown to be permeable to all of the cell's constituents except protein, the maintenance of these differences in composition represents a delicate balance between diffusion and active transport of ions. Many of the latter are energy-dependent and associated with membrane-bound enzyme systems or carriers such as the so-called sodium-potassium dependent, ouabain-sensitive ATPase, which is responsible for at least some of the Na and K movements.

It is evident that the sensitive balance of the intracellular milieu provided by the plasma membrane is subservient to various changes in membrane permeability, membrane-associated enzyme or carrier systems, the electrochemical gradient, or the energy supply. Each of these changes has been demonstrated to occur in various cell injuries and to account for a wide variety of structural and functional alterations of cells in disease states.

The control of intracellular volume, which depends largely on the control of water content, is a fundamental characteristic of mammalian cells (Tosteson, 1964). This control seems to be accomplished through primary modification of electrolyte composition. Water movements are passive according to the osmotic gradient; active transport of water is not believed to occur in mammalian cells. Factors that affect the steady state distribution of water between cells and their environment include differences in hydrostatic pressure, in the chemical activity of water, in electrical potential, in temperature, and in chemical potential. Since the activity of water within the cell and the hydrostatic pressure within the cell are essentially equal to those of the extracellular fluid, water at the normal steady state of the cell is at equilibrium. Because of the presence of a non-diffusible anion,

a

b

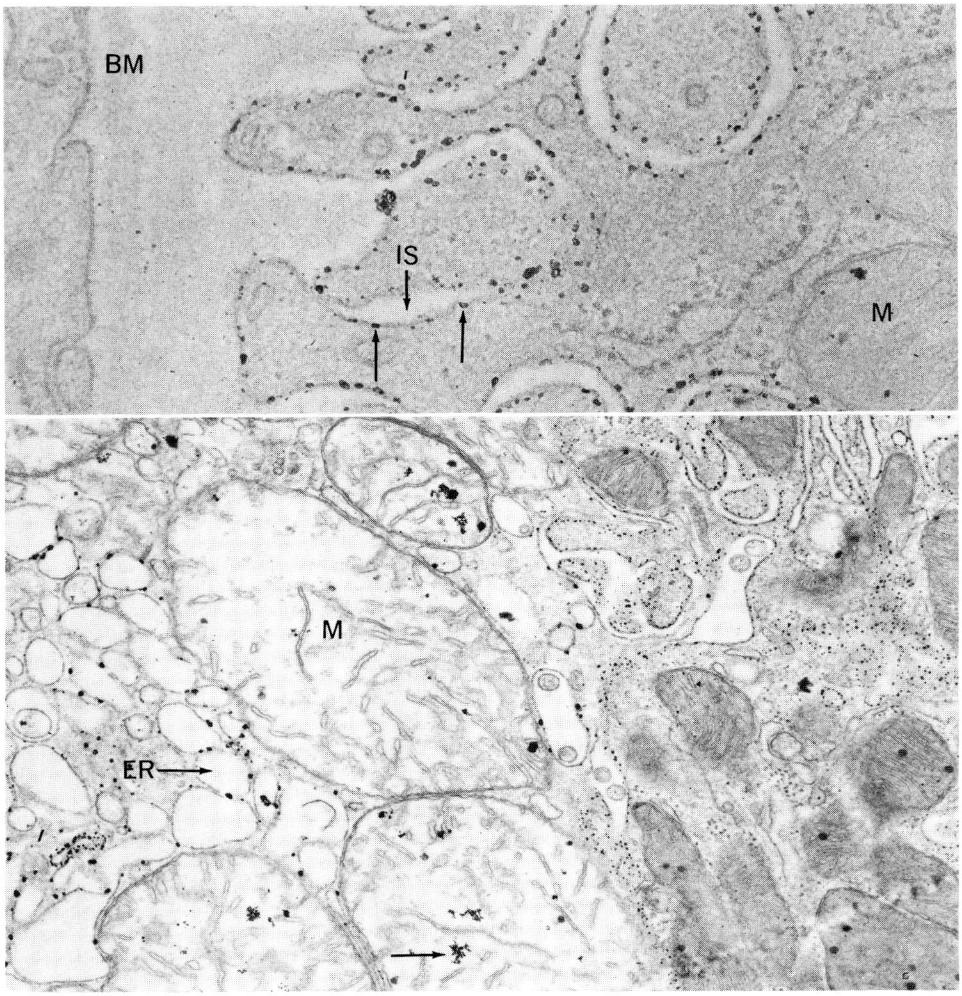

Figure 2-10. **a.** Base of proximal tubule from perfused rat kidney showing localization of sodium binding sites (arrows) displayed with potassium pyroantimonate along the inner surface of the basilar cell membrane. Intracellular membranes such as those of the mitochondrion (M) do not show deposits. IS, intercellular space; BM, basement membrane. (Courtesy of Dr. C. Craig Tisher).

b. Alteration in sodium binding sites after mechanical damage to cell resulting in necrosis. At the right, the normal binding sites are seen along complex cell membrane in the intact cell. At the left, sodium binding sites are seen within the damaged cell along endoplasmic reticulum (ER) and within the mitochondria. (Courtesy of Dr. C. Craig Tisher).

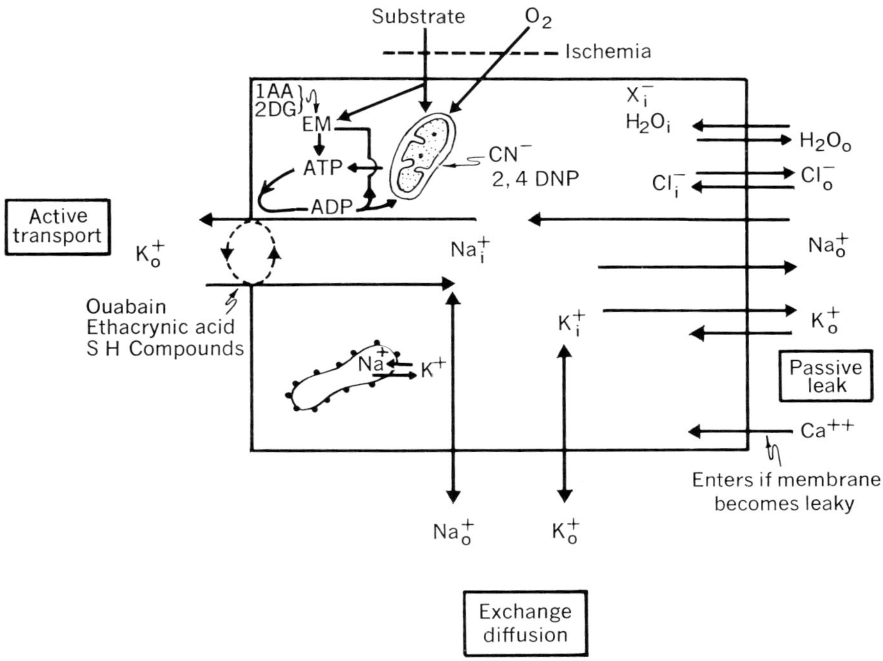

Figure 2-11. Diagram showing some important factors in cell volume regulation in mammalian cells. For explanation see text. (Trump **et al.,** 1971).

chiefly protein, and the presence of charged cations and anions such as sodium, potassium, and chloride, which can traverse the membrane, there is a possibility that the cells might exist at Gibbs-Donnan equilibrium. This can not be the case, however, since if cells were at Gibbs-Donnan equilibrium, the osmolality inside the cell and the intracellular pressure would significantly exceed those in the extracellular fluid. For many years, this problem was resolved by stating that the cell membrane was not permeable to sodium and potassium; however, since the introduction of radioisotopes as tracers, permeability to these ions is readily shown. It now appears that the sodium and potassium transport mechanisms are the key to regulation of intracellular volume, and that small anions such as chloride and bicarbonate exist at equilibrium whereas neither sodium nor potassium is at equilibrium.

If the operation of this mechanism is interfered with by any means, the cells tend to approach Gibbs-Donnan equilibrium by taking on fluid with dissolved solute at a concentration equal to that in the extracellular phase, leading to an increase in intracellular volume and hydrostatic pressure. If this is permitted to continue, cell volume will increase until either the membrane bursts or its volume is constrained by some external force which equals the internal hydrostatic pressure. This increase in cell volume, known as *isosmotic swelling,* is the most important type of volume change observed in all types of injured cells *in vivo* (Trump *et al.,* 1970). It has been especially well studied in the red cell, where many types of hemolysis occur in isosmotic fluid as a result of injury by one or another means to the plasma membrane and its associated transport functions. Such injury could involve direct modification of membrane permeability or of the transport systems within the membrane as well as interference with the supply of energy (possibly ATP) for the transport systems.

It is also possible to observe osmotic types of volume changes if the osmolality of the extracellular fluid is increased or decreased. This occasionally occurs in clinical conditions such as diabetes or severe dehydration on the one hand, or infusion of dilute solutions or distilled water on the other. It is also possible to produce isosmotic swelling by replacing extracellular sodium with a penetrating cation such as potassium.

4. Metaplasia

Metaplasia at the organ or tissue level refers to the appearance of structures which though normal in some loci are abnormal for the sites in question. Ultrastructurally the same definition can be applied to organelles. One of the best examples is the peculiar development of cilia in unusual locations. Though most cells possess centrioles and often at least one cilium, many more cilia can develop along epithelia, such as that lining the kidney tubule, or along bile canaliculi. A striking example is the development of numerous basal bodies and cilia, many of which are abnormal, in olfactory sensory epithelial cells. The stimulus for this development is not known; it probably involves a disorder of ciliary replication since centrioles and presumably cilia have been shown to be at least partly self-replicating and to possess their own DNA. Other examples of ultrastructural metaplasia are the development of cell processes in stimulated cells, as mentioned above, and the induced appearance of numerous pinocytic vacuoles.

E. Mitochondria (Figs. 2-12 to 2-18)

Alterations in the structure and function of mitochondria are quite common in sublethally and lethally injured cells. Understandably, changes in mitochondrial form and function can have important consequences to the general cell economy and mitochondrial adaptations can often be understood as the basis of certain

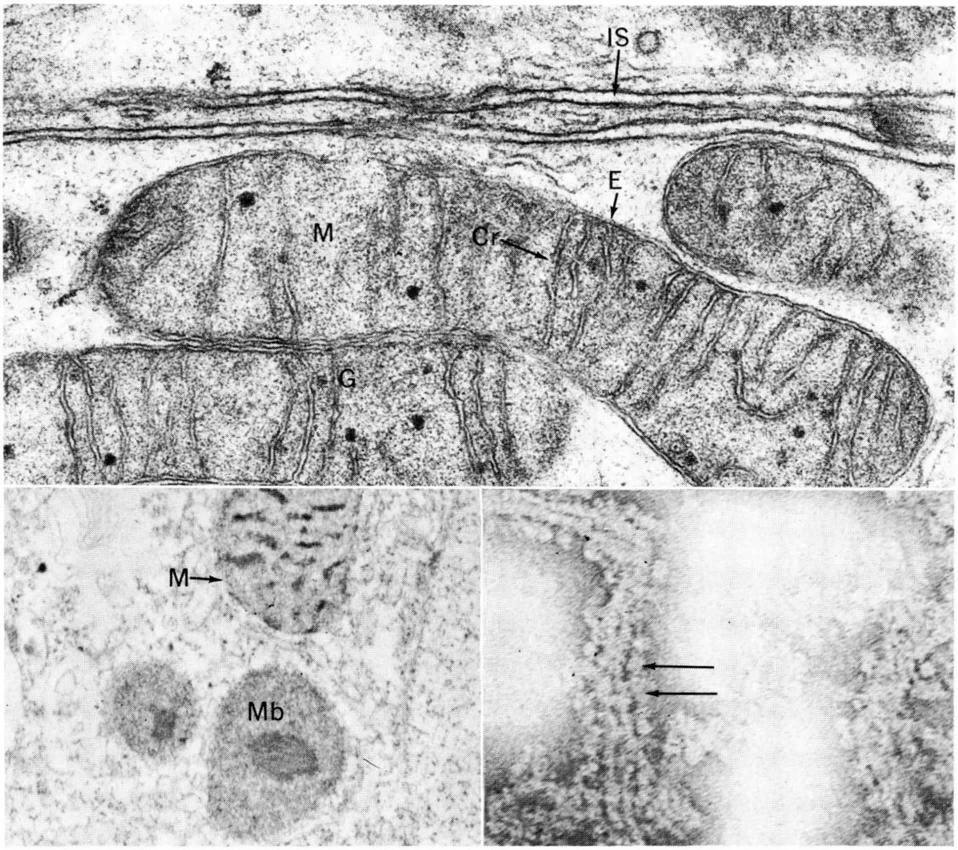

a

b

c

Figure 2-12. **a.** A portion of the cytoplasm of a normal human proximal convoluted tubule cell to demonstrate the characteristic appearance of mitochondria (M). Note the configuration of outer (E), and inner membrane, cristae (Cr), and normal intramatrical granules (G). IS, intercellular space. (Courtesy of Dr. C. Craig Tisher).

b. Mitochondria (M) from a normal rat kidney cell showing localization of cytochrome oxidase activity along inner membranes. The microbodies (Mb) are free of reaction product. Seligman method.

c. Negative stain preparation of a normal mitochondrion showing knob-like particles (arrow) on tubular extensions from the inner membrane. These knobs have been shown to contain the Mg-stimulated ATPase. (Courtesy of Dr. Wolfgang J. Mergner).

sublethal injuries with new steady states. Aspects of normal mitochondrial structure and function are illustrated in Figure 2-12 and reviewed by Parsons (1965).

1. Energy transduction, ion accumulation, and mitochondrial functional states (Fig. 2-13)

Mitochondria move, swell, and contract continually, and it is appropriate to speculate that these movements can exert control over local aspects of the cellular micro-environment, and that accumulation of water and/or ions by mitochondria could provide sensitive and local control and even functional compartmentalization within the protoplasm; compartmentalization of ATP, for example, has been suggested.

The principal function of mitochondria is the supply and storage of energy in the form of high-energy compounds. This can be thought of as resulting from the production of an energized state in the presence of substrate and oxygen. The functional characteristics of mitochondria are properties of the electron transport system and associated coupling factors, both of which reside in intimate association with the cristae and other subunits of the inner membrane.

The mechanism of coupling for ATP synthesis, ion accumulation, and mechanochemical change has not been elucidated. Three theories to explain the phosphorylation-coupling reactions have been proposed. These are: (1) the chemical intermediate theory; (2) the chemiosmotic theory; and (3) the conformation-coupling theory. The most exciting hypothesis from the standpoint of structural-functional correlation is conformation coupling, which asserts that the energy transformation resides in changes in protein conformation within the structure of the mitochondria—a process akin to contraction and relaxation of muscle filaments. From the morphologic standpoint, this theory would imply that the marked morphologic transformations accompanying differences in mitochondrial functional states may well be closely related to the energy coupling mechanism itself.

Mitochondrial structure is closely linked with mitochondrial function. Differences in rate of respiration, phosphorylation, ion uptake, and water uptake are reflected by changes in ultrastructure. These considerations are summarized in Figures 2-14 to 2-18.

2. Mitochondrial swelling (Figs. 2-14, 2-15, 2-18)

Mitochondrial swelling is defined as an increase in mitochondrial size due to uptake of water and thus is to be distinguished from mitochondrial enlargement. It has often been studied in isolated mitochondria by morphologic examination,

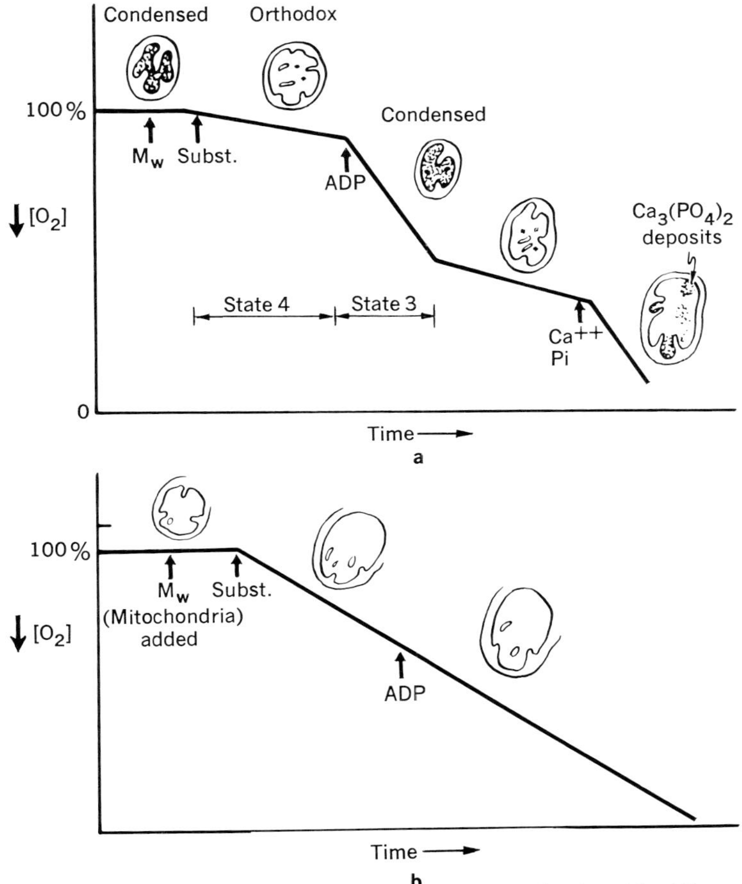

Figure 2-13. **a.** Metabolic transformations in normal mitochondria. When mitochondria are isolated in 0.25 M sucrose, the inner compartment appears condensed. After addition of substrate in the presence of oxygen, they transform to the "orthodox" conformation, State 4. When a phosphate acceptor, ADP, is added, mitochondria enter a phase of rapid respiration and change to the condensed conformation. The cycle can be repeated if substrate and oxygen are present; however, the condensed-to-orthodox transformation is prevented by addition of electron transport inhibitors such as cyanide. If calcium and phosphate are added, mitochondria undergo marked swelling and calcium phosphate accumulates along the inner membrane. Oxygen concentration in the medium is shown along the ordinate.

b. Similar tracing of the behavior of mitochondria from ischemic cells. Swelling of the inner compartment is present at zero time. When substrate is added, further swelling occurs; however, contraction does not occur following addition of ADP. Mitochondria are said to be "uncoupled" and to have lost respiratory control.

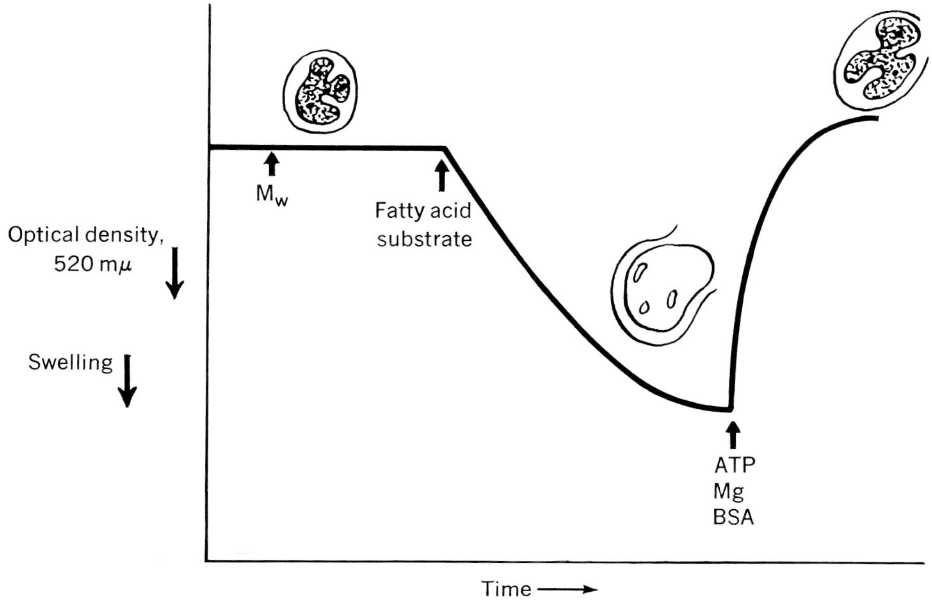

Figure 2-14. Optical density or light scattering trace of a swelling and contraction cycle. This represents "energized" swelling. When isolated, mitochondria have the condensed configuration; however, following addition of a swelling agent in the presence of substrate, high-amplitude swelling of the inner compartment occurs with rupture of the outer membrane. The swelling is readily reversed by addition of ATP, magnesium, and albumin; the mitochondria again become condensed and the optical density increases. Mitochondria may also show "pseudoenergized" swelling in which the inner membrane is permeable even in the absence of substrate. Mitochondria are added at Mw.

(Fig. 2-15) measurement of packed mitochondrial volume (mitocrit), or measurements of light scattering (Fig. 2-14). Light scattering is inversely proportional to the degree of swelling, since a suspension of swollen mitochondria is relatively transparent. Two patterns of mitochondrial swelling are recognized. The first is a large increase in volume: *high-amplitude swelling;* the other, *low-amplitude swelling,* may reflect principally redistribution of water between inner and outer compartments of mitochondria. Mitochondrial swelling can be seen within cells by electron microscopy or by utilizing phase contrast microscopy in conjunction with time lapse cinematography.

Swelling of mitochondria in injured cells is a phenomenon which has been known for many years. It is clear that this increase in mitochondrial volume imparts a granular appearance to the cytoplasm in light microscopic preparations

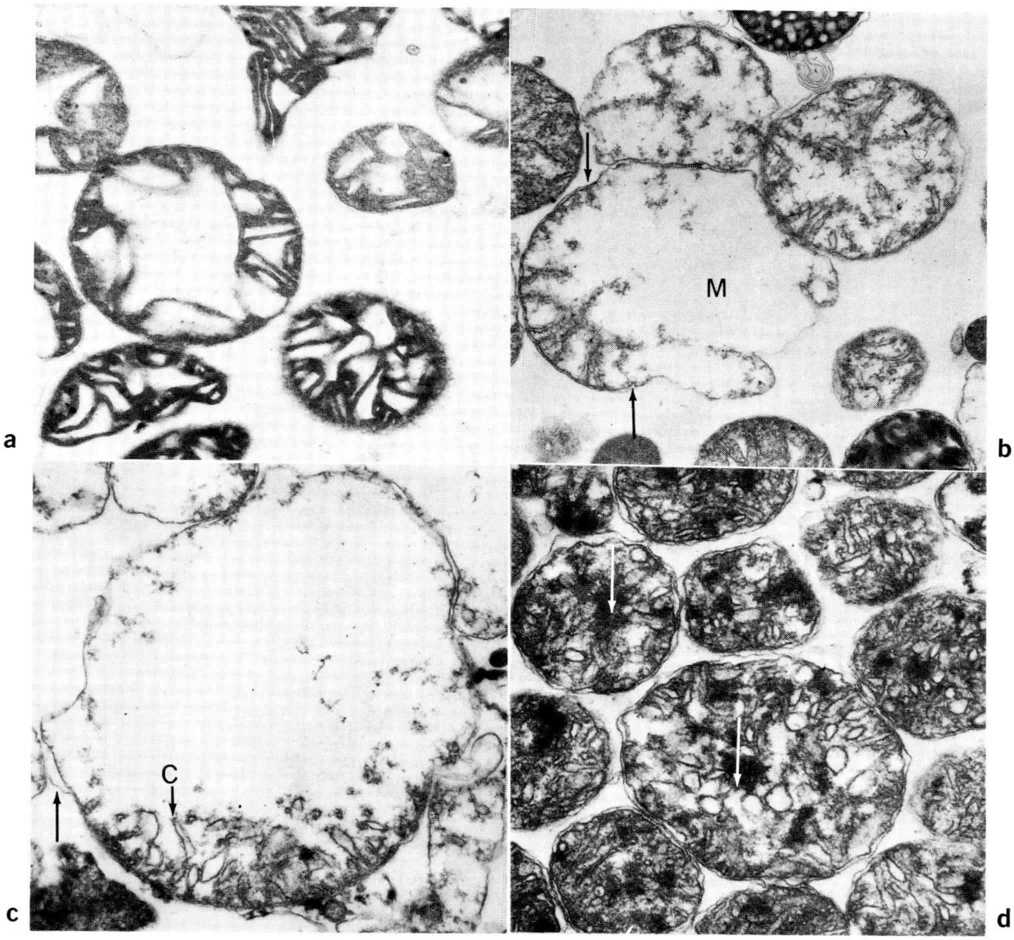

Figure 2-15. Alterations in isolated mitochondria.

a. Mitochondria from control kidney incubated in isosmotic potassium chloride. The normal condensed conformation is maintained.

b. Mitochondria (M) isolated in the same medium but from a kidney that had been ischemic for two hours. High-amplitude swelling occurs, with interruption of outer membrane (arrows).

c. Hypotonic swelling of mitochondrion in distilled water. Note the massive expansion of inner compartment. Cristal residues (C) appear attached along one pole as does a remnant of the outer membrane (arrow).

d. Mitochondria aged in sucrose for 24 hours, showing fragmentation of cristae and appearance of fluffy intramatrical deposits (arrows).

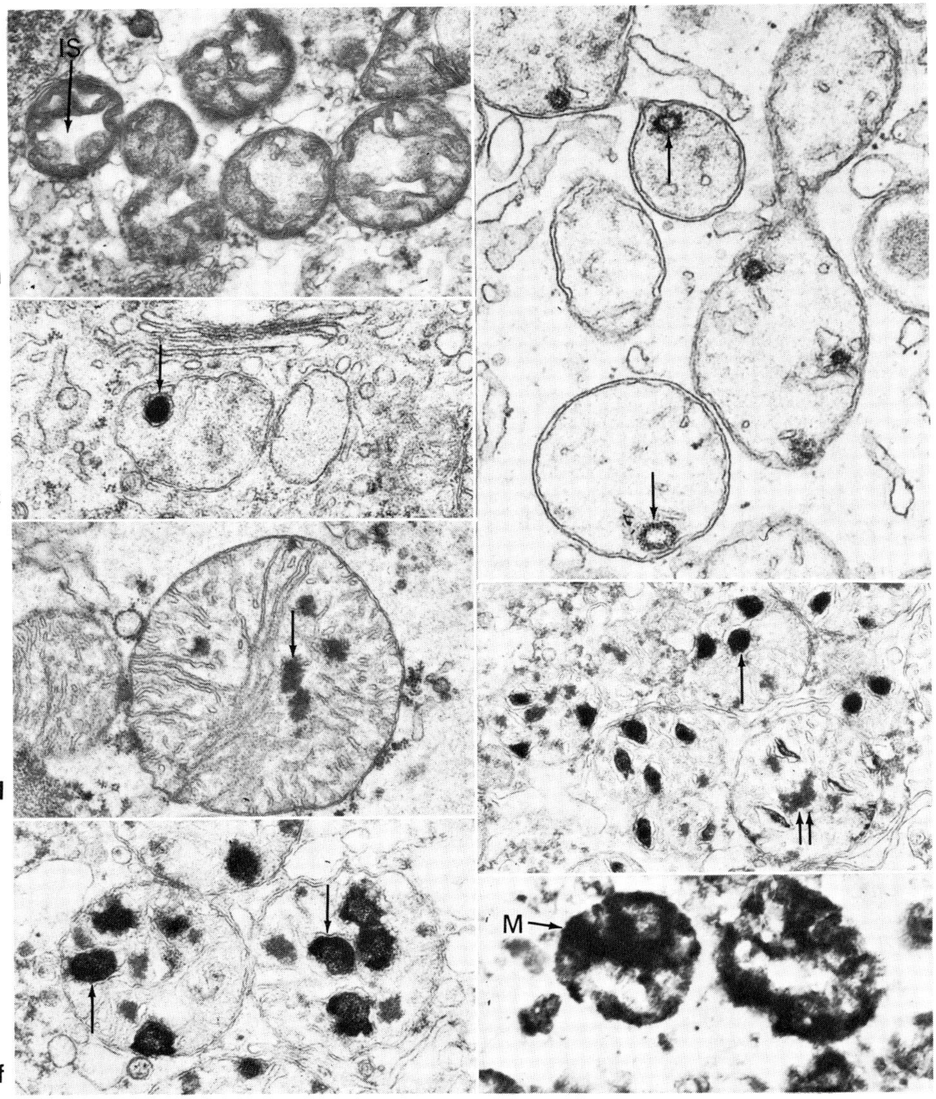

a
b
c
d
e
f
g

Figure 2-16. **a.** Mitochondria in a kidney tubule cell irradiated with ultraviolet light for 4 hours. The cell sap is pale and calcification is seen along the inner membrane in the form of annular deposits of microcrystalline material. The calcium has entered the cell through the damaged plasma membrane. (Courtesy of Dr. Fred L. Ginn).

b. Kidney tubule mitochondria after 2 hours of anoxia. At this late stage there are irregular matrix densities (arrow) and areas of pallor. Matrix granules have disappeared completely.

and is one basis of "cloudy-swelling" or "hydropic degeneration." Mitochondrial movements have also been noted within normal, uninjured cells where mitochondria are seen by time-lapse photography to exhibit periodic swelling and contraction.

Mitochondrial swelling in vitro. Low-amplitude volume changes (less than 20 per cent) in mitochondria accompany transitions between different respiratory steady rates (Fig. 2-14). When mitochondria pass from the energized to the de-energized condition, there is a rapid contraction as measured with optical density techniques. The mechanism of movement of water from inner to outer compartments is thought to relate to changes in protein conformation which in turn are related to mitochondrial functional state in a fashion akin to changes in the actomysin filaments during muscle contraction. In the low-amplitude contracted state, mitochondria appear condensed with very dark matrix and expanded outer compartment, including the envelope and the intracristal spaces; in the expanded state, mitochondria retain their ordinary appearance.

High-amplitude swelling is accompanied by a large change (up to 1000 per cent) in optical density. Morphologically, the increase in volume is confined essentially to the inner compartment. The inner compartment appears to expand by unfolding of the cristae; the outer compartment expands after rupture of the outer membrane. High-amplitude swelling implies an increase in the permeability of the inner membrane to the solute in the medium in which the mitochondria are suspended. At least in the early stages, high-amplitude swelling is reversed by addition of ATP and magnesium.

There are many categories of agents which cause swelling *in vitro.* These include ions, such as calcium; natural products such as fatty acids ("U factor") which can be released from mitochondrial membranes by calcium treatment of mitochondria, during aging, and during mitochondrial change following lethal cell injury; hormones such as thyroxine; and membrane damaging events such as lipid

c. Mitochondria from a kidney tubule cell 6 hours after administration of mercuric chloride, showing homogeneous deposit (arrow) within the intracristal space.

d. Kidney tubule mitochondria 12 hours after injury due to administration of mercuric chloride. At this stage, the mitochondria exhibit low-amplitude swelling with a condensed conformation and expanded outer compartments (IS).

e. Kidney tubule mitochondria 24 hours after administration of mercuric chloride. There are two types of deposits: (a) flocculent intramatrical densities (double arrow), and (b) microcrystalline deposits in apposition to the inner membrane (arrow).

f. Mitochondria in kidney tubule cell 48 hours after mercuric chloride administration. Complete calcification of mitochondrial profiles is seen.

peroxidation or treatment of mitochondria with surface active agents or phospholipases. Prolonged reduction of ATP levels within mitochondria appears to promote breakdown or deterioration of inner membranes with high-amplitude swelling; certain ionophorous antibiotics such as valinomycin promote mitochondrial swelling even in potassium chloride solutions. Although the functional significance of high-amplitude swelling is not completely understood, it seems definitely to be associated with loose coupling during the early stages and, if prolonged, with complete loss of phosphorylating ability.

Mitochondrial swelling and contraction in cells (Fig. 2-16). In intact cells, low-amplitude changes resembling those occurring in the respiratory steady states *in vitro* have been observed in conditions which change the respiratory steady states. Especially important in this regard are such metabolic alterations as changes in the ATP/ADP ratio, usually associated with increased ATP utilization and thus with an effective "ATPase" activity, which need not be enzymatic in nature. Such changes include increased transport of sodium, increased uptake of amino acids, or other ATP-requiring processes, all of which decrease the amount of ATP and reduce the ATP/ADP ratio. Mitochondria then appear condensed with expansion of the outer compartment. Other conditions associated with low-amplitude changes and condensation, indicative of the de-energized state, are those associated with inhibition of the process of energizing mitochondria such as anoxia or treatment with electron transport inhibitors. Early after such treatment most mitochondria de-energize and appear condensed; re-energization is prevented by anoxia or electron transport inhibitors. A delicate balance seems to exist between the de-energized state and high-amplitude swelling, since the integrity of the inner membrane is dependent on ATP. With prolonged anoxia or prolonged treatment with respiratory inhibitors the inner membrane rapidly deteriorates and soon mitochondria pass from a condensed phase to a phase of high-amplitude swelling.

High-amplitude swelling identical with that observed in mitochondria *in vitro* is observed after lethal injuries to cells *in vivo* (Figs. 2-15, 2-16). Initially, high-amplitude swelling occurs during the phase of altered homeostasis. At this phase the changes are reversible. Later, however, the mitochondria lose the ability to contract even if ATP and magnesium are added. If mitochondria are isolated from cells after a lethal injury such as prolonged anoxia, they show much greater permeability to normally impermeant salts such as potassium. Morphologically, high-amplitude swelling in intact cells begins with loss of matrical granules (Fig. 2-16b)—which may herald the loss of maintenance ATP—pallor of the matrix, and appearance of a dense flocculent material within the inner compartment. Later, fluffy densities appear with the matrix. The outer membrane is interrupted permitting expansion, and ultimately the inner membrane also deteriorates, terminating with formation of tubular forms.

3. Progressive changes in mitochondria in lethally injured cells (Figs. 2-15, 2-16, 2-17)

Although it is difficult to make generalizations which apply to all types of injury, the following is a common pattern of reaction in mitochondria following lethal injury to cells with a number of chemical toxins, anoxia, or treatment with electron transport inhibitors.

Phase of altered homeostasis. During the phase of altered homeostasis there is a loss of the matrix granules; they may exhibit a de-energized appearance with condensation of the matrix and later show high-amplitude changes with expanded inner compartments and flocculent material within the matrix (Fig. 2-16) (Trump *et al.,* 1970). Functionally, such mitochondria are characterized by increased swelling response to potassium chloride *in vitro,* loss of respiratory control, and at least partial uncoupling.

Phase of necrosis. Following the point of no return, mitochondria generally show the effects of high-amplitude swelling and dense, fluffy deposits appear within the matrix (Fig. 2-16). Under many conditions, calcium is accumulated (Fig. 2-16a,e,f) (Reynolds, 1965). These calcium phosphate precipitates typically begin to form in apposition to the inner membrane and are often found in small bays surrounded by cristae. As the necrotic phase progresses, the flocculent and crystalline densities increase in size and number. In some instances the mitochondria may be completely replaced by microcrystalline aggregates of calcium phosphate. Ultimately, the inner membrane fragments and gives rise to tubular forms which often resemble cristae. In this phase the mitochondria are incapable of oxidative phosphorylation, although some succinate or NAD-linked oxidations may persist even after irreversible damage.

It is thought that release of fatty acids such as oleic acid is related to the increased membrane permeability and conceivably may be in part responsible for the production of flocculent densities. If mitochondria from lethally injured cells are studied *in vitro,* their functional activity can be at least partially restored by pretreating with serum albumin which binds fatty acids and enables a partial reversal of the respiratory inhibition.

4. Mitochondrial inclusions (Figs. 2-16, 2-17)

Mitochondrial inclusions frequently develop in abnormally functioning cells. Such inclusions may represent insoluble precipitations of ions, abnormal protein

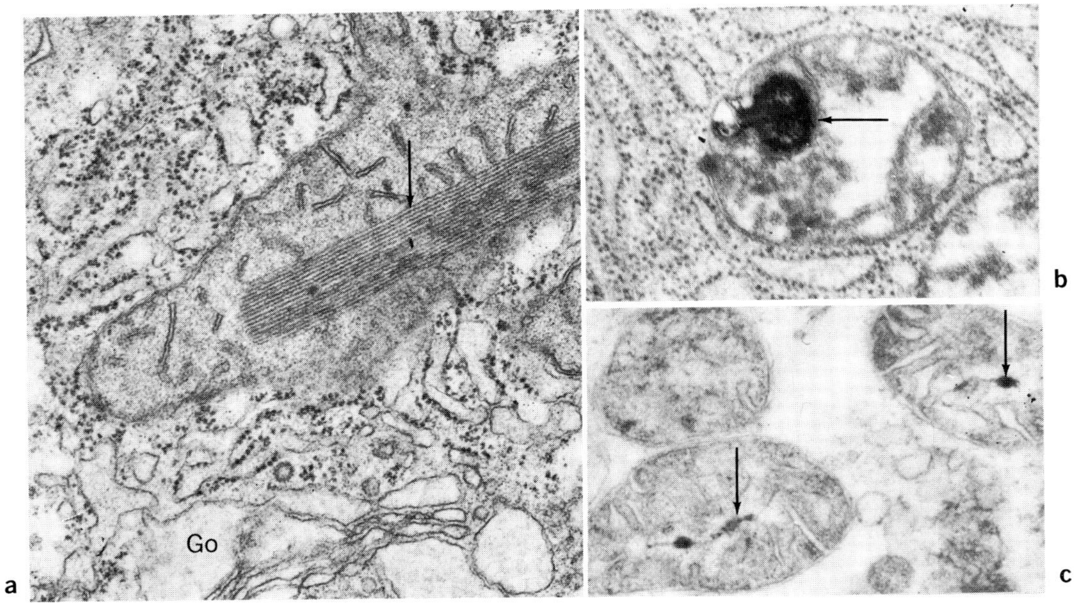

Figure 2-17. **a.** Mitochondrion from human hepatic cell containing a paracrystalline intramatrical inclusion (arrow). Go, Golgi apparatus. (Courtesy of Dr. Edward A. Smuckler).

b. Mitochondrion from a kidney tubule cell after the administration of Janus green B showing a lamellar intramatrical inclusion.

c. Mitochondria from the Meadow mushroom containing intramatrical accumulations of DNA. (Courtesy of Dr. F. Stephen Vogel).

depositions, rearrangements of membranes or other phospholipids forming lamellar inclusions, focal changes in the conformation of matrix proteins, or accumulations of nucleic acids.

Accumulation of ions. Ion accumulation in association with phosphorylation intermediates or via the mechanisms common to phosphorylation is an important function of mitochondria; it represents a common way in which the energized state is discharged through energized reactions supported by either ATP or substrate and oxygen. Mitochondria can accumulate a variety of divalent cations in addition to calcium. Among them are magnesium, barium, manganese, and strontium. Often the phosphate is taken up simultaneously, resulting in formation of insoluble phosphates within the mitochondrion. If both calcium and ADP are simultaneously presented to a mitochondrion, calcium will be preferentially accumulated; not until all calcium has been removed from the medium will ADP be phosphorylated. Thus if mitochondria are continually exposed to high concentrations of calcium they will not phosphorylate ADP and will ultimately be destroyed. This may significantly contribute to the irreversible injury that occurs in mitochondria *in vivo* when extracellular fluid contains higher than normal concentrations of calcium. This occurs, for example, in hyperparathyroidism, or in conditions where the permeability of the cell membrane is altered, resulting in calcium leak into the cell and reversal of the cytoplasmic Na/K ratio.

Nucleic acid. Accumulations of nucleic acid visible even by light microscopy occur in certain mitochondria (Fig. 2-17). In trypanosomes, for example, the so-called kinetoplast represents an accumulation of mitochondrial DNA at one end of the large mitochondrion. The mitochondrion within this protozoan can undergo reversible changes in size as a function of availability or non-availability of oxygen.

Other types. Various other materials are included within mitochondria but unfortunately most of these are presently of unknown significance (Fig. 2-17). These include: the presence of fibrils, often helically arranged, within the intracristal space in mitochondria in human alcoholics; large distorted mitochondrial granules in cases of calcification of the kidney; formation of dense bodies within the intracristal spaces called *corpora intracristam;* various crystalline and paracrystalline structures.

5. Abnormalities in mitochondrial growth and replication

There is now increasing evidence that mitochondria are self-replicating and independent, to some extent, of nuclear control (see review by Scarpelli, 1970). They contain DNA and synthesize some proteins by mechanisms which are at least partially autonomous. They may be responsible in part for the so-called cytoplasmic inheritance factors.

Certain mitochondrial changes in disease are best understood in terms of alterations in mitochondrial growth and replication. These often seem to lead to the production of large, abnormally shaped mitochondria (Fig. 2-18), which may have inclusions easily visible by light microscopy and sometimes called megamitochondria (mitochondrial giants). These enlarged mitochondria are to be distinguished from mitochondrial enlargement due to swelling, in which the increased size is mainly caused by uptake of water. Megamitochondria can be observed in liver cells in alcoholism, as large, round eosinophilic inclusions. These megamitochondria may be larger than the cell nucleus and are quite distinct from the so-called alcoholic hyalin, a change within the cytoplasmic ground substance as mentioned below. Other conditions associated with enlarged liver mitochondria in-

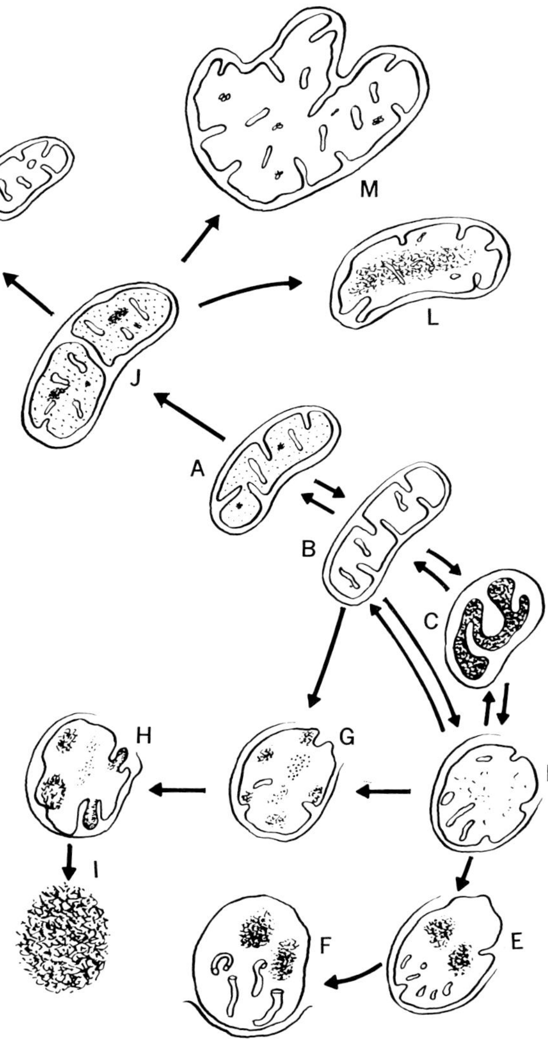

Figure 2-18. Diagram of progressive mitochondrial changes in cell injury.

a. Typical normal mitochondrion.

b. The mitochondrial granules are lost, presumably due to decrease in ATP.

c. Condensed mitochondrion in which the matrix is contracted, possibly the result of condensation of matrix proteins following changes in ADP/ATP ratio. Increased levels of ADP often produce contraction.

d. This shows high-amplitude swelling after ion and water movements into the mitochondrion with rupture of the outer membrane.

clude treatment with copper chelating agents, essential fatty acid deficiency, vitamin E-selenium deficiency, cirrhosis, and non-hemolytic jaundice. Mitochondrial enlargement is also seen in kidney tubules in tubular necrosis, and in tissue culture cells under abnormal growth conditions. The pathogenesis of the enlargement may involve fusion of mitochondria or failure of mitochondrial fission. Quantitative studies on mitochondrial mass in cells with megamitochondria indicate that the total mitochondrial volume may remain constant, which implies that there are fewer larger mitochondria.

In addition to heterogeneity in size, mitochondria may show extreme pleomorphism with scalloping of mitochondrial margins, protrusions of one mitochondrion into another, and formation of crystal-like patterns within the mitochondria. Pleomorphism has been seen in neoplastic cells.

Variation of mitochondrial number can also be observed. Simple starvation of the rat produces a marked decrease in mitochondrial number within a few days. Following re-feeding, mitochondrial division and growth occur (Scarpelli, 1970).

F. Cytocavitary Network (Figs. 2-19 to 2-30)

1. Historical background

The application of the electron microscope to the study of cells has revealed that the cytoplasm contains a variety of membrane systems which permeate virtually the entire cytoplasm (Fig. 2-19, 2-21) (Goldblatt, 1969). Various parts of this system have been referred to in the past by terms such as endoplasmic reticulum, cytomembranes, Golgi apparatus, lysosomes, microbodies, and nuclear en-

e. Fluffy deposits which probably represent aggregations of denatured proteins are seen; at this stage mitochondria are severely damaged, and P/O ratios approach zero.

f. Tubular forms have arisen from the inner membrane.

g. Deposits of apatites occur following calcium and phosphate accumulation by mitochondria.

h. The calcium deposits are in annular patterns adjacent to the inner membrane.

i. The entire mitochondrion has calcified.

j. Beginning mitochondrial division with a septum separating the inner compartment into two phases, each of which contain clumped mitochondrial DNA in the matrix.

k. The division is completed.

l. A megamitochondrion which may arise from defective mitochondrial division or

m. A paracrystalline aggregate in the mitochondrial matrix, as seen in human livers. from fusion.

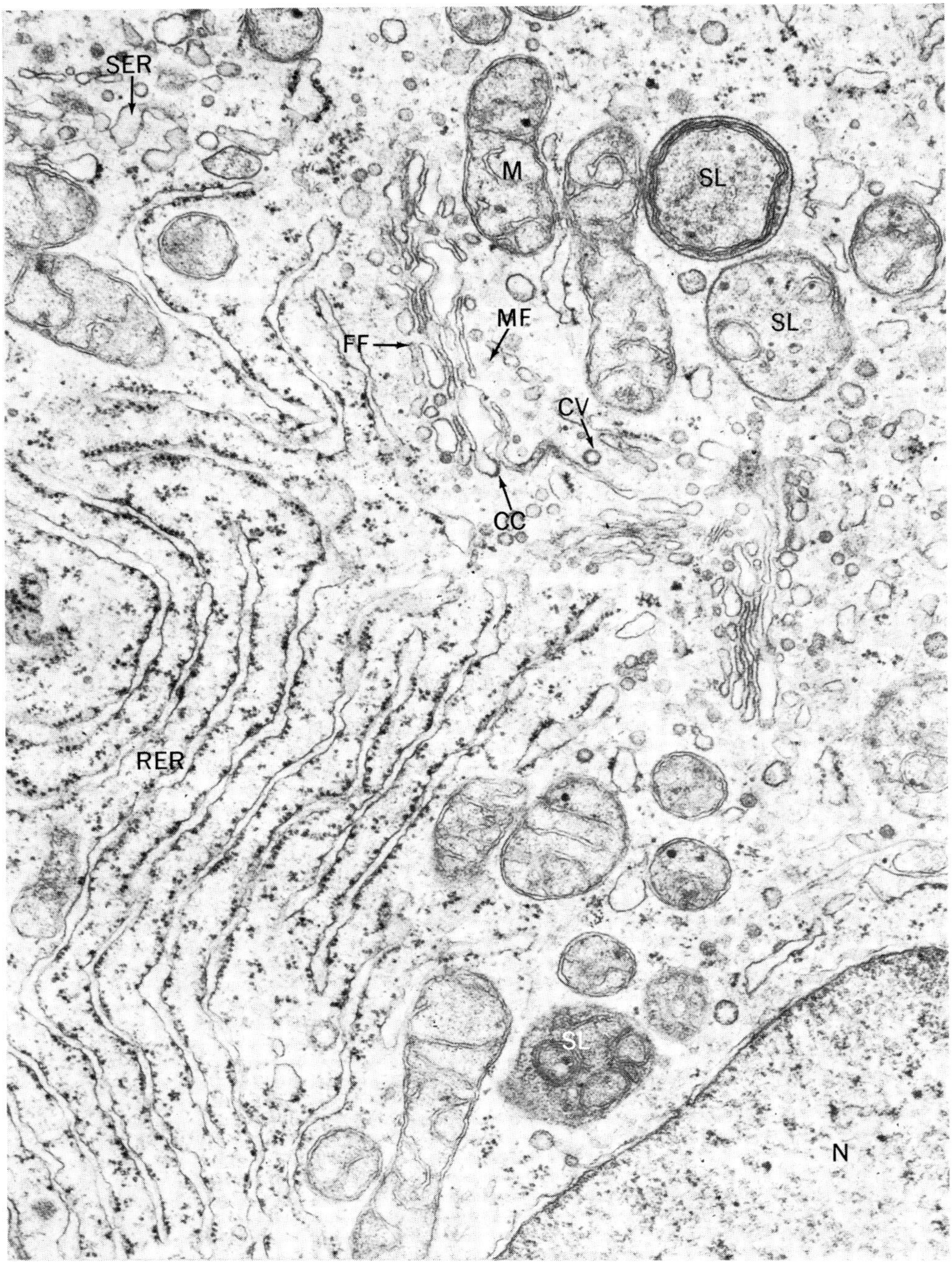
SER
M
SL
SL
MF
FF
CV
CC
RER
SL
N

velope. There has been, however, considerable difficulty in arriving at precise definitions of various portions of this membrane system and, with few exceptions, they have been made only under a set of rather limited conditions. It is now evident that all of these components form part of a membranous system in the cell which is involved in many aspects of cell metabolism and which forms a functionally interconnected system of cavities that are separated from the cell sap by membranes. We shall refer to this system as the "cytocavitary network."

2. Architecture of the cytocavitary network; membrane movements

The space of the cavity is topologically equivalent to the extracellular space and the membrane is topologically equivalent to the plasma membrane. Transport between various portions of the system, as well as from the cell sap to the lumen

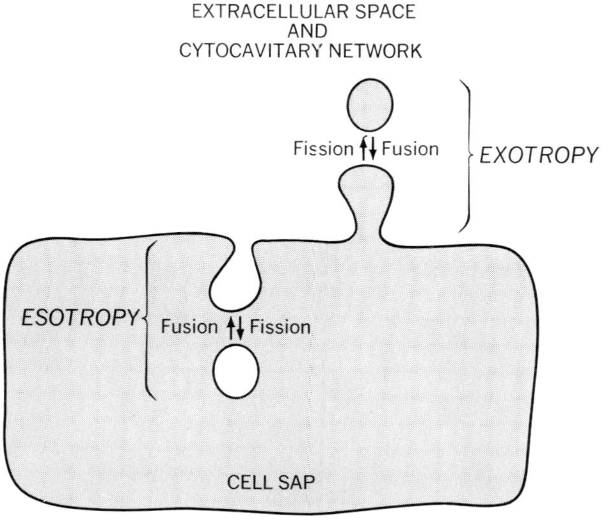

Figure 2-20. Diagram illustrating concepts of esotropy and exotropy. For explanation see text.

Figure 2-19. Region of Golgi apparatus in normal human kidney tubule cell. The cisternae of rough-surfaced endoplasmic reticulum (RER) are in transition to Golgi apparatus at the forming face (FF). Some coated vesicles (CV) and coated caveoli (CC) are present in the Golgi region. Note the vesicles along the maturing face (MF) of the Golgi apparatus and the adjacent digestive vacuoles (SL) containing debris. Mitochondria (M) and cytoplasmic filaments can be seen. SER, smooth-surfaced endoplasmic reticulum; N, nucleus.

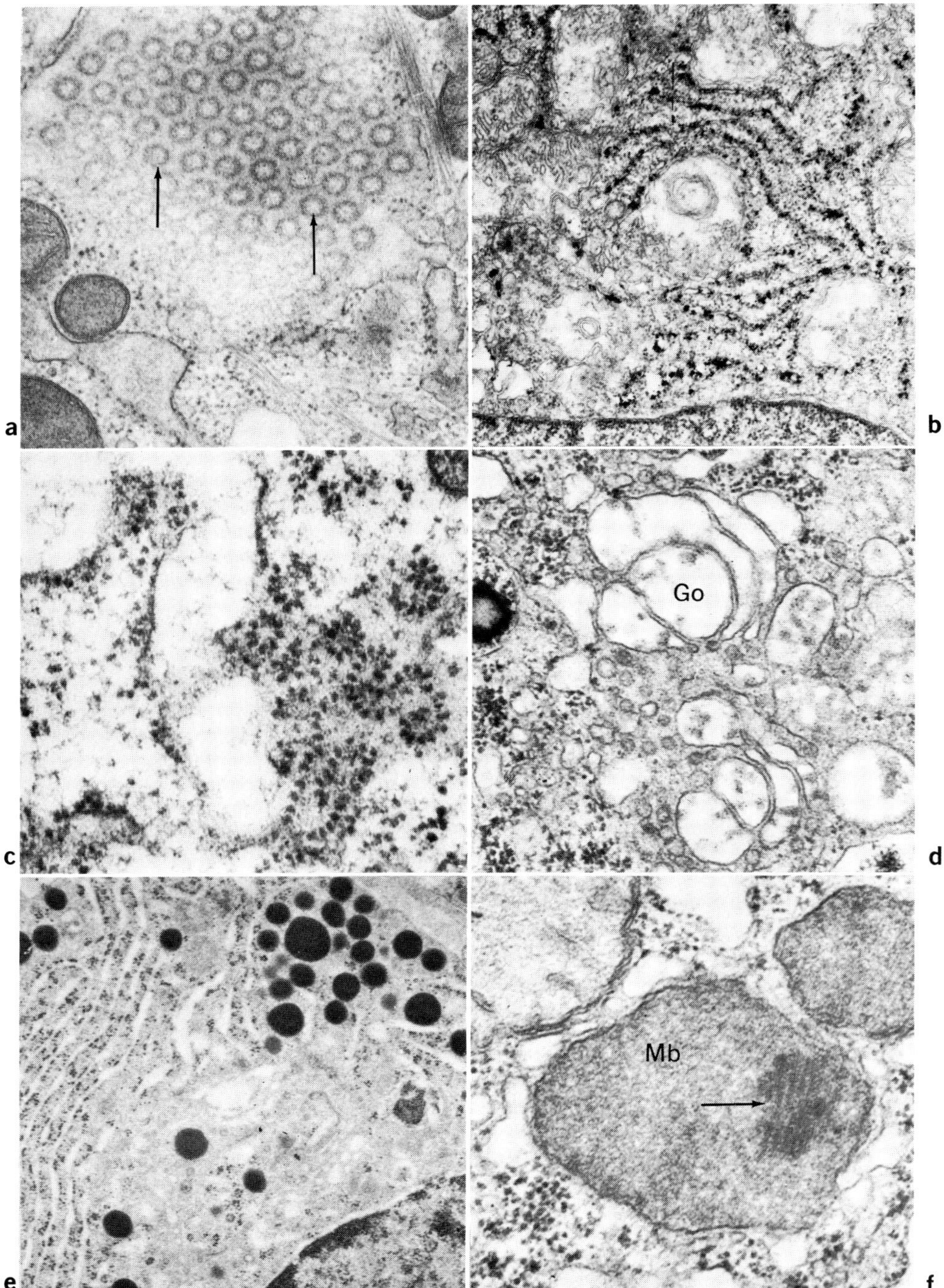
a
b
c
Go
d
e
Mb
f

or the extracellular space often occurs by means of vesicle formations and fusions. Although these may initially seem complicated, they can be reduced to two geometrically simple processes termed *esotropy* and *exotropy* (Fig. 2-20).

Esotropy (Greek—a turning in) refers to a turning in of the membrane toward the cell sap followed by fission to form a new membrane-bound cavity. The cavity is topologically equivalent to the extracellular space or the space of the cytocavitary network. When the phenomenon occurs in the reverse direction (reverse esotropy), a vesicle fuses with the membrane, bringing the vesicle contents into continuity with the extracellular space or with the space of the cytocavitary network. Examples of forward esotropy include pinocytosis, elaboration of transport vesicles from the ER at the forming face of the Golgi apparatus, elaboration of secretory vesicles from the maturing face of the Golgi apparatus, and formation of microbodies. Examples of reverse esotropy include fusion of secretory granules with the cell membrane, fusion of Golgi vesicles with phagosomes, and fusions between various secondary lysosomes.

Exotropy (Greek—a turning out) refers to a turning out of the membrane toward the extracellular space or toward the space of the cytocavitary network. This is often followed by fusion and formation of a new membrane-bound structure. In this case, however, the vesicle contains cell sap or structures such as viruses or mitochondria that are contained within the cell sap. The polarity of the membrane of the new vesicle is identical with that of the cell itself, e.g. the glycocalyx is directed outwardly. In reverse exotropy, fusion of an exotropic structure brings the portions of cell sap into contact. Exotropy into the endoplasmic reticulum appears to be a common mechanism of autophagocytosis. Many viruses have appropriated this mechanism, acquiring their outer envelope by exotropy into the

Figure 2-21. **a.** Surface view of annulate lamellae in HeLa cell. The pores are indicated by arrows.

b. Hepatic parenchymal cell. Glucose 6-phosphatase activity within the endoplasmic reticulum is demonstrated by the Wachstein-Meisel lead phosphate technique (arrows).

c. Regenerating kidney tubule cell 2 days after the administration of mercuric chloride, showing a surface view of the rough endoplasmic reticulum. Numerous chains of polysomes are present (arrow).

d. Golgi region (Go) from hepatic parenchymal cell of a protein-deficient rat. The Golgi elements are dilated. (Courtesy of Dr. William D. Bradford).

e. Secretory granules (arrow) are present in the region of the Golgi apparatus in this cell from the anterior pituitary gland.

f. Microbody (Mb) or peroxisome from a normal rat. The paracrystalline core or nucleoid (arrow) is characteristic of rat microbodies but is not seen in human cells.

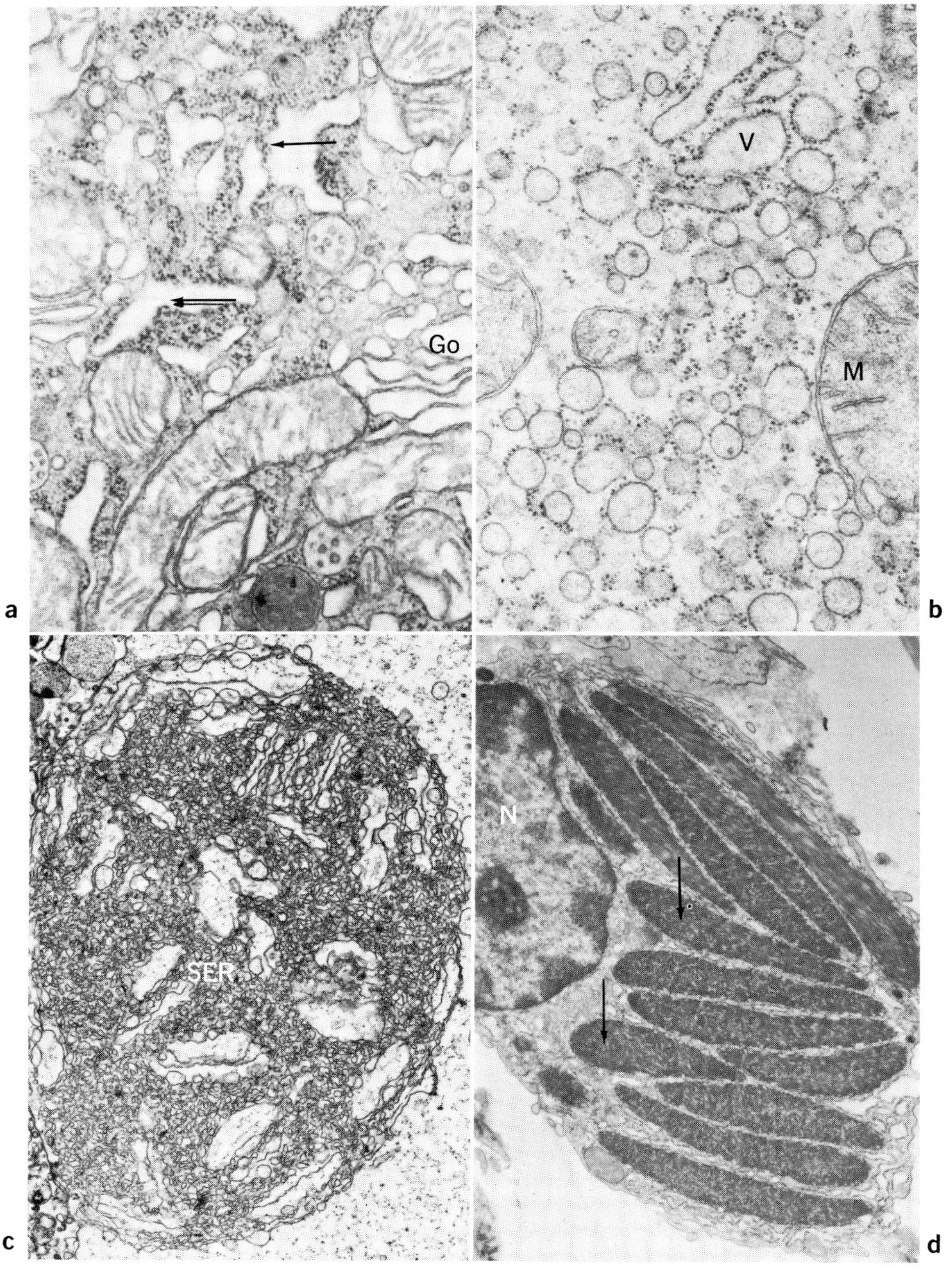
a
Go
b
V
M
c
SER
d
N

ER, into the space of the nuclear envelope or by budding from the surface plasma membrane directly. At the extreme, mitotic division could be considered a gross example of exotropy. Examples of reverse exotropy include viral entry into cells, where the viral envelope fuses with the cell membrane and, at the cell level, fusion of cells to produce syncytial giant cells.

Fusions between exotropic and esotropic vesicles have not been reported. Although much remains to be learned about the precise basis of these membrane movements, available evidence strongly indicates that they are dependent on high-energy compounds such as ATP.

3. The cytocavitary membrane

Membrane structure. Membranes of at least two size classes are found in the cytocavitary network (Arstila and Trump, 1968). The thinner class is in the order of 50-60 Å in thickness and is found in the endoplasmic cisternae, the microbodies, the forming face of the Golgi apparatus, and the nuclear envelope. The thicker membranes, 80-90 Å thick, are found at the maturing face of the Golgi apparatus and in digestive vacuoles, phagosomes, multivesicular bodies, residual bodies, and secretory vacuoles.

Transition between the two types occurs in the Golgi apparatus, and it is possible that during membrane flow through the Golgi region, additional materials such as cholesterol are added to the membrane.

Changes in molecular architecture. Many functions of the endoplasmic cisternae are dependent on the normal conformation of the membrane itself and on the functional proteins within it. These in turn are dependent on normal protein-protein and protein-lipid interactions within the membrane (Trump *et al.*, 1970). These relationships are well shown when fragments of endoplasmic cisternae are treated with phospholipase C, an enzyme found in *Clostridium welchii,* which releases approximately 80 per cent of membrane phospholipid as diglyceride and

Figure 2-22. a & b. Effects of ischemia on the endoplasmic reticulum. After 30 minutes of ischemia **(a)** there is marked dilatation of the endoplasmic reticulum (arrow) and Golgi apparatus (Go) in the cytoplasm of this Purkinje cell. After one hour of ischemia **(b)** one sees fragmentation of the ER cisternae (V) and dissociation of polysomes.

c. Proliferation of smooth endoplastic reticulum (SER) in a kidney tubule cell 12 hours after administration of mercuric chloride.

d. Plasma cell showing a Russell body, consisting of accumulation of paracrystalline material (arrows) within ER cisternae. (Courtesy of Dr. William O. Dobbins III).

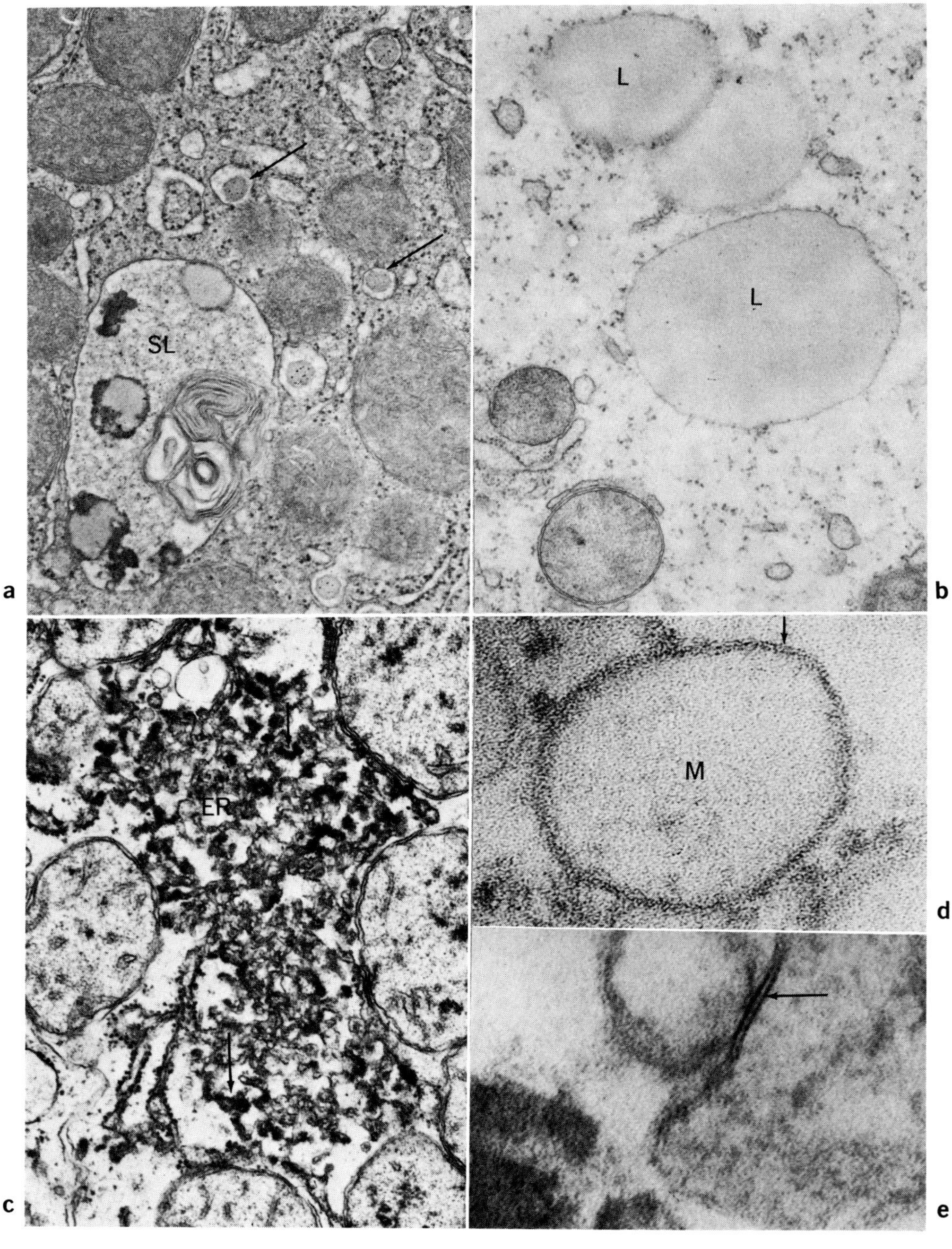
SL
L
L
ER
M
a
b
c
d
e

inactivates glucose 6-phosphatase. At the same time membrane structure is altered and the thickness of the membrane increases by approximately 60 per cent. The released diglycerides seem to accumulate in the center of the membrane, in the clear zone between the dense laminae. The striking feature of this model is that if phospholipids are again added to the modified membranes, the glucose 6-phosphatase activity can be restored and the membrane structure returned to a normal configuration. This emphasizes the role of lipid-protein interactions in both membrane structure and function.

Endoplasmic membranes, like cell membranes, may be altered through peroxidation of the fatty acids of membrane lipids (see p. 93). When the endoplasmic membranes are peroxidized in the test tube, characteristic changes occur (Figs. 2-23c,e, 2-24). They include detachment of ribosomes from the surface of the membranes, widening of the trilaminar membrane and accumulation of dense material along the outer surfaces of the membrane. Later, there is collapse of cisternae and aggregation of cisternal profiles, perhaps through binding of the dense material. Similar changes are seen in intact liver cells after administration of carbon tetrachloride, or in kidney cells after administration of mercuric chloride. Since detachment of ribosomes is the earliest morphological change in both peroxidation of microsomes in the test tube and after carbon tetrachloride poisoning in the liver, it is tempting to consider that membrane peroxidation is responsible for this.

Detachment and scattering of ribosomes occur in a number of other cell injuries, probably reflecting modifications in the ribosome-membrane interaction. For example, agents such as detergents, that directly modify lipid interactions, are known to detach ribosomes from the endoplasmic membrane. Detachment and scattering of polysomes are not necessarily irreversible changes, and a normal environment can sometimes be restored with restoration of normal polysomes.

Figure 2-23. **a.** Cytoplasm of a liver cell from a female rat after the administration of ethionine, which reduces ATP levels by approximately 80 percent. A large lysosome (SL) is present; triglyceride droplets (arrows) accumulate within the cisternae of the endoplasmic reticulum as a result of the lack of ATP.

b. Large lipid droplets (L) in the cytoplasm of a choline-deficient rat.

c. Cytoplasm of a hepatic parenchymal cell after the administration of carbon tetrachloride. Clusters of collapsed endoplasmic reticulum appear (ER). The densities (arrows) are characteristic of peroxidation lesions.

d & e. Effect of peroxidation on the unit membrane. In the fragment of endoplasmic reticulum from a control rat (**d**), the spacing of the unit membrane is closer than in that of a peroxidized membrane (**b**) at the same magnification.

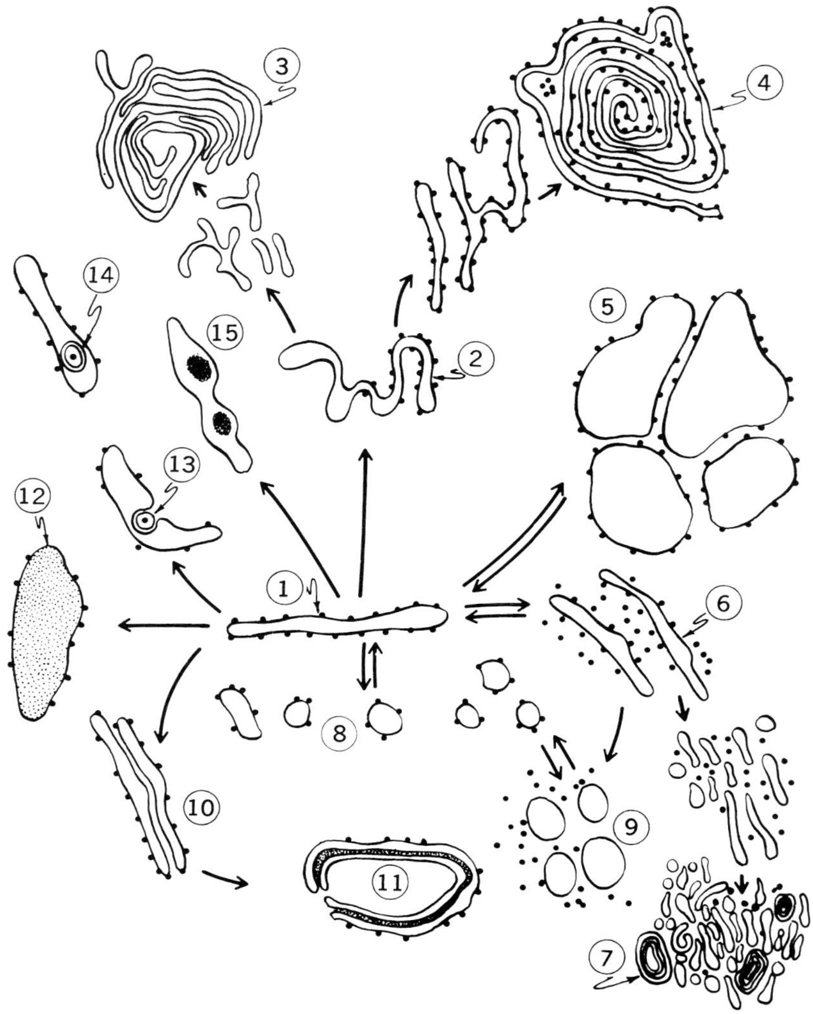

Figure 2-24. Conformational changes in rough endoplasmic reticulum. (1) normal conformation; (2) stimulated synthesis of rough and smooth ER membranes results in (3) proliferations of smooth ER, as after phenobarbital-induced detoxification, and (4) complex proliferations of rough endoplasmic reticulum; (5) dilatation of endoplasmic cisternae is caused by mild injuries with changes in ion and water movements; (6) degranulation (loss of polysomes from the endoplasmic reticulum) is a common response to injury; (7) peroxidation results in changes of membrane conformation and accumulation of densities; (8) and (9) progressive fragmentation of ER results in smooth vesicles and detached polysomes; (10) and (11) paired cisternae are formed after treatment with certain hormones including cortisone; (12) materials such as glycoproteins may accumulate with ER cisternae; (13 and (14) exotropy of naked virions into the endoplasmic reticulum cisternae results in an enveloped virus within ER; (15) lipoproteins may accumulate in ER.

Changes in membrane conformation. The endoplasmic cisternae are capable of dramatic transformations in injured cells (Smuckler and Arcasoy, 1969). These are summarized in Figure 2-24. When a cell is lethally injured by anoxia, the cisternae rapidly fragment into vesicles (Fig. 2-22a,b) and lose their attached ribosomes. The next stage of breakdown presumably involves dissolution of the endoplasmic membranes to form lipoprotein subunits, which in turn give rise to their component lipids and proteins. The lipids may ultimately reassociate into various types of bilayer configurations such as the myelin figures referred to above.

Another type of transformation involves dilatation of the cisternae (Figs. 2-22a, 2-24, 2-37a), the membrane remaining intact. This dilatation may be extreme, and often occurs with influx of sodium and water into the cell.

Stimulation of endoplasmic membrane synthesis, as with the administration of drugs such as phenobarbital or dilantin, leads to dramatic increases in cisternal number and length in liver cells. This cisternal redundancy eventually results in large proliferations, whorls, and glomerular arrangements (Fig. 2-22c). Concomitant with the increase in membrane synthesis, one can detect parallel increases in a number of hepatic detoxifying enzymes, which constitute an integral part of the membrane structure. In some conditions, abnormally retained secretory products may accumulate in endoplasmic reticulum cisternae (Fig. 2-22d). Changes in membrane conformation related to esotropy or exotropy are common and are discussed below.

Alterations in metabolic activities. An important metabolic activity of the endoplasmic reticulum involves the detoxification system just mentioned, which catalyzes the hydroxylation of several types of compounds, including drugs, steroid hormones, and carcinogenic dyes (Ernster, 1970). The system involves NADPH (the reducing agent), a flavoprotein (NADPH cytochrome-C reductase), cytochrome P-450, and molecular oxygen, and results in the incorporation of one oxygen atom into the reaction product, ROH, and the other into H_2O. A similar system involved with steroid hydroxylation is found in adrenal cortex mitochondria. When animals are treated with compounds capable of undergoing hydroxylation, enhancement of the liver microsomal hydroxylating activity occurs, with a net synthesis of enzyme components; this is accompanied by formation and accumulation of new membranes of endoplasmic cisternae. The system is interesting in that it exhibits cross-reactions between drugs, for it has been clearly shown that hydroxylation of one drug can be enhanced by the *in vivo* administration of another. Cross-reactivity between different drugs is shown in the excessive hydroxylase activity of human alcoholics. Whether or not these metabolizing activities are always helpful is not clear. In some instances the opposite is true, for increased metabolism following induction may speed the toxic response to agents such as carbon tetrachloride and may result in metabolism of carcinogenic agents to the more proximate compound (see Chapter 6).

4. Abnormalities in intracellular digestion

The term lysosome was originally used by de Duve and his associates to refer to a class of cytoplasmic particles limited by a membrane and containing acid hydrolytic enzymes which are capable of rapidly digesting many components of the cell (see reviews by de Duve and Wattiaux, 1966, and Dingle and Fell, 1969). The enzymes exhibit the property of structure-linked latency (Fig. 2-25); when the particles are intact the substrate cannot gain access to the enzyme, and measured enzyme activities are low. If the membrane is damaged, substrate gains access to enzyme and the enzyme activity can be measured. In a homogenate the extent of this damage can be measured as an increase in free enzyme activity and can be regarded as an estimate of lysosomal integrity. If the damage is more severe, the enzymes may escape completely from the lysosomes, and enzyme activity can be measured in the supernatant after centrifugation at 100,000 g for thirty minutes.

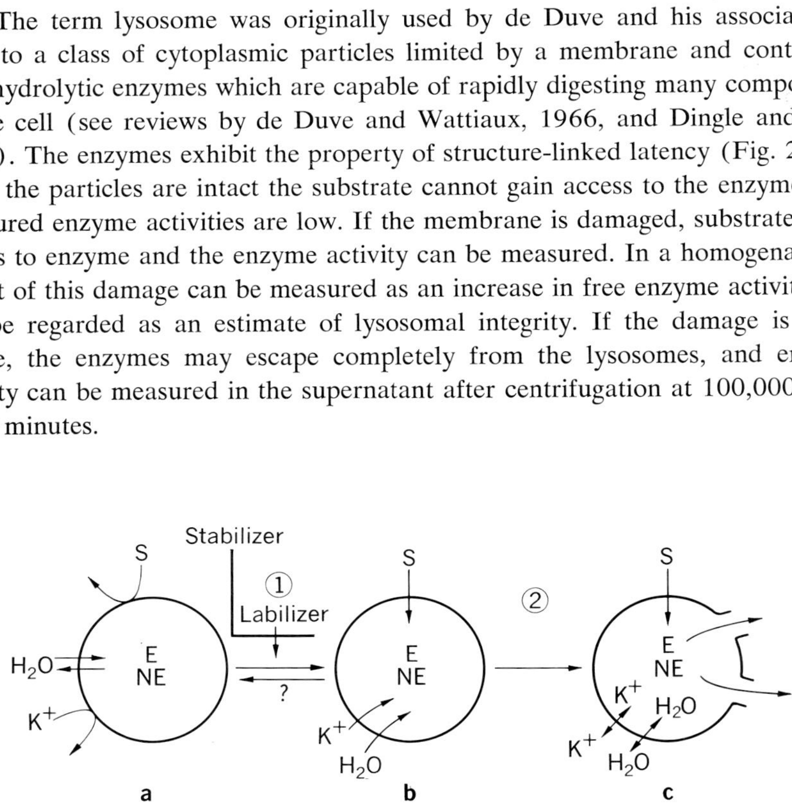

Figure 2-25. Structure-linked latency in lysosomes. In step 1, after treatment with a "labilizer," the permeability of the lysosomal membrane is increased, allowing access of substrate to enzyme. In step 2, damage to the membrane permits release of enzymes. A is a normal lysosome. B is a lysosome with increased permeability; influx of ions and water presumably results in swelling at this stage. C represents a severely damaged lysosome with escape of enzymatic and non-enzymatic contents and equilibration with the cell sap. E, enzymes (acid hydrolases); NE, non-enzymatic components (basic protein, leukocidin, ferritin, polysaccharides, substances introduced via pinocytosis); Labilizers: low pH, mechanical damage, ATP deficiency, Vitamin A, testosterone, polyene antibiotics, progesterone; Stabilizers: cortisone, cholesterol, chloroquine, acetylsalicylic acid; S, substrates that range in size from β-glycerophosphate to macromolecules such as DNA and protein.

While the concept of the lysosome as defined by its content of acid hydrolases has been an extremely useful one, it is now apparent that lysosomes represent special cases of secretory and digestive vacuoles which blend imperceptibly between acid hydrolase-containing and non-acid hydrolase-containing structures and indeed transform from the one type into the other. In the present chapter, therefore, they are considered the part of the cytocavitary network that is chiefly concerned with intracellular digestion. Intracellular digestion is a process of importance in a wide variety of normal and pathologic cellular reactions.

Heterophagy and Autophagy. Heterophagocytosis refers to the esotropic uptake of particles such as macromolecules or macromolecular complexes from the surface of the plasma membrane. Often this uptake is referred to as endocytosis, or pinocytosis. This results in the appearance of the *heterophagosome,* which carries ingested particles toward the cell center. The heterophagosome acquires acid hydrolases by fusion with Golgi-derived vesicles or by fusion with pre-existing digestive vacuoles to form a new digestive vacuole (Fig. 2-27a). The material within may then be hydrolysed to either indigestible debris or soluble intermediates such as small dipeptides or amino acids, which can be reutilized or released from the cell. The phenomenon of *autophagocytosis* is similar to heterophagocytosis (Figs. 2-26, 2-27b). In this instance the vacuole appears to form by exotropy into a cisterna of endoplasmic reticulum or other portion of the cytocavitary network (Arstila and Trump, 1968). This results in the enclosure of a portion of cytoplasm, such as a mitochondrion, in a double-walled sac. Enzyme is added by fusion of endosecretory vesicles or digestive vacuoles with the outer membrane of the sac in the double-walled stage. The inner membrane thickens to resemble the membrane of other digestive vacuoles. Both autophagy and heterophagy are apparently energy-requiring processes which utilize ATP or other high energy intermediates, but forces involved in these membrane movements are not fully understood.

Certain endocrine cells, such as those of the anterior pituitary, secrete hormones to the extracellular space. In conditions where secretion is shut off, the hormone is transferred to the lysosome system where it is destroyed. Thus, the direction of this secretory step can provide control over release of secretory material.

Although most material within digestive vacuoles is digested, some debris remains. This debris is largely lipid, a fact probably related to the relative lipase deficiency of the digestive vacuoles. The debris often becomes auto-oxidized and forms pigmented autofluorescent materials which are termed *lipofuscin* or *aging pigment* (Fig. 2-28b). The debris-filled bodies are called residual bodies. In some cells, the residual bodies are known to fuse with the plasma membrane and dis-

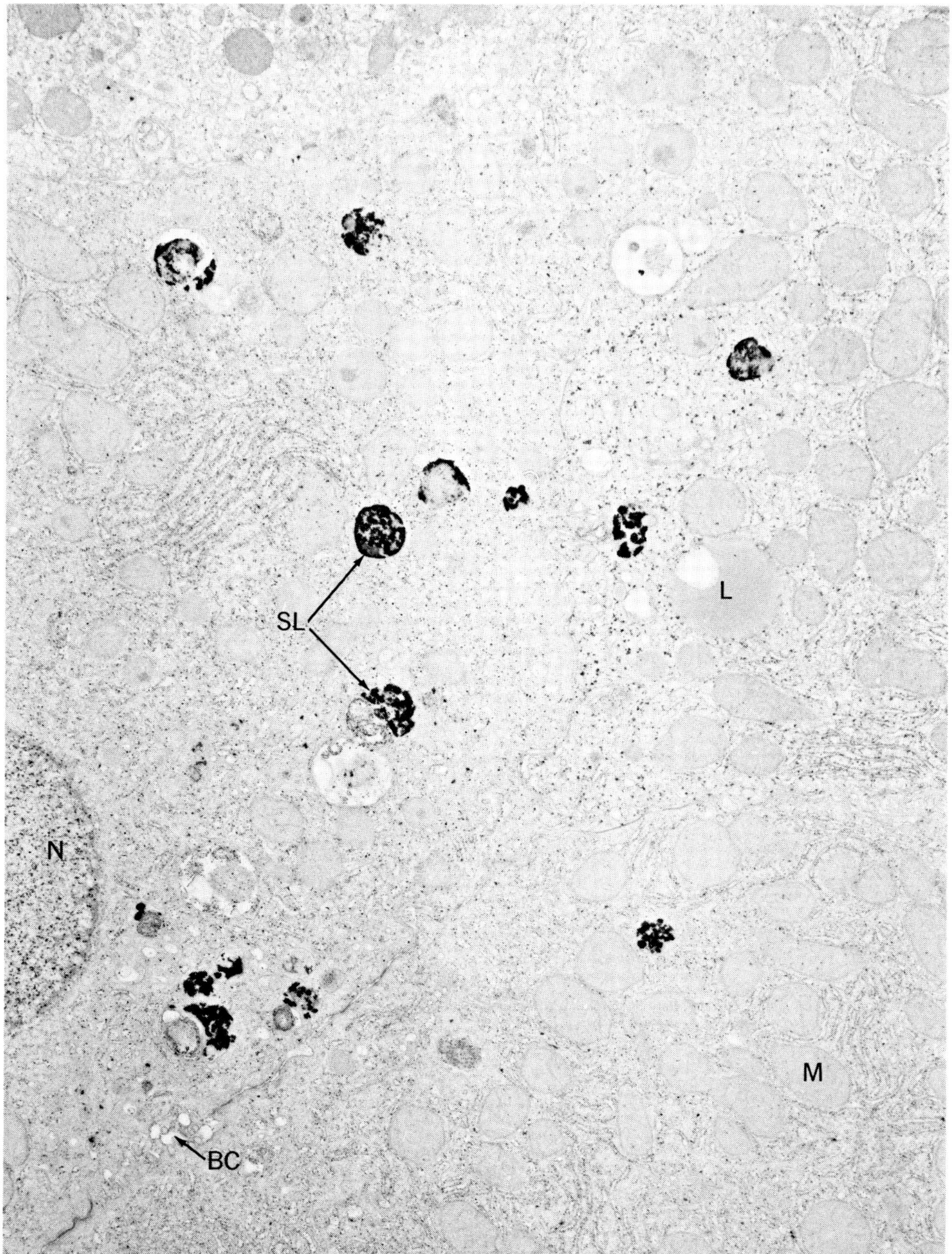
SL
L
N
M
BC

charge the debris; in others, however, this probably cannot occur and lipofuscin-filled residual bodies tend to accumulate (Fig. 2-28b). The neuron is such a cell; neuronal lipofuscin or aging pigment increases in a linear fashion with age. Neurons become, as it were, filled with the debris of a lifetime.

In addition to acid hydrolases, digestive vacuoles contain certain non-enzymatic components. These include iron in the form of ferritin or hemosiderin (Fig. 2-28a), polysaccharides (Fig. 2-28c), complex glycoproteins, glycogen (Fig. 2-28d), plasminogen activator, an antibacterial substance known as phagocytin, and some heat-stable hemolysins.

The digestive vacuole system in cell economy and protection against disease. Although it is difficult to separate the normal from the pathologic functions of the digestive vacuole system, it is useful to consider those functions in normal cells which exert a protective effect, on the one hand, in relationship to cell injury on the other.

Heterophagy. The role of heterophagy in nutrition is, of course, best exemplified in unicellular forms such as amoeba which derive their nutrition solely in this way. By contrast the role of heterophagy in nutrition of mammalian cells is poorly understood, but its mechanisms are present in many cells and are often important to the animal as a whole. For example, the cells lining the proximal convoluted tubules of the kidney have well-developed systems for heterophagy and are continually reabsorbing proteins from the lumen which have passed through the glomerulus (Ericcson, 1965). This is of considerable importance in the conservation of body protein. When the glomerulus is diseased, as in glomerulonephritis, much more protein leaks through the glomerulus and much more is reabsorbed by the tubules (Fig. 2-30b). Heterophagocytosis of microorganisms by leukocytes constitutes an important defense mechanism against infection (Fig. 2-29) (see Chapter 4). In this instance, the specific granules of the leukocyte fuse with the phagosome, releasing digestive enzymes and other antibacterial substances into it. It has recently been suggested that antigen processing via heterophagy by macrophages is an essential preliminary step in the stimulation of immunoglobulin synthesis by antibody-producing cells. A more controversial area is the possible role of heterophagic uptake in memory transfer and in the uptake of interferon. Certain endocrine secretory cells such as thyroid epithelium, take

Figure 2-26. Cytoplasm of several hepatic parenchymal cells one hour after administration of glucagon which induces autophagocytosis. The dense black deposits in the autophagic vacuoles (SL) are due to the presence of lead phosphate deposited there by cytochemical reaction which demonstrates the presence of acid phosphatase in the vacuoles. N, nucleus; BC, bile canaliculus; M, mitochondrion; L, lipid droplets.

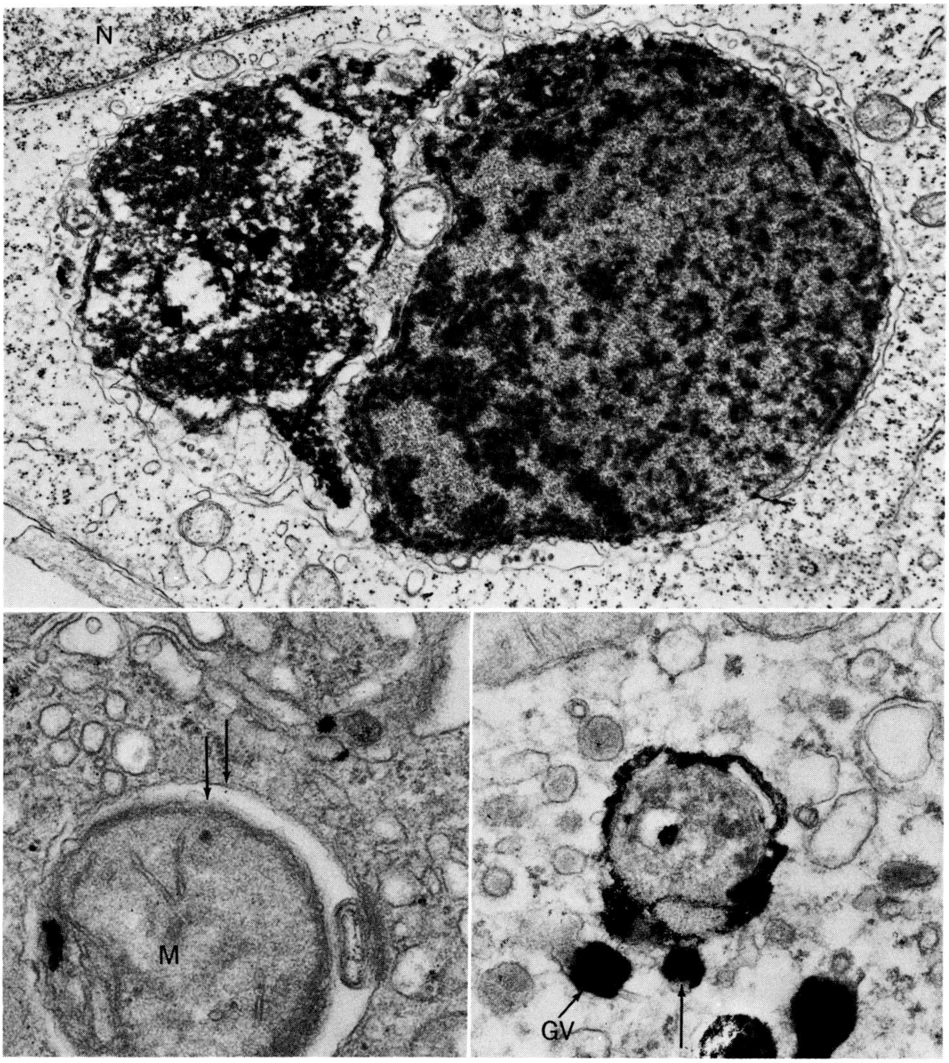

a
b
c

Figure 2-27. **a.** Giant heterophagic vacuole in a HeLa cell 12 hours after infection with herpes virus. The digestive vacuole contains debris from necrotic cells that have been phagocytosed. N, nucleus.

b. Newly formed autophagic vacuole in rat liver one hour after administration of glucagon. Note the double limiting membrane (arrows). The vacuole contains a mitochondrion (m) and a focus of acid phosphatase reaction product probably representing phagocytized Golgi vesicles. Gomori lead phosphate technique.

c. Autophagic vacuole one hour after the administration of glucagon, showing apparent fusion of an acid phosphatase-containing vesicle (arrow) with the outer wall of an autophagic vacuole. Note the nearby Golgi vesicle (GV) with acid phosphatase activity.

up colloid via heterophagy before processing and then releasing it into the bloodstream. Heterophagy is also apparently at work in the newborn intestine during suckling to reabsorb maternal immunoglobulins present in milk. A general mechanism for the turnover of necrobiotic cells is heterophagy by scavenging phagocytes.

Abnormal uptake of soluble materials is often reflected by the appearance of intracellular vacuoles which represent distended phagosomes and digestive vacuoles. A striking example is the watery vacuolization of the proximal tubule following the administration of mannitol or sucrose to patients. This condition has been termed *osmotic nephrosis* (Fig. 2-30a). Insoluble and/or indigestible material is often retained within the digestive vacuoles of phagocytes. This is the basis of tattooing and of anthracosis. In tattooing these pigments are retained for a lifetime in the digestive vacuoles of cutaneous macrophages, and in anthracosis inhaled carbon is retained for years in pulmonary phagocytes.

Autophagy. Autophagy provides an obvious means for organelle turnover. In the liver cell, for example, it is estimated that the rate of mitochondrial turnover (half-life ten days) could be accounted for by autophagocytosis, and at least some of hepatic glycogen turnover occurs within autophagic vacuoles (Hers, 1965). Autophagocytosis may also serve as a mechanism of nutrition under unfavorable conditions such as general starvation or specific dietary deficiencies. Accepting the reduction in number of organelles, the cell seems to behave as if it will utilize its own substance in order to maintain homeostasis.

Some of the most dramatic examples of increased autophagy occur in association with involutionary processes such as the atrophy of the mammary gland after lactation, the atrophy of the secondary sex organs in elderly persons, and the atrophy of functional units in organs such as the liver or kidney that accompanies progressive ischemia. In all such cases organ remodeling is accompanied by the appearance of large autophagic vacuoles which ultimately become pigmented residual bodies.

Autophagy seems also to have important relations to differentiation and cell division. Phytohemagglutinin-stimulated lymphocytes exhibit numerous autophagic vacuoles. Large numbers of autophagic vacuoles are observed in the regenerating liver after hepatectomy. It has been suggested that autophagocytosis could be related to cell division functioning in the destruction of antimitotic materials.

Role of digestion in injured cells. A variety of sublethal injuries results in the formation of increased numbers of autophagic vacuoles (Figs. 2-26, 2-27). Pathogenetic factors include damage to membranes in organelles, decreased nutrition, regeneration of cells, neoplasia, and damage by bacterial products. It

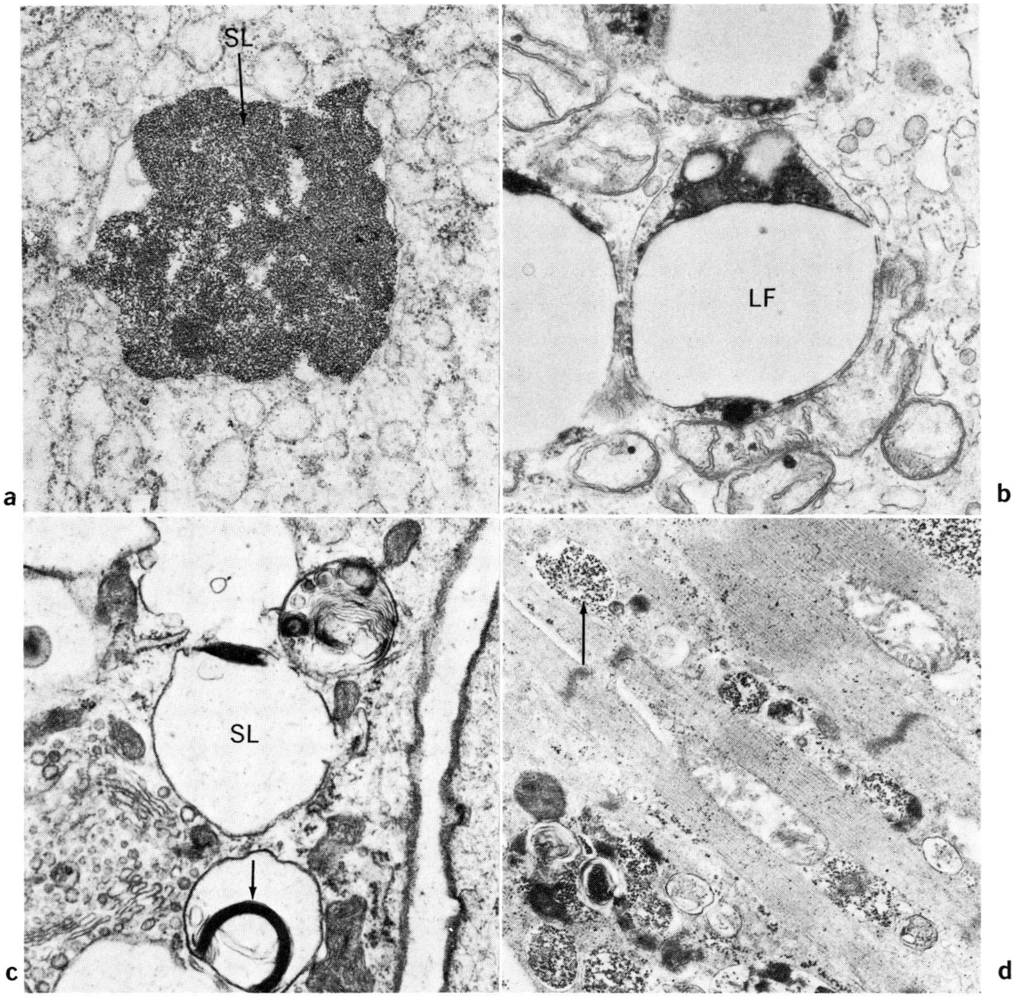

Figure 2-28. **a.** Hepatic cell from a patient with hemosiderosis. A large lysosome (SL) is almost filled with fine dense granules of ferritin and hemosiderin. Similar granules are scattered in the cell sap.

b. Kidney tubule cell from human patient. Large accumulations of lipofuscin (LF) are seen in several lysosomes.

c. Visceral epithelial cell of the glomerulus from a patient with neurovisceral lipidosis. Large lysosomes (SL) are filled with lipid debris forming myelin figures (arrow) and with acid mucopolysaccharides which appear pale in these preparations.

d. Heart-muscle cell from a patient with Pompe's disease. Glycogen-filled lysosomes (arrows) are present in the sarcoplasm. M, mitochondrion. (Courtesy of Dr. Doyle Graham).

appears that damage to organelle membranes, which occurs as a non-specific feature of many diseases, is especially effective in promoting the formation of autophagic vacuoles. One known pathogenetic factor involved in membrane damage is the lipid peroxidation which occurs experimentally in animals deficient in antioxidants such as vitamin E; numerous autophagic vacuoles result promptly from such deficiencies. Allison (1968) has recently proposed a hypothesis of carcinogenesis which is based on autophagic destruction or alteration of chromosomes to produce mutations. It is true that certain chemical carcinogens, especially the polybenzenoid hydrocarbons, are concentrated in lysosomes, but this theory of carcinogenesis is yet to be established.

Inadequate autophagic digestion may result from enzyme deficiencies or de-

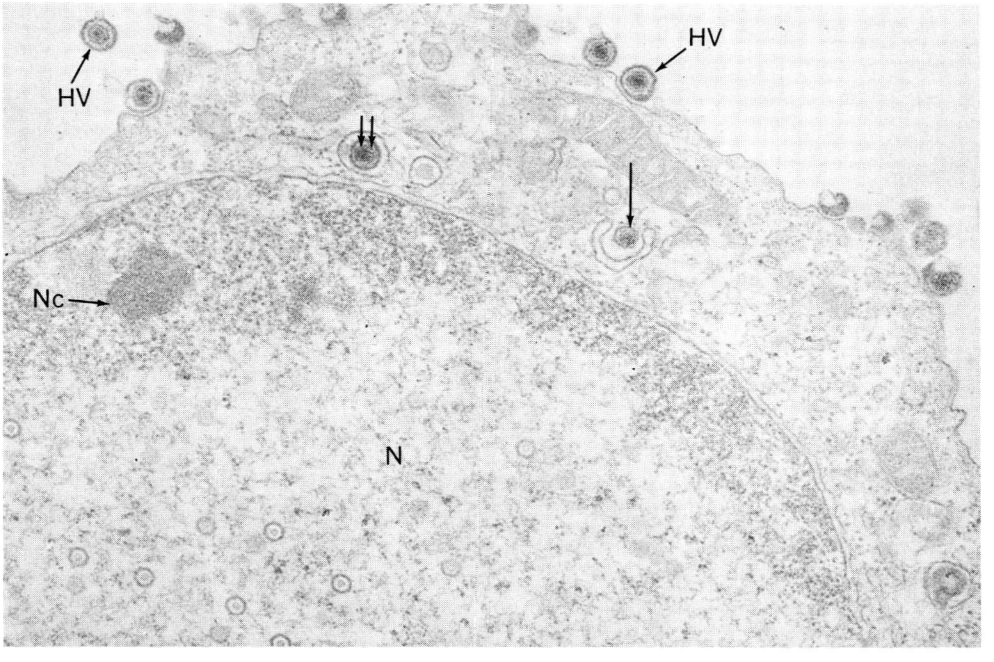

Figure 2-29. Section of cultured fibroblast 36 hours after infection with herpes virus (HV). Note the naked virions in the nucleoplasm (N) and the clumping of nuclear chromatin. The nucleolus is partially stratified. Virions are present within the cell sap, and one virion is apparently in the process of exotropy into the endoplasmic reticulum (arrow). One is also present at the cell surface; some of these may be in the process of uptake by the cell. (Courtesy of Dr. William D. Bradford).

letions (see below). Certain toxic compounds such as Trypan Blue and Triton WR-1339 are concentrated within lysosomes and result in inactivation of one or more enzymes. This can lead to functional alterations of particular importance in developing embryos, where administration of such compounds may result in congenital malformations.

Suicide-bag hypothesis. It has been proposed that the event which sends the cell beyond the point of no return is the bursting of hydrolase-laden vacuoles and consequent destructive release of enzymes. Although there is little doubt that digestive vacuoles do in fact break during the necrotic phase and release hydrolases in the cell sap, it has been difficult to support this hypothesis as it was originally stated. Changes characteristic of lethally altered cells do not usually begin to appear in the region of the cell rich in acid-hydrolase containing structures. In fact, the presence of intact digestive and endosecretory vesicles can be demonstarted well into the necrotic phase (Trump and Ginn, 1969). Under certain conditions, however, it does appear that the suicide-bag hypothesis may pertain. Perhaps the best example is the use of photosensitive dyes which can be concentrated within lysosomes and then, following exposure to light, will catalyze a photooxidation of the lysosomal membrane, resulting in the bursting of lysosomes and cell death.

Changes in lysosomal enzymes. In some cells, stimulation of pinocytic uptake of digestible materials induces the synthesis of increased amounts of acid hydrolases. This apparently represents genetic induction and can be inhibited by inhibitors of RNA or protein synthesis.

On the other hand, since there are many enzymes present in the digestive vacuoles, one could postulate a series of diseases in which each of the enzymes is deficient or absent (Hers, 1965) (Fig. 2-28c,d). Some such diseases have been identified. In general, these diseases result in accumulation of materials within ambidigestive vacuoles in various cells throughout the body (see chapter 7). In other instances, storage diseases may result from synthesis of abnormal materials which cannot be digested by the normal enzymes. Many of these storage diseases exert their most serious effects on neurons. These diseases may be susceptible to therapy by replacement of the missing enzyme in at least some organs, applying the principle which allows the mixing of contents between heterophagic and autophagic vacuoles. It has been shown in Pompe's disease (Type II glycogen storage disease), for example, that parenterally administered γ-glucosidase will be taken into the liver cell and will result in removal of glycogen from the vacuoles.

Lethal digestion has been proposed as a process involving conversion of an innocuous to a harmful substance by digestion. A possible example of the process

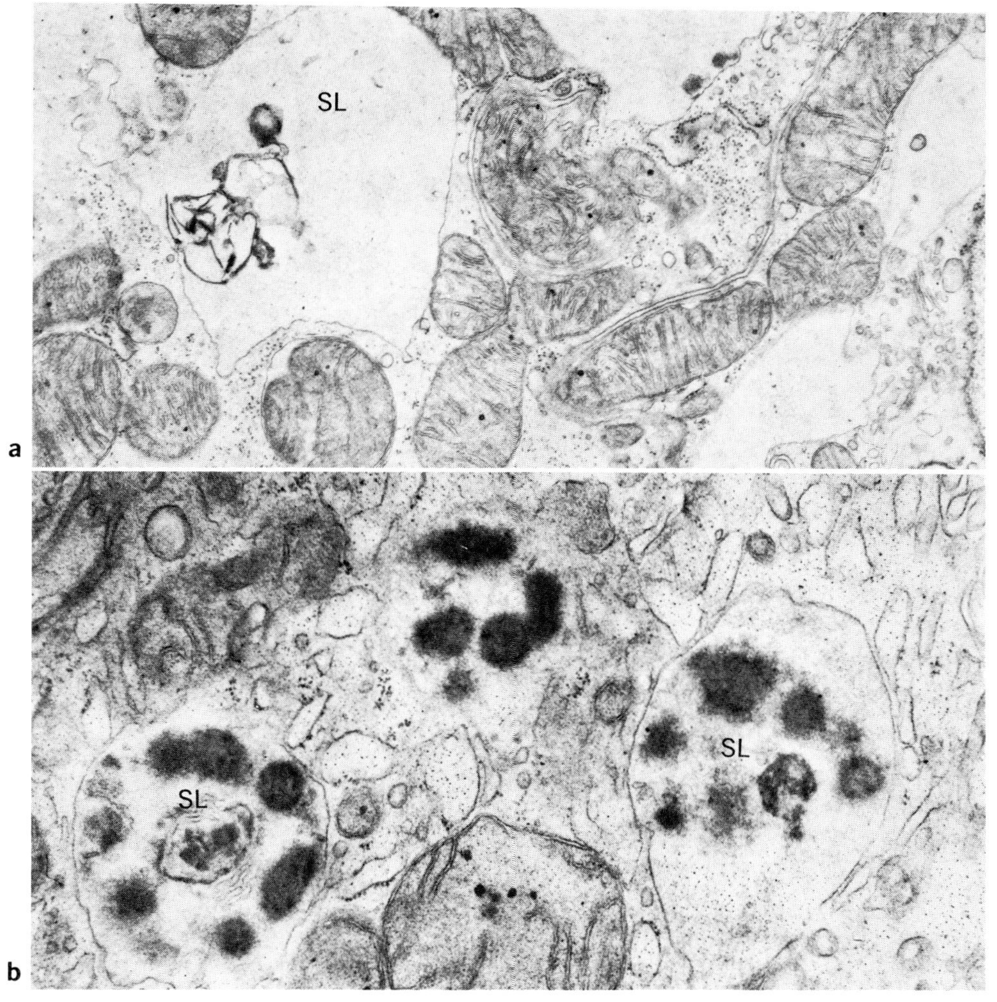

Figure 2-30. **a.** Proximal tubule cell of the rat after administration of sucrose. Marked enlargement of lysosomes (SL) characterizes hydropic or sucrose nephrosis.

b. Kidney tubule cell from a child with glomerulonephritis. Reabsorbed proteins accumulate in the proximal tubule lysosomes (SL).

would be esotropic uptake of virus. Uncoating of the virus in lysosomes may release the infectious nucleic acid which would then be free to infect the host.

Intracellular transport. An example of increased transport of material to the lysosomes for storage is provided by ferritin and hemosiderin storage in the liver cell. Apoferritin is synthesized, in part, on the rough endoplasmic reticulum and transported through that system to the Golgi apparatus and then to the lysosomes where storage and turnover occur. In conditions associated with increased levels of iron in the bloodstream, iron taken up by the liver cell may be added to the apoferritin which is in the cytocavitary network, to form ferritin, which is relatively immune to attack by lysosomal enzymes and hence accumulates within all hepatic lysosomes. If this continues, the liver becomes loaded with iron, and much of the ferritin becomes converted to an insoluble, rather poorly characterized iron-containing protein called *hemosiderin.* In periods of iron depletion, iron is released from ferritin within the lysosomes and re-enters the bloodstream. In two disease states, hemochromatosis and hemosiderosis, abnormal amounts of ferritin and hemosiderin are stored within hepatic lysosomes (Fig. 2-28a). Since ATP is necessary for transport within the ER and through the Golgi system, ATP deficiency results in defective transport of lysosomal enzymes and non-enzymatic components.

Hydrolase release from cells. Lysosomal enzymes are released from cells in the acute inflammatory reaction and appear to be responsible for some of the changes in capillary permeability at the site of inflammation. Leukocyte granules also contain leucocidin, which can act on other leukocytes producing degranulation and loss of digestive enzymes. Inadequate release of lysosome contents can result in accumulation of residual bodies or lipofuscin pigment. Neurons and muscle cells have poorly developed systems for secretion of lysosome contents and thus accumulate aging pigments.

Abnormal fusions. An abnormality possibly related to abnormal fusion comprises a group of diseases in various animals including Aleutian trait in the mink, partial albino cattle, and the Chediak-Higashi syndrome in humans. Aleutian mink trait, the best studied of these syndromes, results from an alteration of one gene and possibly one enzyme. In many cells, primary and secondary lysosomes, secretory granules, and pigment granules are bizarre in shape.

Abnormalities in peroxisomes. Microbodies, one type of peroxisome, represent a distinct group of storage vacuoles which form as diverticula of the cytocavitary network (de Duve and Bauduin, 1966). These vacuoles have been found in a variety of different cell types, especially in the hepatocytes and renal proximal tubular cells of vertebrates and in some protozoa (Hruban and Rechcigl, 1969). Morphologically, microbodies are typified by their thin (65-70Å), single, limiting membrane, their finely granular inner matrix, and in some species by an electron-dense core and/or a so-called marginal plate (Fig. 2-21f). The core may be either amorphous or paracrystalline. The term *marginal plate* refers to an electron dense plate about 85 Å thick which is separated from the limiting membrane by a narrow space. Microbodies are known to contain a number of peroxidative enzymes such as catalase, urate oxidase, D-amino acid oxidase, and, in some instances, enzymes associated with glycogen metabolism such as malate synthetase. Because the function of these enzymes is mainly peroxidative, microbodies are sometimes referred to as *peroxisomes*. Although their biological function has not yet been completely elucidated, these enzymes are known to participate in the metabolism of uric acid, and there are strong indications that they are involved in carbohydrate oxidation, in gluconeogenesis, in energy production, and in the oxidation of reduced NAD. They may also participate in the metabolism of lipids, bile acids, and prostaglandins.

At present little is known about the role of microbodies in the pathogenesis of cellular injury (Hruban and Rechcigl, 1969). The structure and number of microbodies are known to change after the administration of a wide variety of chemical compounds such as salicylates, chlorophenoxyisobutyrate (CPIB), lithocholic acid, and taurocholic acid. Since all of these compounds are known to decrease serum cholesterol levels, it has been postulated that microbodies may participate in the breakdown of cholesterol and may therefore play a role in the susceptibility to atherosclerosis. An interesting hypothesis regarding a possible role of catalase in cellular injury was proposed by de Duve, who suggested that this enzyme may form a safety device for oxidation of hydrogen peroxide in case of accelerated production. Since free hydrogen peroxide is a potent inducer of lipid peroxidation, the excess of catalase within microbodies could thus serve as an important inhibitor of intracellular lipid peroxidation.

G. Cytoplasmic Ground Substance

1. Normal structure and function

The cytoplasmic ground substance comprises the continuous phase of cytoplasm and consists of a gel-like material in which are suspended structures such as microtubules (Fig. 2-31), cytoplasmic filaments, glycogen deposits, free ribosomes, and possibly, in some instances, lipid droplets. It has been difficult to study because of its lack of formed materials.

Rapid changes in viscosity of this compartment have been noted in movies of injured cells, for example in the sap within membranous blebs at the cell surface. Increased Brownian motion of cytoplasmic particles, such as mitochondria, denotes changes in protoplasmic viscosity. The proteins of the cell sap may play a role in cell volume regulation through ion binding, contraction, or other conformational change.

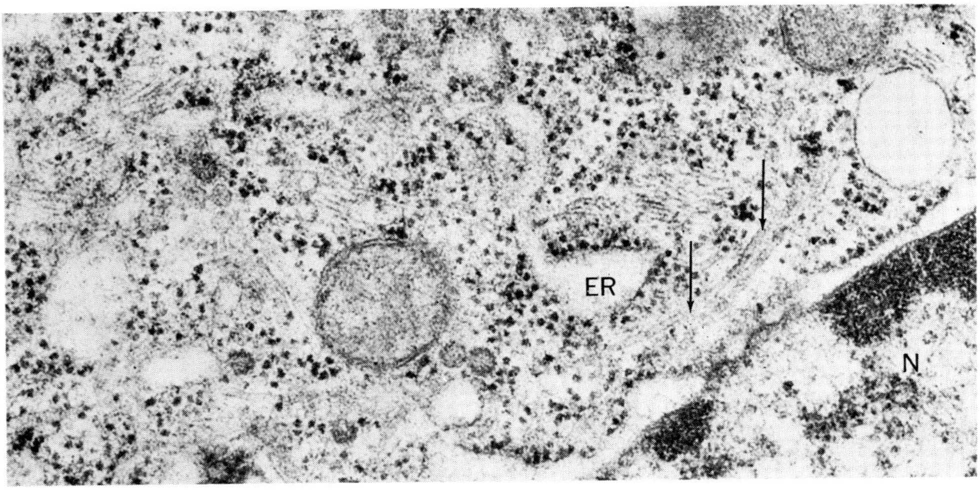

Figure 2-31. Ehrlich ascites tumor cell photographed to illustrate microtubules (arrows) in the cytoplasm. ER, endoplasmic reticulum; N, nucleus.

2. Modifications in injured cells

Alcoholic Hyalin (Fig. 32c). The term *alcoholic hyalin* designates a type of degeneration within hepatic cells originally described by Mallory in patients with alcoholic cirrhosis. It consists of cytoplasmic clumps of eosinophilic hyaline material which form multiple droplets and irregular meshworks distributed predominantly in the perinuclear cytoplasm of hepatic cells. By light microscopy, masses of alcoholic hyalin appear acidophilic and irregular in outline; they stain with dyes reacting with phospholipid. With the electron microscope, hyalin is characteristically found in areas which normally contain large amounts of rough endoplasmic reticulum and is associated with disarray, fragmentation, and disappearance of the rough endoplasmic reticulum. It is composed largely of a meshwork of fibrils approximately 80-100 Å thick. The pathogenesis of alcoholic hyalin is not clear; one current hypothesis states that it is derived from membranes of the endoplasmic reticulum. It should be differentiated from megamitochondria (see p. 41), which are also seen in the liver cells of alcoholics. Somewhat similar in appearance are aggregates of filaments which occur in the cytoplasm of aging neurons (Fig. 2-32d).

Changes in myofilaments. Changes in the size and number of myofilaments have been observed in both atrophy and hypertrophy of muscle. Especially striking is the toxicity of plasmocid for muscle; this quinoline derivative causes complete dissolution of I-band components including actin filaments; Z lines also disappear. In the human muscle disease known as Zenker's hyaline degeneration, changes in the ground substance consisting of decreased density and loss of fibrils seem to account for the characteristic light microscopic appearance.

Changes in density. Cell sap has been observed to exhibit marked changes in electron density after cell injury. A diffuse increase in density producing so-called dark cells and suggesting selective dehydration of individual cells has been observed in many non-specific types of injury where it is often associated with dilatation of the endoplasmic reticulum. Decrease in density of the cell sap may occur in conditions causing acute dilatation of the cisternae of the endoplasmic reticulum (Fig. 2-37a).

Another form of coagulation of cell sap can occur when there is denaturation of the cytoplasm as in thermal burns or laser irradiation.

In glycogen storage diseases other than Pompe's disease, increased numbers of glycogen rosettes are noted within the cell sap.

Fatty change. Although certain accumulations of triglyceride seem to occur within the endoplasmic reticulum (Fig. 2-23a) (see page 85), it cannot be excluded that triglycerides may also accumulate in another compartment, possibly within the cytoplasmic ground substance (Fig. 2-23b). A definitive, limiting membrane cannot be identified around most large lipid droplets.

Microtubules. Microtubules are generally defined as cylindrical structures (180-300 Å in diameter) with electron-dense walls and a less dense interior (Fig. 2-31). A relationship between microtubules and intracellular movements seems well established: chromosomal movements during mitosis and the motion of spermatozoa are examples. Microtubules have also been postulated to take part in the transport of water and small ions and in the formation of a skeletal support in epithelial cells. It is not known how microtubules develop.

The role of microtubules in cellular injury is for the present poorly understood. They are rather labile structures, which completely disappear after the use of certain fixatives or at low temperatures. On the basis of their association with cellular movements, one might speculate that abnormalities in their growth or function could seriously hamper cell function in general. Similarly, disappearance of the microtubules in axons could seriously impair transport of materials along the axon. A role for microtubules in constraining so-called saltatory movements of cell particles has been defined. Saltatory movement refers to rapid, back-and-forth linear movements of cytoplasmic particles such as mitochondria or lysosomes. In the presence of colchicine, which induces fragmentation of microtubules, these cytoplasmic movements become disordered. Colchicine and vin-

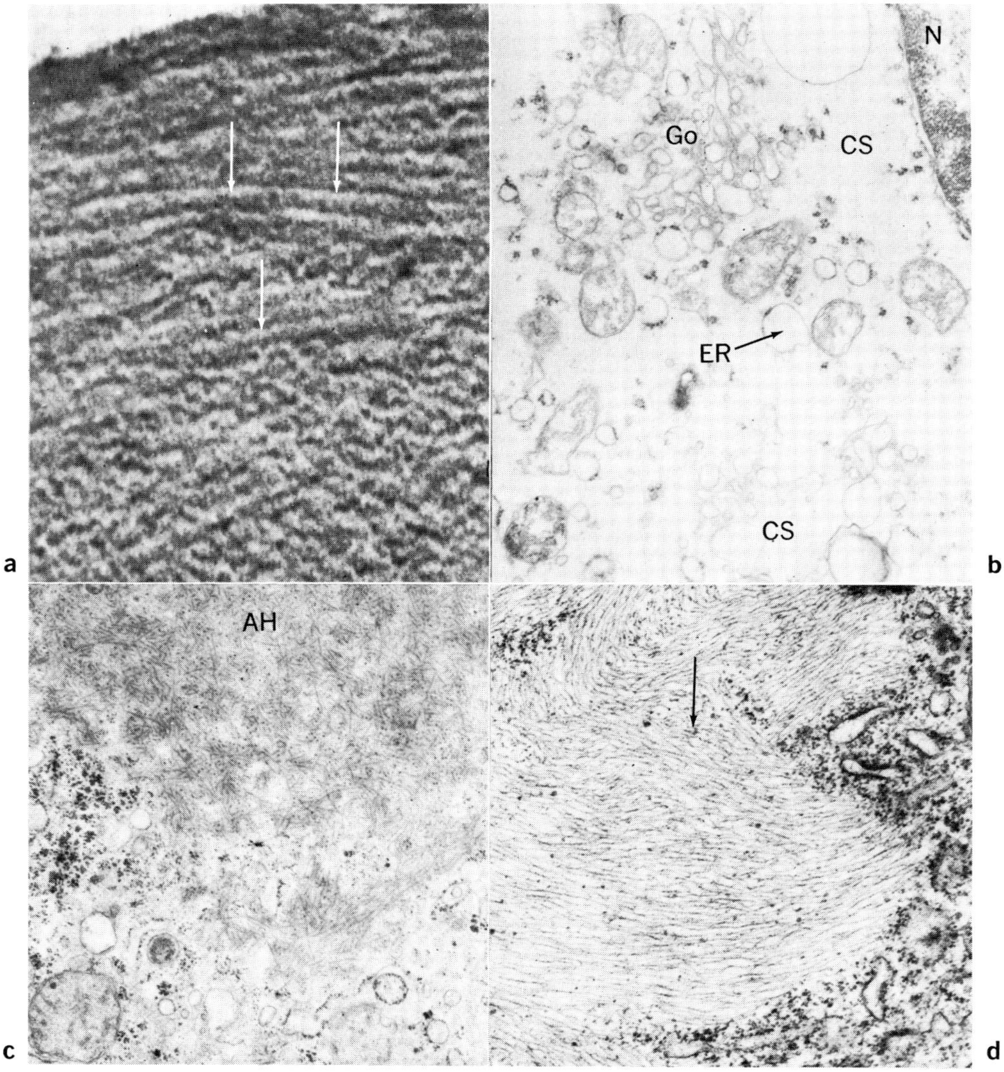

Figure 2-32. **a.** Freeze etched preparation of an erythrocyte from a patient with sickle cell disease. Alignment of linear microtubular forms of hemoglobin (arrow) is clearly seen. (Courtesy of Dr. Larry Lessin).

b. Astrocyte from the cerebellum of a rat after 30 minutes of anoxia. The nuclear (N) chromatin is clumped, the cell sap (CS) is expanded, and the endoplasmic reticulum (ER) dilated. Go, Golgi apparatus.

blastine also affect the microtubules of the mitotic spindle, and its application results in mitotic arrest at metaphase.

Hemoglobin. Mammalian erythrocytes may exhibit several types of pathologic change in components of the cell sap. In certain types of hemolytic anemia, especially those induced by phenylahydrazine or other drugs associated with oxidative denaturation of hemoglobin, precipitates called *Heinz bodies* occur within the red blood cell. These consist of relatively insoluble products of hemoglobin denaturation. It has also been suggested that these precipitates may form during the normal process of red cell senescence, leading to red cell destruction. The initial morphologic lesion in Heinz body development is the formation of an apparently crystalline structure, which usually appears in the region of mitochondria and grows by coalescence and condensation, finally coming to lie just beneath the cell membrane. These structures result in considerable distortion of cell shape and deformation of the plasma membrane. It is thought that such changes within the cytoplasm of red cells render the cells relatively rigid, increasing the chances of injury as cells pass through limited spaces such as the splenic cords. The resulting injury to the cell membrane presumably predisposes to hemolysis by accelerating erythrophagocytosis.

A striking conformational change in the cell sap occurs during red blood cell sickling in sickle cell anemia (Murayama, 1966). In well-oxygenated blood from patients with this disease, the red cells are morphologically indistinguishable from normal erythrocytes. When the oxygen tension is reduced, however, the cells shrink and crumple into sickle or holly leaf shapes. The only chemical difference between normal and sickle hemoglobin lies in the substitution of valine for glutamic acid at the sixth position in the two beta chains. This single amino acid substitution has two major effects: first, it causes deoxygenated hemoglobin, or S, to be much less soluble than deoxygenated normal hemoglobin or either form of oxyhemoglobin; second, a new molecular conformation ensues which predisposes to neat molecular packing. Other physical characteristics confirm the parallel alignment of hemoglobin molecules. Electron microscopic study reveals microtubular paracrystalline structures (Fig. 2-32a) which, on further study, are found to represent hollow cables, each formed of six hemoglobin monofilaments.

c. Hepatic cell cytoplasm from a patient with alcoholic cirrhosis. An accumulation of alcoholic hyalin is present (AH). This deposit is formed by a tangle of fine filaments within the cytoplasm. See also Figure 2-3e. (Courtesy of Dr. Oscar A. Iseri).

d. Neurofibrillary tangle in a neuron exposed to vincristine sulfate for 9 days, showing an accumulation of partially oriented fibrils. See also Figure 2-3f. (Courtesy of Dr. Peter W. Lampert).

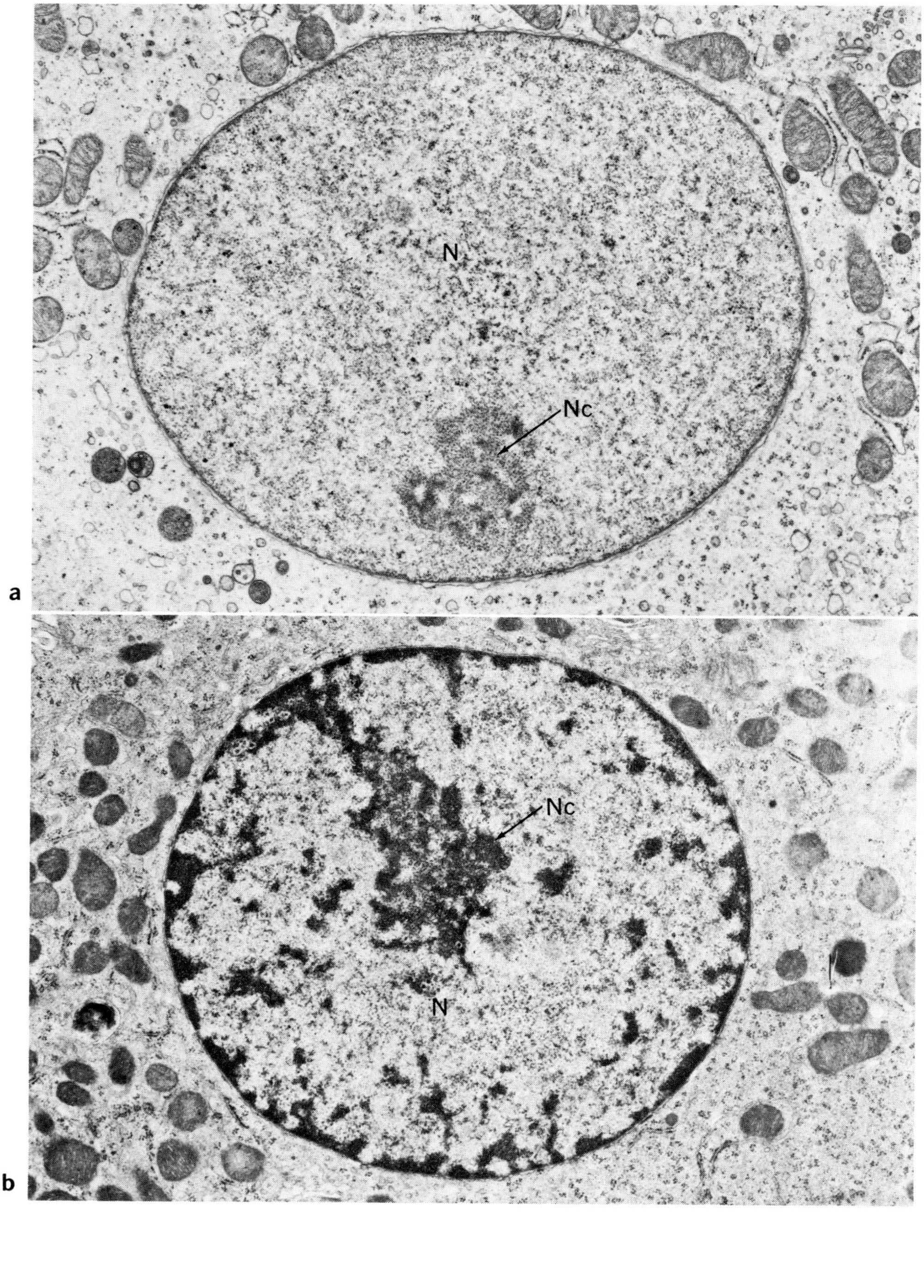
N
Nc
a
Nc
N
b

H. Genetic Transcription and Protein Synthesis

Although various steps of protein synthesis and genetic transcription take place in different parts of the cell, these parts are considered as a system because of the important interrelationships which they exhibit. The system comprises the nucleus, the nucleolus, the membrane-bound polysomes within the cytoplasm, and the free polysomes within the cell sap.

1. Alterations in the nucleus

There are marked variations in the structure and functional activities of the nucleus during different phases of the mitotic cycle (Fig. 2-38). During interphase, some regions of the chromatin called heterochromatin remain condensed. They are essentially inactive in RNA synthesis, which presumably takes place on the expanded portions of the chromatin (euchromatin). Chromatin fibrils are attached to the nuclear envelope adjacent to the nuclear pores and may have some effect on inducing formation of the latter structures.

The nucleus also contains other granules called interchromatin granules, perichromatin granules, perichromatin fibrils, and coiled bodies. The functional significance of all the granules is still poorly understood, although they may function as carriers of RNA (Fig. 2-33a, b).

The nucleus is separated from the cytoplasm by a nuclear envelope continuous with the endoplasmic reticulum from which it appears to form after mitosis is completed. At the nuclear pores the two membranes come together with obliteration of the perinuclear cisterna. This cisterna may markedly enlarge in injured cells. It seems clear that the pores serve as semipermeable barriers between nucleus and cytoplasm and may be the pathway for transfer of RNA or other macromolecules to the cytoplasm.

The significance of nuclear alterations in cell injury depends on the stage of the cell cycle at the time of injury. In postmitotic cells it seems quite clear that interference with nuclear function is not immediately lethal for the cell. Thus it cannot explain the progression to cell necrosis after acute injury such as infarc-

Figure 2-33. **a.** Kidney tubule cell fixed with osmium tetroxide. Note the even distribution of the nuclear chromatin and interchromatin granules. N, nucleus; Nc, nucleolus.

b. A similar kidney tubule cell after fixation with glutaraldehyde followed by osmium. The chromatin is clumped along the nuclear envelope and around the nucleolus (Nc). N, nucleus.

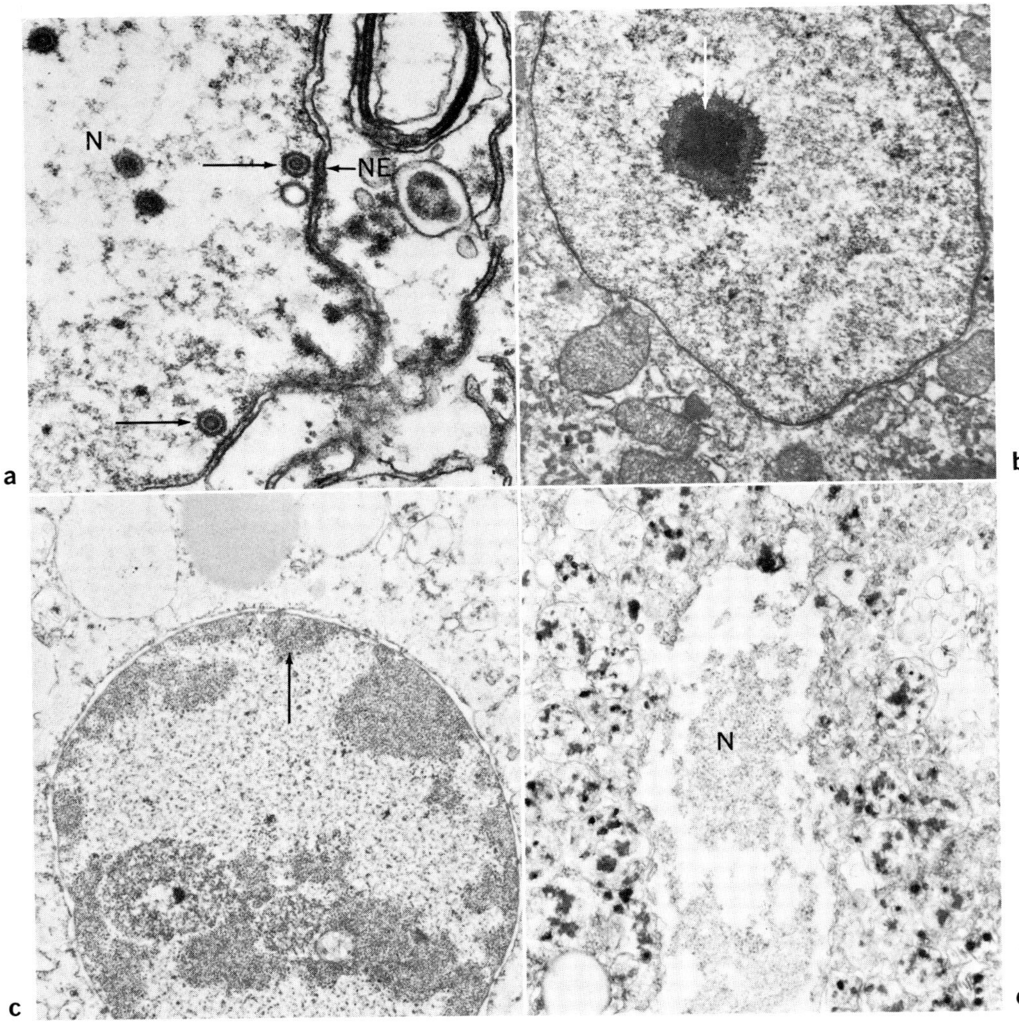

Figure 2-34. **a.** HeLa cell 48 hours after infection with Herpes simplex virus showing the appearance of naked virions (arrows) or nucleocapsids in the nucleus (N). Within the nucleus there is dissolution of chromatin. Note also thickening and apparent reduplication of nuclear envelope (NE). (Courtesy of Mr. Bernard Poeschel).

b. Lead-induced nuclear inclusion (arrow) in a rat kidney tubule cell. (Courtesy of Dr. Robert Goyer).

c. Clumping of chromatin (arrow) and partial dissolution of the nucleolus in an Ehrlich ascites cell after treatment with mercuric chloride for 2 hours. (Courtesy of Dr. Kauno Laiho).

d. Karyolysis of the nucleus (N) in a kidney tubule cell 24 hours after the administration of mercuric chloride. (Courtesy of Dr. Thomas Gritzka).

tion. In fact, there are numerous experiments in the literature employing suitable cell types which indicate that the entire nucleus may be removed from a cell by microdissection without killing the cell until several days have passed.

There is, on the other hand, a series of nuclear changes in lethal and sublethal reactions to injury, which is of importance not only in recognizing the effects of cell injury but also in understanding their pathogenesis.

Changes in aggregation and distribution of chromatin (Fig. 2-34). Following diverse types of cell injury the chromatin fibrils, which are normally distributed diffusely in the nucleoplasm of most cells, become aggregated or clumped along the nuclear membrane and around the nucleolus. This process can easily be observed in living cells by phase-contrast microscopy, and, by alternately lowering and restoring the pH of the medium, it can be produced and reversed several times without interfering with the subsequent mitotic activity of the cell. The clumping of nuclear chromatin exposes large areas of interchromatin substance in which fine filamentous materials can be clearly seen. The interchromatin granules seem to separate from the chromatin and appear in linear aggregations at the interface between chromatin and interchromatin substance.

The phenomenon of chromatin aggregation and condensation proceeds very rapidly after injurious stimuli and is one of the earliest responses of the cell to injury. As necrosis proceeds in the cell these aggregated chromatin fibrils condense further, become focally rarefied, and finally disappear; this is presumably the result of attack by DNase and cathepsins from lysosomes. Eventually the nucleus contains little or no DNA and at this point is said to exhibit karyolysis. In karyolytic nuclei the nuclear envelope often remains relatively intact. The change known as pyknosis is equivalent to clumping of chromatin and, in nuclei with smaller volumes, the masses of condensed chromatin may occupy the entire nucleus giving it a uniform basophilic appearance.

Nuclear inclusions. Various types of nuclear inclusions have been described in injured cells.

Pseudoinclusions (Fig. 2-35a) represent deep cytoplasmic indentions into the nucleus which, because of the plane of section, appear to reside within the nucleoplasm. These can be easily identified by the nuclear pores in the envelope surrounding them. Pseudoinclusions increase in number as the nuclei become irregular and are often observed to occur in cells undergoing rapid turnover.

True inclusions are abnormal depositions or accumulations which actually lie within the nucleoplasm. Perhaps the most characteristic of these are inclusions formed by virus particles (Fig. 2-34a) which may be striking because of their crystalline array. Intranuclear inclusions may also occur in the nuclei of renal tubules in heavy metal poisoning with bismuth or lead (Fig. 2-34b). Many other

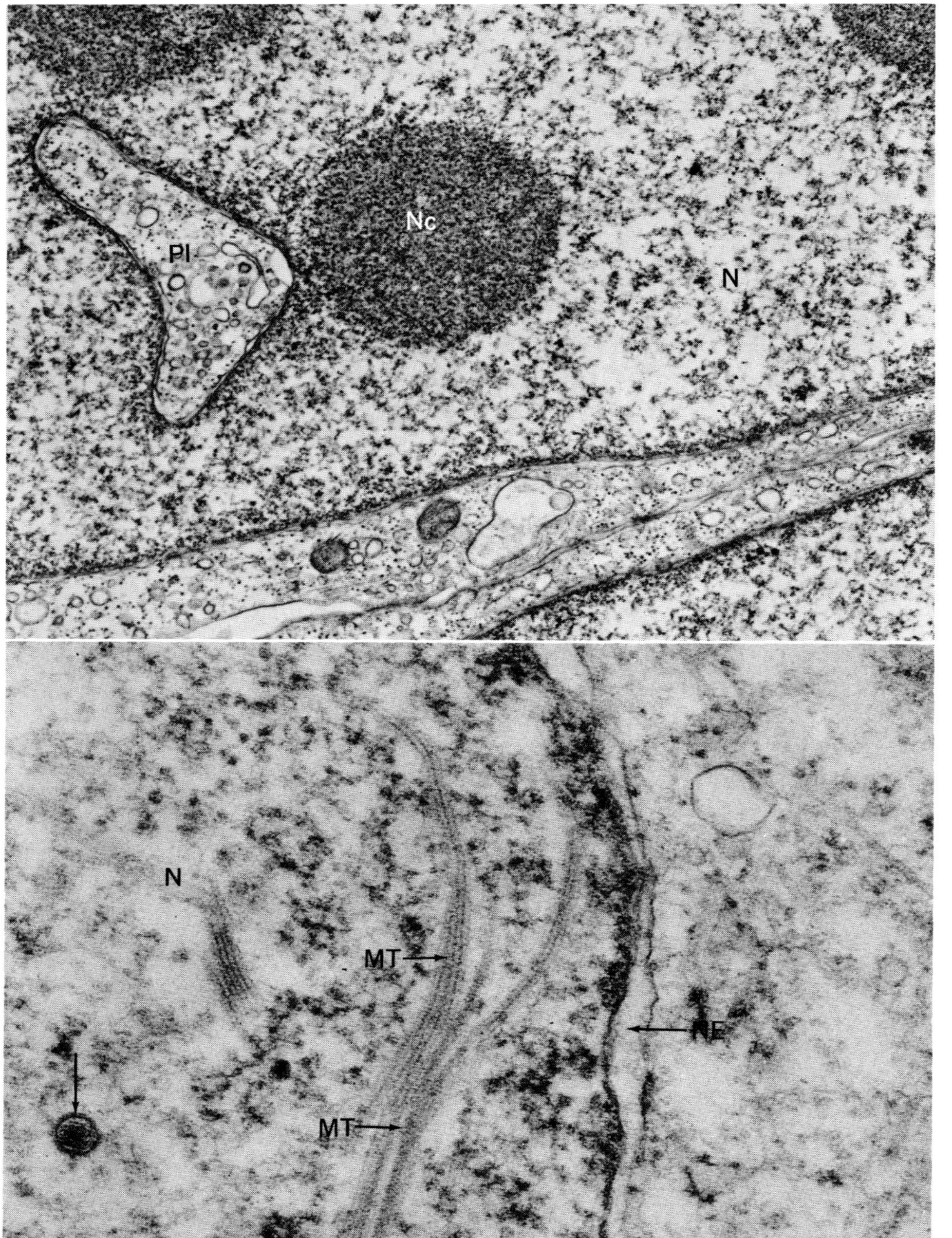

a

b

kinds of accumulation of vesicles, glycogen, concentric lamellar bodies, fibrillar structures, vacuoles, and tubular (Fig. 2-35b) or filamentous inclusions have been described but are of unknown significance.

2. Alterations in the nucleolus (Fig. 2-36)

Nucleoli in most cells have at least three distinct regions: (1) those containing dense ribosome-like particles 150-200 Å in diameter, (2) those containing filaments 80-100 Å in diameter, and (3) those containing intranucleolar chromatin fibrils identical with the fibrils in the nucleoplasm (Bernard and Granboulan, 1968). The ribosome-like particles and the 80-100 Å filaments both seem to represent RNA and protein. The fibrils are arranged in an open skein-like structure sometimes termed the *nucleolonema,* whose open regions (nucleolar vacuoles) contain the chromatin fibrils of the intranucleolar chromatin which, with the condensed chromatin in the periphery of the nucleolus (nucleolus-associated chromatin), probably represent the nucleolus organizer. Nucleoli have a constant relationship to specific chromosomes and tend to be constant in number and position for a given species.

In recent years it has been established that both the 28S and the 18S components of ribosomal RNA are synthesized in the nucleolus. This synthesis proceeds via the RNA polymerase reaction and is sensitive to actinomycin D.

Numerous carcinogenic and antimetabolic agents induce changes in the structure and function of the nucleolus, which may be related to their metabolic effects. Among these are actinomycin D, lasiocarpine, aflatoxin, and ultraviolet irradiation, all of which interfere with DNA-dependent RNA synthesis. These agents cause segregation or stratification of the nucleolar components into regions composed of particles, RNA-protein fibrils, and chromatin fibrils, respectively, plus an altered RNA-protein component or dense plaque (Fig. 2-36c,d). They also arrest the production of RNA subunits within the nucleolus (and elsewhere in the nucleus).

Ethionine, which traps adenine in the formation of s-adenosyl-ethionine, in a sense produces and inhibits RNA and protein synthesis, an effect opposite to

Figure 2-35. **a.** HeLa cell showing pseudoinclusion (PI) of the nucleus (N). Note that the pseudoinclusion is surrounded by a typical double-layered nuclear envelope and contains cytoplasmic structures.

b. Nuclear microtubules (NT) in cultured fibroblasts 36 hours after infection with Herpes simplex virus. Note a virion (arrow) within nucleoplasm. NE, nuclear envelope. (Courtesy of Dr. William D. Bradford).

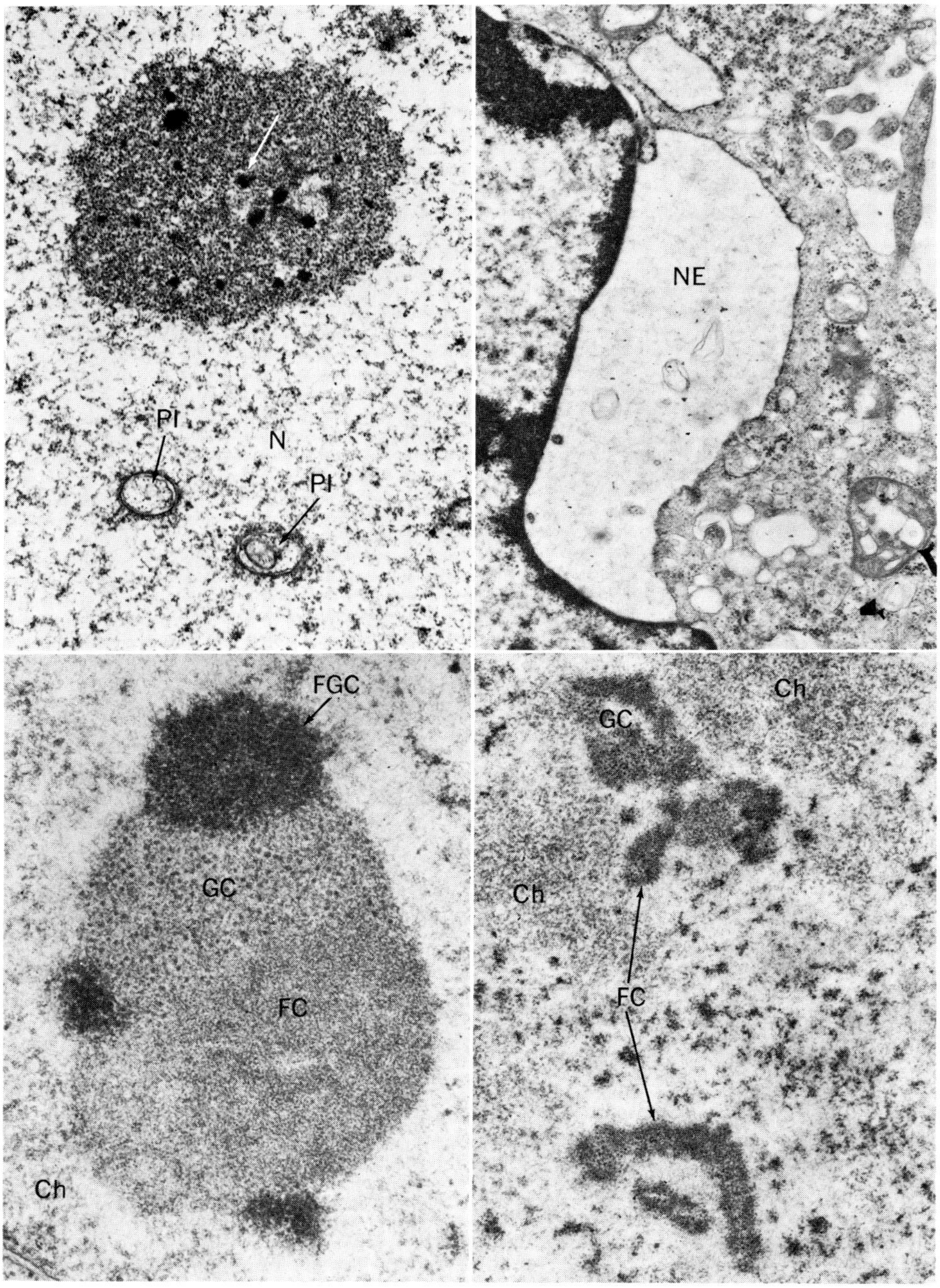
a
PI
N
PI
b
NE
c
FGC
GC
FC
Ch
d
GC
Ch
Ch
FC

segregation. Components of the nucleolus are widely dispersed (Fig. 2-36d), but can be reaggregated after the administration of adenine (Shinozuka *et al.,* 1968).

3. Alterations in protein synthesis

The effects of inhibition of protein synthesis are highly dependent on the phase of the cell cycle. Thus, postmitotic liver parenchymal cells, kidney tubular cells, or striated muscle cells can survive virtually complete inhibition of protein synthesis for relatively long periods of time. It is therefore unlikely that acute necrotizing injuries, which commonly show early effects on protein synthesis, exert their lethal action by this means.

Changes in the ribosome-membrane association are common early events after a variety of lethal or sublethal cell injuries. Detachment of polysomes from the membrane is usually associated with their breakdown and appearance of monosomes in the cell sap (Fig. 2-37). At least in some instances, the sedimentation properties of the monosomes may be markedly altered as well. This detachment from the membrane is apparently always associated with defective protein synthesis *in vivo* or *in vitro,* although in some cases it has been possible, at least partially, to repair the defect by the use of artificial messengers such as polyuridylic acid. The precise mechanisms involved in the membrane detachment have not been worked out; it was mentioned above, however, that conditions known to modify membrane structure are especially prone to promote such detachment (see p. 51). It is highly probable that the membrane attachment is of great significance to polysome function. There are, for example, indications that the membrane may contain some type of message and that the endoplasmic electron transport system may be involved in the generation of high energy intermediates

Figure 2-36. **a.** Nucleolar changes in a HeLa cell nucleus 12 hours after infection with Herpes simplex virus. The nucleolus has a spotty moth-eaten appearance with highly condensed areas (arrow). Two pseudoinclusions (PI) are present at the left.

b. A perinuclear vacuole, caused by massive dilatation of the nuclear envelope (NE) appears in an Ehrlich ascites cell 2 hours after treatment with cyanide and iodacetic acid. The chromatin is densely clumped.

c. Segregation of the nucleus of a rat liver cell after administration of actinomycin D. FGC, fibrillar granular component (plaque); GC, granular component; FC, fibrillar component; CH, chromatin. A fourth apparent nucleolar zone at the lower left is a subcomponent of the fibrillar zone. (Courtesy of Dr. Peter J. Goldblatt).

d. Nucleolus of a rat liver cell 12 hours after administration of ethionine to a male rat. The various components are disintegrating. GC, granular component; FC, fibrillar component; CH, chromatin. (Courtesy of Dr. Peter J. Goldblatt).

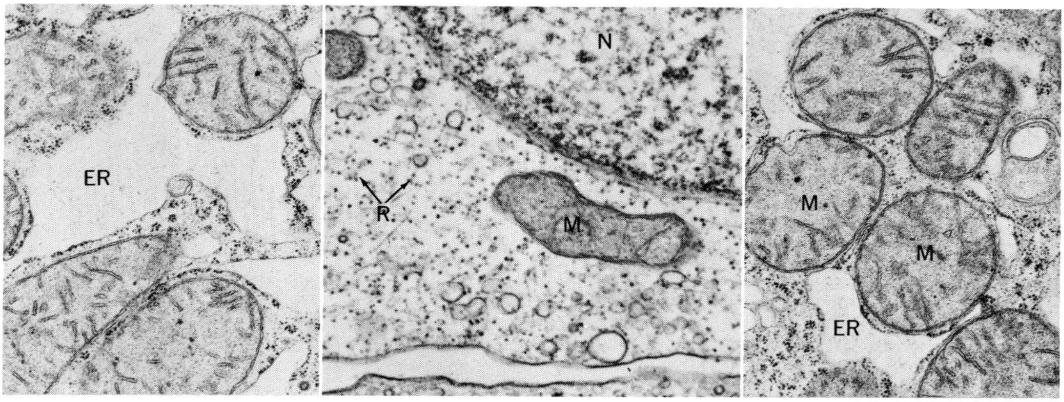

Figure 2-37. **a.** Hepatic parenchymal cell 4 hours after administration of carbon tetrachloride. Marked dilatation of the endoplasmic reticulum (ER) is seen. Polysomes appear intact and mitochondria (M) show no change.

b. HeLa cell 6 hours after infection with Herpex simplex virus showing dissociation of polysomes into ribosome monomers (R). M, mitochondrion; N, nucleus.

for driving protein synthesis. At the same time, it should be noted that membrane detachment is not a prerequisite for protein synthesis inhibition. The antibiotic cycloheximide, for example, which inhibits at the ribosome level, does not promote dissociation and in fact tends to stabilize polysomes against the dissociation that can be induced by other protein synthesis inhibitors such as puromycin.

4. Variation in susceptibility to injury in different phases of the cell cycle (Fig. 2-38)

Through the use of synchronized cell cultures, it has been possible to study variations in sensitivity to toxic agents throughout the division cycle (Baserga and Wiebel, 1967). This variation is extremely important in clinical medicine because it constitutes a possible basis of current cancer chemotherapy and radiotherapy and helps substantially to explain the undesirable side effects of these methods of treatment.

Variations in sensitivity to injury in different mitotic phases is especially evident following injury by ionizing irradiation or radiomimetic agents such as the nitrogen mustards, which are so-called alkylating agents. Cells in early G1 and G2 phases are the least sensitive, and cells in M, late G1, or early S phase are the most sensitive. For a variety of cells, irradiation prolongs the interphase period and delays the entry of cells into mitosis by prolonging the time in G2. Characteristic cytologic changes are observed in the nucleus during cell division, including chromosome breaks, bridge formation between chromosomes at anaphase, and chromosomal fragmentation. In contrast, some cells such as lymphocytes and spermatogonia apparently undergo an immediate, cytolytic type of death after irradiation.

In another category are agents exhibiting differential effects during the cell

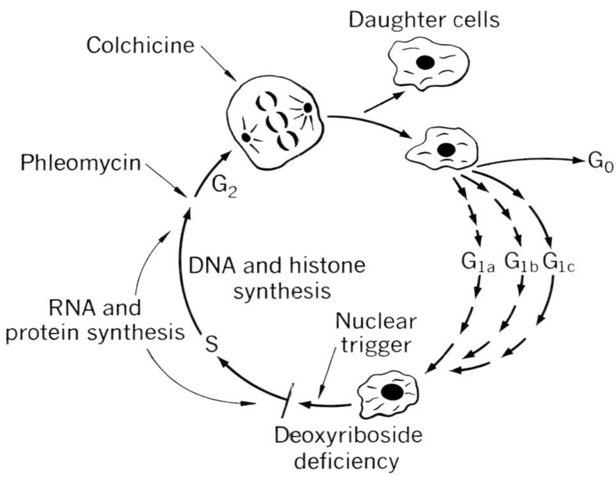

Figure 2-38. Concepts of the cell cycle in relation to cell injury. The replication of animal cells is a highly ordered sequence of molecular events requiring the expression of specific genetic information at certain steps in the cycle. S phase, an interval lasting 6-7 hours in many cells, is concerned with the synthesis of a complete complement of DNA and histones; progression through this interval requires the timely synthesis of RNA as well as DNA and proteins. The G_2 interval, mitosis and cell division, require approximately 2-3 hours and are concerned with the formation of newly synthesized chromatin into chromosome pairs and the distribution of the condensed chromosomes into the daughter-cells. Progression into the G_2 interval requires the completion of DNA synthesis and the antecedent synthesis of RNA and protein. In HeLa cells phleomycin blocks the cell cycle near the end of the DNA synthesis period. Colchicine and other agents active against the microtubules block the progression of cells through metaphase. Cells with different replication times vary mainly in the duration of the G_1 interval and are depicted in the diagram as G_{1a}, G_{1b}, G_{1c}, and G_o. During this interval the cell expresses the phenotypic character of its particular differentiated state. Depending on intracellular and extracellular factors, cells progress through G_1 and become triggered for nuclear replication and histone synthesis (From Mueller, 1969).

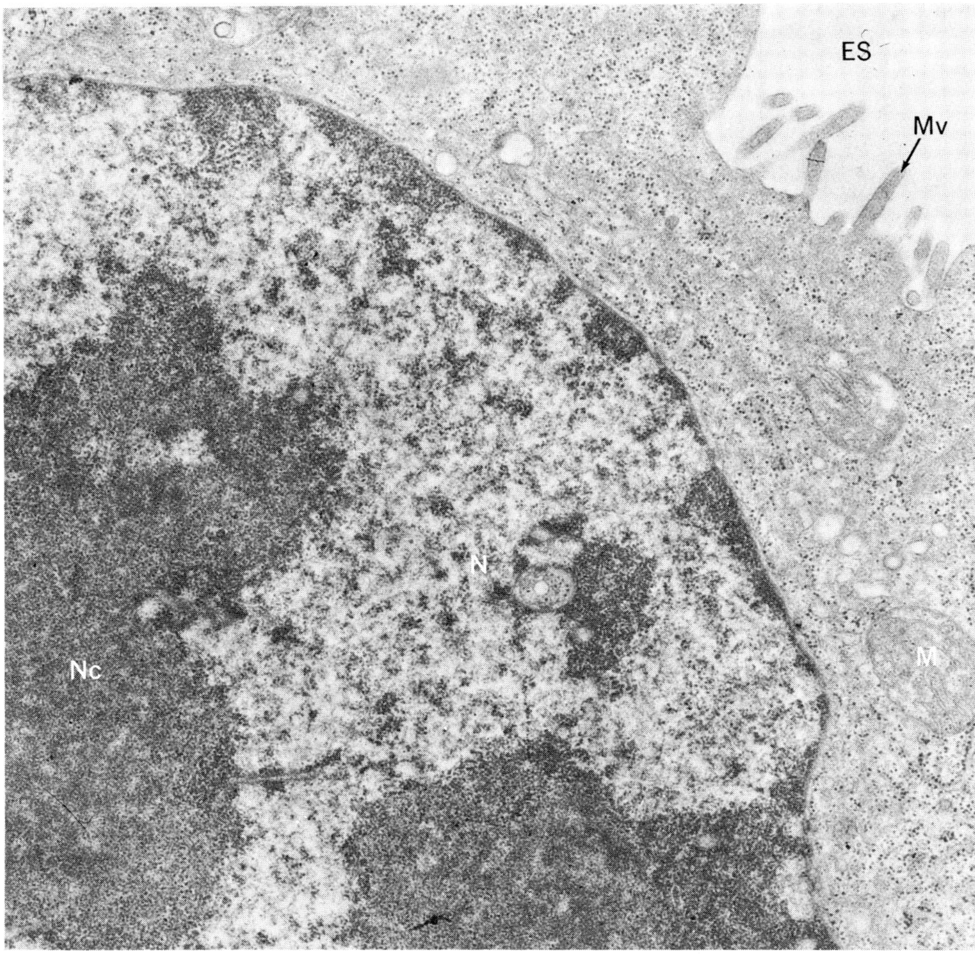

Figure 2-39. This Ehrlich ascites tumor cell has the characteristics of an undifferentiated cell. The nucleus (N) is large in comparison with the cytoplasm, and contains massive nucleoli (Nc). In the cytoplasm are numerous free ribosomes, scant endoplasmic reticulum, inconspicuous mitochondria (M), and the surface membrane is thrown into prominent surface microvilli (Mv). ES, extracellular space.

cycle, the so-called spindle poisons, which include colchicine, griseofulvin, vincristine, and vinblastine. All these agents interfere with the formation of the mitotic spindle, possibly by binding with specific microtubule proteins, thus stabilizing or blocking the process of mitosis in metaphase. The spindle poisons have been used in studies of chromosomes (karyotype analysis) which require the collection of large numbers of chromosomes for morphologic characterization.

It is interesting that some features of the M phase are quite similar to the phase of altered homeostasis after cell injury. During mitosis the cells become rounded, and there is evidence of marked alteration in cell membrane permeability. Existing supplies of high energy compounds are used up and there is little or no further synthesis. The stress of the M phase often proves lethal to the cell whose programmed march through S and G_2 has been interfered with.

5. **The undifferentiated cell** (Figs. 2-39, 2-40)

Undifferentiated cells are important in many pathologic reactions. Such cells occur in regenerating epithelia or mesenchyme, many types of hyperplasia, embryonic tissue and hamartomas, elements of the hematopoietic system, and neoplasia (Haguenau, 1969). The structural and functional characteristics of undifferentiated cells are distinctive and differ little from one cell type to another. Even the cells of highly malignant neoplasms share these same essential features.

Undifferentiated cells are usually rounded or have only a few irregular cytoplasmic processes. Their shape depends on their environment and on the types of adjacent structures. They do not show typical membrane specializations of differentiated cells, such as microvilli or cilia. They are characterized by a high ratio of nuclear to cytoplasmic volume, and the cytoplasm is quite basophilic and pyroninophilic due to the high concentration of RNA in the form of numerous polysomes which are predominantly free within the cell sap. Relatively few profiles of rough endoplasmic reticulum are present. The mitochondria are inconspicuous, probably reflecting the fact that cells usually have well-developed systems for aerobic and anaerobic glycolysis. Digestive vacuoles or lysosomes are usually not prominent, although early in regeneration in some organs such as the liver and kidney, large autophagic vacuoles may occur. Not all other types of endoplasmic storage and secretory vacuoles are prominent. The nuclei are large, often because they are polyploid, and various abnormalities of mitotic division may occur. Nucleoli are numerous, large, and full of particles representing ribosome precursors and perhaps other forms of RNA.

These features of undifferentiated cells probably reflect the fact that the transcription and translation systems are primarily directed toward the task of division. If differentiation occurs after division is completed, the appearance of the specialized organelles characteristic of the particular cell type can be readily followed. In the case of malignant neoplasms, differentiation usually does not occur and the progeny continue into S phase.

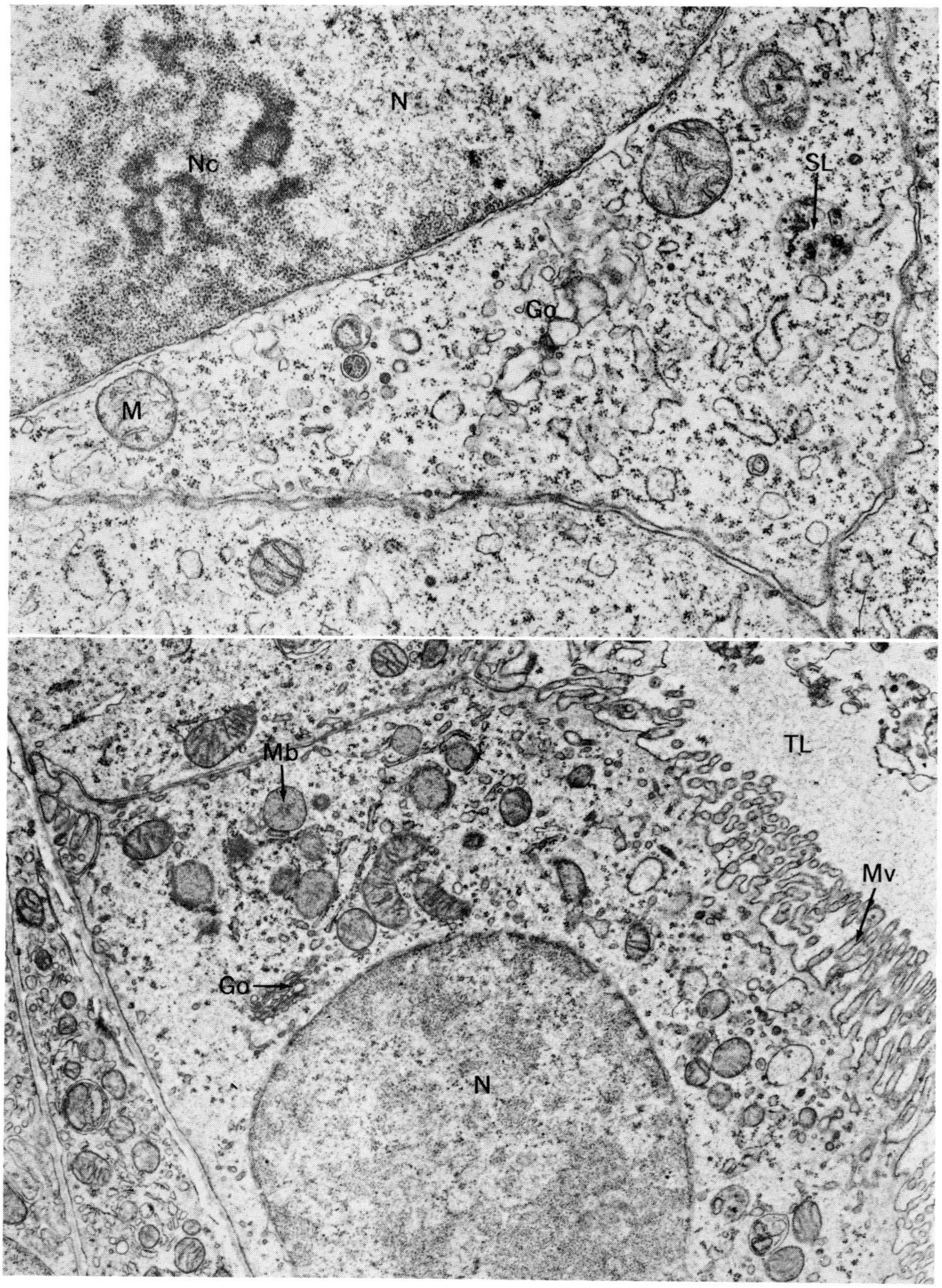
N
Nc
SL
Go
M
a
Mb
TL
Mv
Go
N
b

I. Integrated Aspects of Cellular Reaction to Injury

In this section the interrelations between organelle changes in injured cells will be considered. The effects of injury on cells are complex; accordingly, it is necessary to attempt a synthesis of available data, recognizing the tendency toward oversimplification. Much work remains to be done in this area.

1. Cellular adaptations to sublethal injury

The cell can often adapt to sublethal injury by attaining a new steady state through which it is able to maintain homeostasis even in the face of continued injury (Fig. 2-41). In this section we will consider some of these adaptations.

Hypertrophy. Cellular hypertrophy refers to increased size of cells resulting from an increase in the mass of structural components. Ultrastructurally, it is often reflected by an increase in the size and number of organelles such as mitochondria, endoplasmic reticulum, and ribosomes; that is, hypertrophy of the cell may be represented by both hypertrophy and hyperplasia of organelles.

Administration of many lipid-soluble drugs such as phenobarbital is followed by induction of detoxification enzymes and synthesis of endoplasmic reticulum membrane in the liver. The liver cells undergo hypertrophy. This can be thought of as a protective adaptation on the part of the liver cell, as it substantially augments drug detoxifying ability.

Hypertrophy has been particularly well studied in muscle cells where it represents a response to an increased work load. In hypertrophied cardiac muscle cells there is an increase in the amount of sarcoplasmic reticulum, ribosomes, and numbers of myofilaments, all of which increase the work capacity of the muscle cell. The mitochondria sometimes show a relative deficiency of cristal membranes, which has been said to explain the increased susceptibility of hypertrophied heart muscle to cardiac failure.

Figure 2-40. Stages of regeneration of rat kidney tubule cells after the administration of mercuric chloride.

a. Regenerating cell after 2 days. This cell has taken on the appearance of an undifferentiated cell and looks much like the cell in Figure 2-39. There is a large nuclear-cytoplasmic ratio and a prominent nucleolus (Nc) containing many ribosome precursors. Many ribosomes are lying free in the cell sap. Mitochondria are scarce, as is endoplasmic reticulum. SL, secondary lysosome; Go, Golgi apparatus; M, mitochondrion.

b. After 7 days the cell is redifferentiating. Mitochondria are elongated and much more numerous. A regular brush border of microvilli (Mv) is forming at the luminal surface, the Golgi apparatus (Go) is more closely organized, and microbodies are appearing. TL, tubular lumen; N, nucleus.

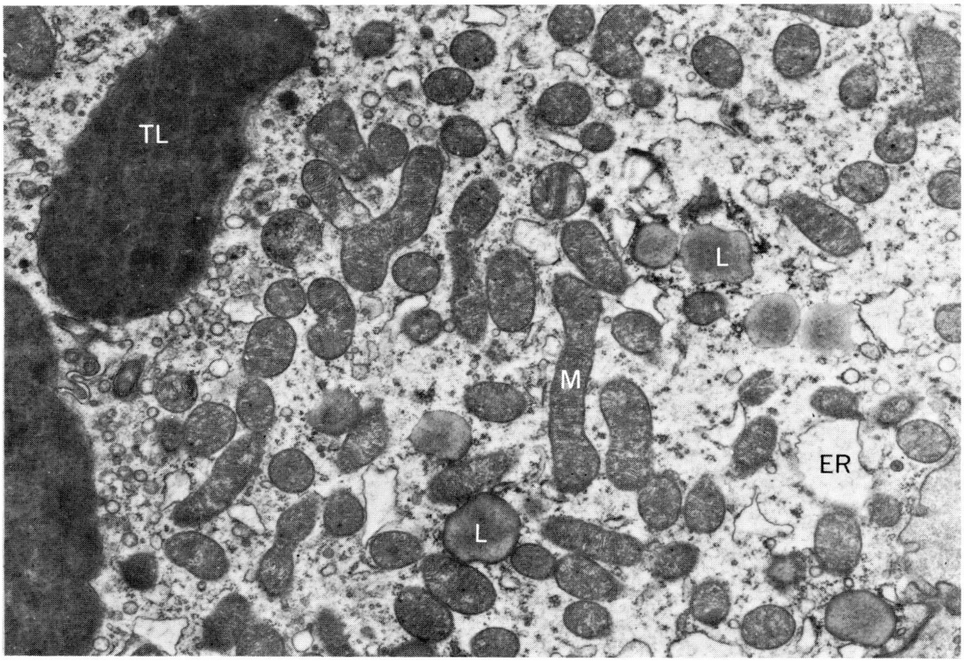

Figure 2-41. Distal tubule cell from a rat poisoned with mercuric chloride. Sublethal alterations have led to a new steady state in which the tubular lumens (TL) are occupied by dense casts. The endoplasmic reticulum (ER) is dilated, and lipid droplets (L) have accumulated. Mitochondria (M) appear normal.

Atrophy. This term refers to decreased size of cells resulting from various factors, including decreased work load, decreased nutrition, hypoxia, or decreased hormonal stimulation. The decrease in cell mass implies continued turnover of cell components, often related to the increased numbers of autophagic vacuoles that are typically found in cells undergoing atrophy. The debris within these vacuoles may be converted to residual bodies, resulting in numerous granules of lipofuscin pigment; in the heart this imparts a brown color to the muscle and the process is termed *brown atrophy.* Additional changes in atrophic muscle include breakdown and decrease in number of myofilaments, fragmentation of the endoplasmic reticulum, and swelling and degeneration of mitochondria.

Virus-cell interaction. These interactions are discussed in Chapters 4 and 6. It is sufficient at this time to point out that, although many viruses are rapidly lethal to cells, other viruses have achieved variable degrees of adaptation. Totally inapparent endosymbiotic infections, latent infections, slow virus infection, and malignant transformation of cells with disappearance of virus are examples. Depending on the type of virus and the type of infection, structural abnormalities in the infected cells may accompany these functional changes. In many DNA viruses, large nuclear inclusions, often containing crystalline aggregates of virions, are typically seen. In RNA viruses, sites of virus production (viral "factories") often result in cytoplasmic inclusions. In both cases membrane changes in the cell may be numerous. These include viral specified changes in plasma membrane composition in the case of influenza virus, extensive fusion and redundancy of the nuclear envelope in herpes virus, proliferations of endoplasmic reticulum associated in vaccinia virus replication, and large filamentous cytoplasmic inclusions in measles virus. Virions can also be found within lysosomes, perhaps resulting from fusions with virion-containing cisternae or vacuoles, or as a result of direct exotropy of virions from the cell sap into the lysosome.

Fatty changes in cells (Figs. 2-23a,b, 2-42). The accumulation of lipid within the cell cytoplasm is a common sublethal reaction to injury which often represents an altered steady state. Although the appearance of the cells is greatly

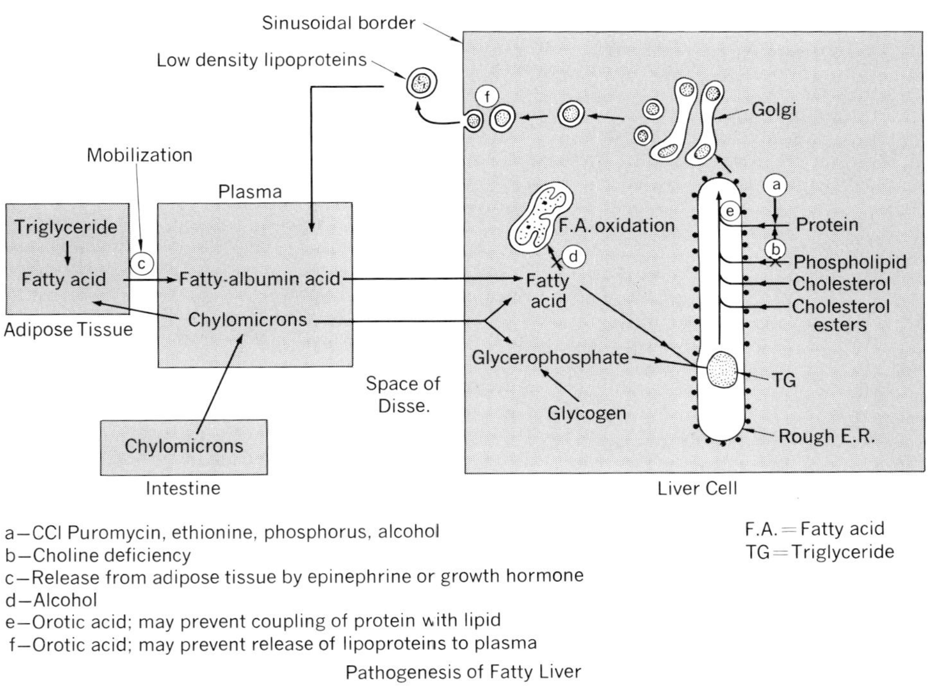

Figure 2-42. Pathogenesis of fatty liver. See text. Modified from Lombardi, 1965.

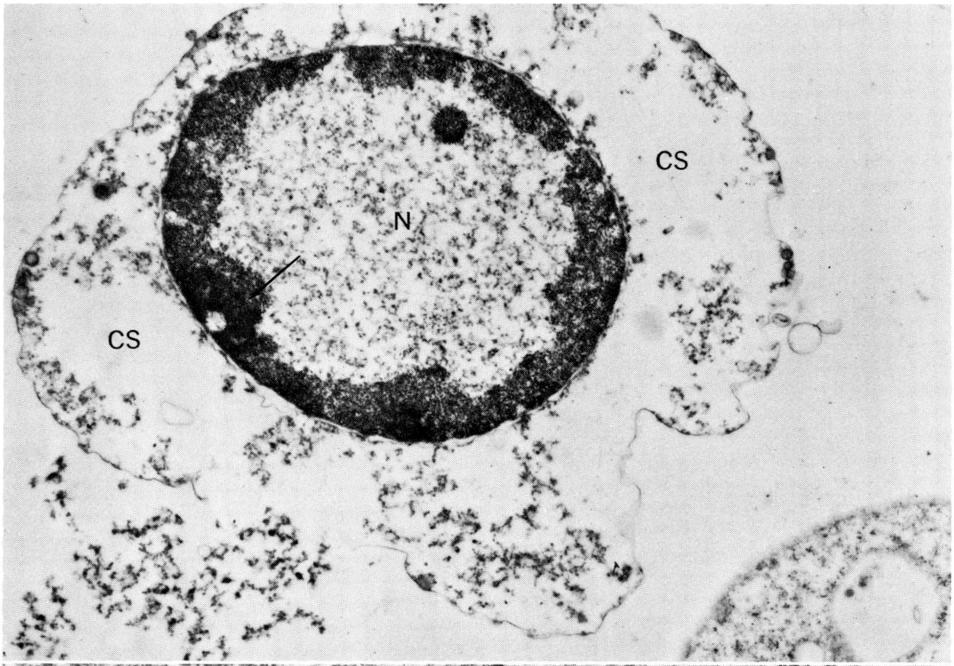

a

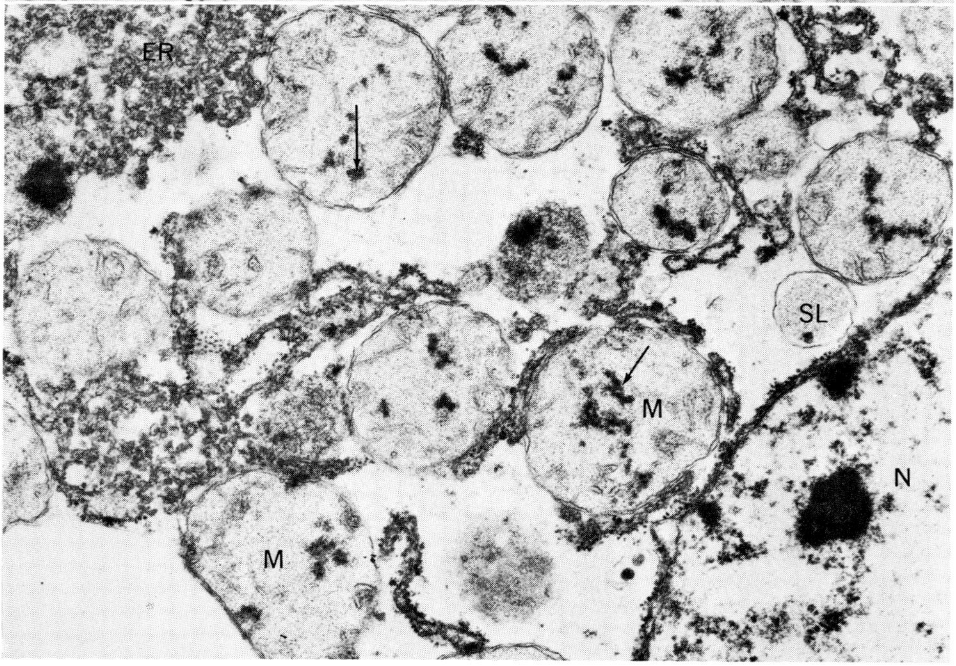

b

changed, cells can exist with large amounts of triglyceride lipid for long periods of time. We know most about fatty changes occurring to the liver cells, where they are a common accompaniment of many human diseases, including chronic alcoholism. Some of the important aspects of lipid metabolism in the liver are shown in Figure 2-42. Lipids reach the liver mostly as alimentary chylomicrons or fatty acids from adipose tissue and are either utilized within the liver or secreted as lipoproteins. The liver is the principal source of serum lipoproteins which are the transport form of all lipids. The small triglyceride droplets that appear within the endoplasmic reticulum and the Golgi complex reflect the formation of lipoprotein particles (Lombardi, 1965).

There is good evidence that any imbalance between supply, utilization, and secretion of lipid by the liver cell can result in a fatty liver (Fig. 2-42). For example, it has been suspected that in some conditions interference with fatty acid oxidation by mitochondria will increase the fatty acid pool and result in accumulation of lipid. Similarly, interference with phospholipid metabolism, as in choline deficiency, or interference with protein synthesis, as after administration of many hepatotoxins, results in imperfect lipoproteins and consequent accumulation of triglycerides within the liver. If the delivery of lipid to the liver is increased, as in conditions of fat mobilizaton, the metabolic capacity of the liver may be exceeded, and triglyceride will accumulate.

In most conditions resulting in fatty liver, the stored lipid is in the form of triglycerides which exist as droplets of moderate density within the cell sap. Their precise location has not been identified; but, because of the high, surface free energy of lipid droplets, it seems rather unlikely that they exist in a free state within the cell sap. They may be surrounded by a monolayer of phospholipid, the hydrophilic ends directed toward the cell sap. In a sense, therefore, lipid droplets exist within the hydrophobic portion of a lipid bilayer, resembling an intramembranous fat deposit. Support for this interpretation comes from experiments with phospholipase-treated microsomes which reveal accumulations of the trilaminar unit membrane.

Figure 2-43. **a.** Necrotic Ehrlich ascites tumor cell after treatment with the sulfhydryl reagent, p-chloromercuribenzoate. The chromatin of the nucleus (N) is severely clumped (pyknosis), and organelles have completely dissolved. The cell sap (CS) is expanded and pale.

b. Portion of a hepatic parenchymal cell after the administration of carbon tetrachloride. The endoplasmic reticulum (ER) is collapsed and flocculent densities have appeared. Mitochondria (M) show high-amplitude swelling of the inner compartment and fluffy densities are present (arrow). The nucleus (N) is divested of chromatin (karyolysis). SL, lysosome.

2. Reactions of cells to lethal injury (Figs. 2-43 to 2-46)

As discussed in the introduction, lethal injury to cells consists of two main phases: a reversible phase of altered homeostasis and an irreversible phase that starts when the cell passes the point of no return. The latter phase, traditionally called necrosis, is characterized by a series of reactions, chiefly autolytic, involving breakdown of cell components.

In Figures 2-44 and 2-45, the integrated aspects of intracellular events occurring after anoxia or chemically induced injury with carbon tetrachloride are shown. As the cell represents the outcome of rather complex interactions between functioning organelles and subcellular systems, it is evident that a series of reac-

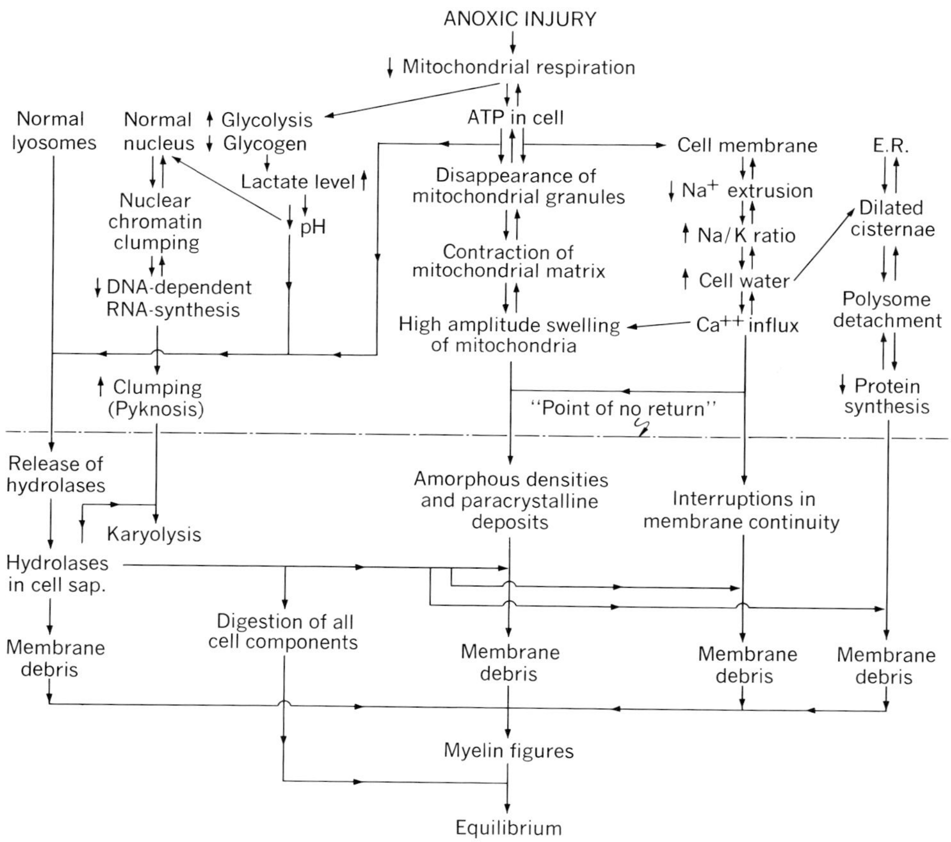

Figure 2-44. Diagramatic representation of the events in a cell after anoxic injury.

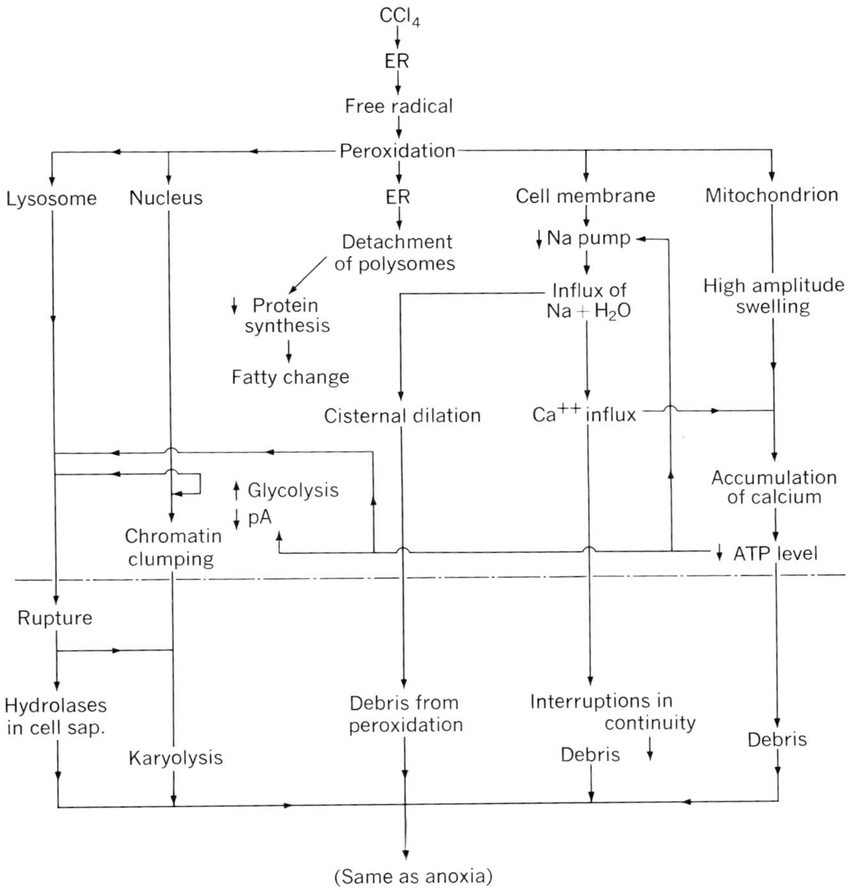

Figure 2-45. Diagramatic representation of the events in a cell after treatment with carbon tetrachloride.

tions such as those following a lethal injury will affect the cell's numerous feedback control mechanisms and result in similarly complex reactions.

Anoxic injury is perhaps the simplest and at present the most fully understood form of lethal injury. In anoxia, which often is produced by ischemia, the initial interaction is to inhibit mitochondrial respiration and oxidative phosphorylation. This immediately stops much of the supply of the ATP to the cell and tends to increase the ADP/ATP ratio. In many cells, inhibition of mitochondrial respiration is followed by stimulation of anaerobic glycolysis which may for a time sustain the ATP levels. In most cells, however, this can occur only for a

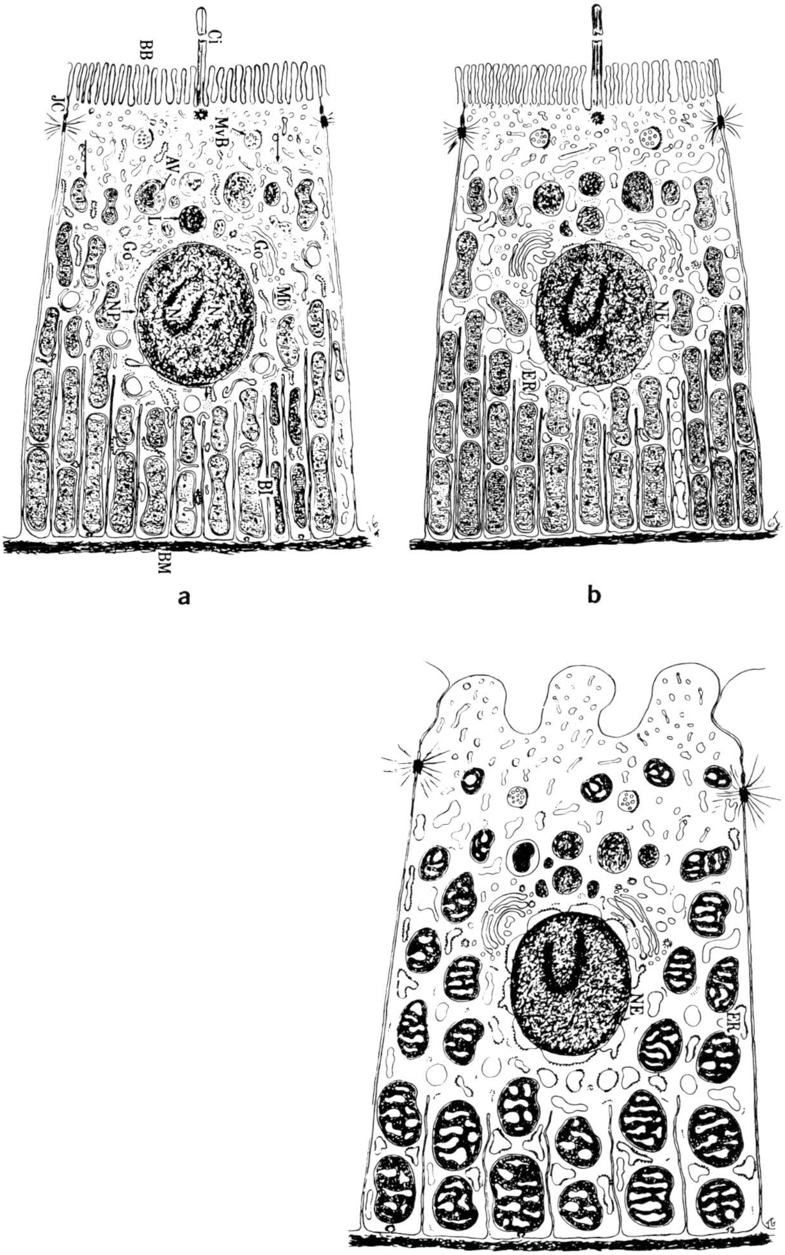

a

b

c

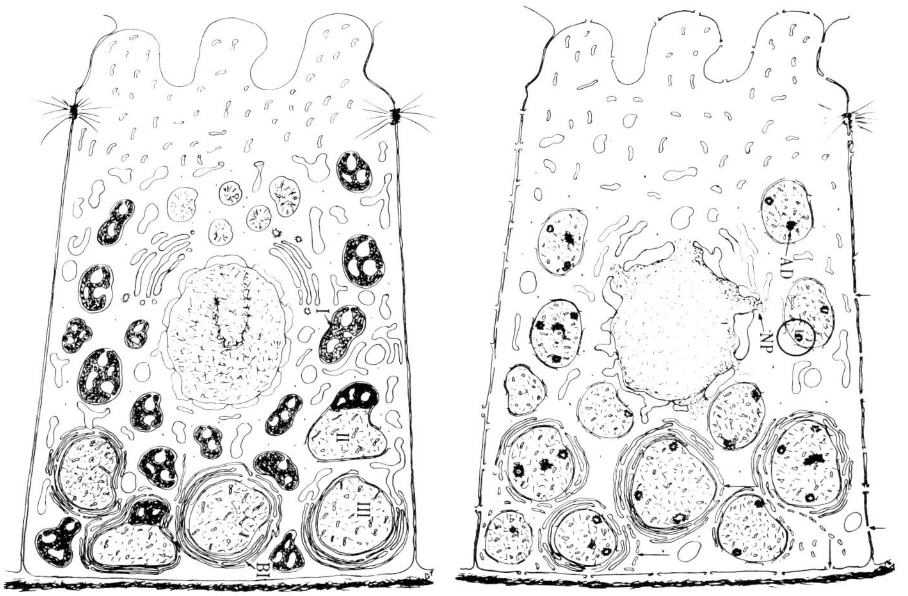

d **e**

Figure 2-46. This series of diagrams depicts stages of loss of cell volume regulation leading from a normal to a necrotic cell.

a. A normal renal tubule cell. Ci, cilium; BB, brush border; JC, junctional complex; L, secondary lysosomes; AV, autophagic vacuoles; Go, Golgi apparatus; N, nucleus; Nc, nucleolus; NP, nuclear pores; Mb, microbodies; arrows, face-on view of rough-surfaced endoplasmic reticulum; BI, basilar invaginations; BM, basement membrane.

b. The only change visible is dilatation of the endoplasmic reticulum (ER) and nuclear envelope (NE).

c. Condensation of the mitochondrial inner compartment with relative expansion of intracristal spaces and swelling of the cell sap. The brush border swells and becomes distorted.

d. Some mitochondria (I) are still condensed like those in c. Others (II) have a condensed portion and a portion in which the matrix is greatly expanded, while some (III) show only expansion of the inner compartment. Basilar infoldings often form circumferential wrappings around mitochondria. Polysomes are infrequent or absent. Lysosomes are pale; the nucleoplasm is dispersed and indistinct.

e. The state of necrosis. All mitochondria are swollen and contain two types of densities: an amorphous type (AD) and a microcrystalline density in apposition to the inner membranes (encircled areas). Interruptions occur in the continuity of the plasma membrane and basilar infoldings (arrows). The nucleus is disintegrating. Nuclear pore (NP). From Ginn **et al.,** 1968.

limited period; ATP supplies are rapidly depleted since they are used for important homeostatic functions such as the activities of the cell membrane. Changes in the ADP/ATP ratio have immediate consequences for the mitochondria: matrix granules are rapidly lost and the matrix contracts severely. The contracted state of the mitochondria may be a very transient phase since it is dependent on continued integrity of the mitochondrial inner membrane. When this integrity is lost, high-amplitude swelling of the inner compartment ensues, probably augmented by the influx of calcium or other swelling agents through the damaged cell membrane.

The decreasing supply of ATP seriously affects cell membrane function (Trump *et al.*, 1970). An early change, discussed above, is a decrease in the rate of sodium extrusion, which tends to increase the sodium-potassium ratio within the cell and is accompanied by influx of cell water. This begins to produce cell swelling. This early change in cell volume serves to involve the cisternae of the endoplasmic reticulum which appear to form a "sink" for the early influx of sodium, chloride, and water. When severe, this produces a vacuolar change within the cell known as *cloudy swelling* which is visible with the light microscope. As cell membrane function is further violated, increased influx of calcium occurs, further augmenting the high-amplitude mitochondrial swelling through release of factors such as fatty acids (U factor).

Decreased mitochondrial respiration also has early effects on other components within the cell. Acceleration of the rate of anaerobic glycolysis leads to an increase in cell lactate levels and a reduction in cellular pH. Early, reversible clumping of nuclear chromatin can probably be attributed to the pH change, which also tends to labilize lysosomal enzymes, though they may not actually be released prior to the point of no return. In the endoplasmic reticulum there is dissociation and breakdown of polysomes from the membrane surface, accompanied by decreased ability for protein synthesis and change in the polysome patterns as seen by ultracentrifugation.

Cells can only tolerate markedly decreased ATP levels for a limited time which varies with the cell in question. Ultimately the cell loses the ability to recover, even if the oxygen supply is restored. This loss is most likely related to irreversible damage to the mitochondrial inner membrane and closely follows the onset of high-amplitude swelling. Depending upon the type of injury, mitochondria develop flocculent amorphous densities or paracrystalline accumulations of calcium-containing materials related to hydroxyapatite. Calcium continues to accumulate even if the ability to phosphorylate is markedly depressed. The lysosomal membranes lose their integrity, and hydrolases are released into the cell sap, further stimulating the breakdown of cell membranes. Finally all membranes are converted to debris and to myelin figures, and the cell approaches chemical equilibrium with the environment.

A second general type of integrated reaction to injury occurs after exposure of liver cells to carbon tetrachloride, which has been an important compound in providing a model for studying cell reactions to injury. Carbon tetrachloride apparently interacts initially with the endoplasmic reticulum, where it is metabolized to form free radicals (Recknagel, 1967). The free radicals appear to stimulate lipid peroxidation throughout the cell with damage to cellular membranes, and at an early phase glucose 6-phosphatase, a membrane-bound enzyme of the endoplasmic reticulum, is rapidly inactivated. Detachment and dissociation of polysomes occur quickly, and the rate of protein synthesis decreases rapidly. The decreased protein synthesis results in accumulation of triglycerides within the cell. From this point on, the changes are similar to those after anoxia. The mitochondria and cell membrane show early evidence of change, and there are rapid decreases in cellular ATP levels and influx of sodium, water, and calcium; the mitochondria readily accumulate calcium. As seen in the diagram, the subsequent changes can be interpreted in a fashion similar to those described for anoxia.

Anoxic and carbon tetrachloride injury provide useful models for understanding the complexity of cell interactions following lethal injury. It should be emphasized, however, that these are examples of specific injuries to specific cell types. In other cases, slight differences from these models are common. For instance, rapidly dividing cells may be modified when nucleic acid or protein synthesis is interfered with; postmitotic cells are not seriously damaged by this treatment, but will succumb rapidly to changes in ATP synthesis and membrane transport.

References

Allison, A. (1968), The role of lysosomes in the action of drugs and hormones, Adv. in Chemotherapy, *3*:253.

Arstila, A. U., and Trump, B. F. (1968), Studies on cellular autophagocytosis. The formation of autophagic vacuoles in the liver after glucagon administration, Amer. J. Path., *53*:687.

Barber, A. A., and Bernheim, F. (1967), Lipid peroxidation: Its measurement, occurrence, and significance in animal tissues, *in* Advances in Gerontological Research, Vol. 2, pp. 355-403, Academic Press, New York.

Baserga, R., and Wiebel, F. (1969), The cell cycle of mammalian cells, *in* Inter. Rev. of Exp. Path., Vol. 7, pp. 1-30, G. W. Richter and M. A. Epstein, Eds., Academic Press, New York.

Bernhard, W., and Granboulan, N. (1968), Electron microscopy of the nucleolus in vertebrate cells, *in* The Nucleus, pp. 81-149, A. J. Dalton and F. Haguenau, Eds., Academic Press, New York and London.

Branton, D., and Park, R. B. (1968), Papers on Biological Membrane Structure, Little, Brown and Co., Boston.

Cohn, Z. H. (in press), Endocytosis and the vacuolar system of cells, *in* Cell Membranes: Biological and Pathological Aspects, G. W. Richter and D. G. Scarpelli, Eds., Williams and Wilkins Co., Baltimore.

de Duve, C., and Baudhuin, P. (1966), Peroxisomes (Microbodies and related particles), Physiol. Rev., *46*:323.

de Duve, C., and Wattiaux, R. (1966), Functions of lysosomes, Ann. Rev. Physiol., *28*:435.

Dingle, J. T., and Fell, H. B. (Eds.) (1969), Lysosomes in Biology and Pathology, Part I, pp. 3-508, North Holland Publishing Co., Amsterdam.

deReuck, A. V. S., and Knight, J. (Eds.) (1963), Ciba Foundation Symposium, Cellular Injury, Little, Brown and Co., Boston.

Dourmashkin, R. R., and Rosse, W. F. (1966), Morphologic changes in the membranes of red blood cells undergoing hemolysis, Amer. . Med., *41*:699.

Dowben, R. M. (Ed.) (1969), Biological Membranes, Little, Brown and Co., Boston.

Ericsson, J. L. E. (1965), Transport and digestion of hemoglobin in the proximal tubule. II. Electron microscopy, Lab. Invest., *14*:16.

Ernster, L. (in press), Enzymatic properties of membrane-associated cell fractions as related to drug metabolism, *in* Cell Membranes: Biological and Pathological Aspects, G. W. Richter and D. G. Scarpelli, Eds., Williams and Wilkins Co., Baltimore.

Farber, E., and Magee, P. N. (Eds.) (1965), Biochemical Pathology, Proc. 1st Int. Symp. in Biochem. Path., Seven Springs, Champion, Pa., pp. 1-242, Williams and Wilkins Co., Baltimore.

Ginn, F. L., Shelburne, J., and Trump, B. F. (1968), Disorders of cell volume regulation. I. Effects of inhibition of plasma membrane adenosine triphosphatase with ouabain, Amer. J. Path., *43*:1041-1071.

Goldblatt, P. J., Sullivan, R. J., and Farber, E. (1969), Induction of partial nucleolar segregation in hepatic parenchymal cells by actinomycin D following inhibition of ribonucleic acid synthesis by ethionine, Lab. Invest., *20*:283.

Goldblatt, P. J. (1969), The endoplasmic reticulum, *in* Handbook of Molecular Cytology, A. Lima-de-Faria, Ed., North Holland Publishing Co., Amsterdam.

Haguenau, F. (1969), Ultrastructure of the cancer cell, *in* Biological Basis of Medicine, Vol. 5, pp. 433-486, E. E. Bittar and N. Bittar, Eds., Academic Press, New York and London.

Hers, H. G. (1965), Inborn lysosomal diseases, Gastroenterology, *48*:625.

Hruban, Z., and Rechcigl, M., Jr. (1969), Microbodies and related particles, *in* Inter. Rev. Cytology, Suppl. 1, pp. 1-251, G. H. Bourne and J. F. Danielli, Eds., Academic Press, New York.

Lombardi, B. (1965), Considerations on the pathogenesis of fatty liver. *in* Biochem. Pathology, E. Farber and P. N. Magee, Eds., Proc. 1st Int. Symp. in Biochemical Path., Seven Springs, Champion, Pa., pp. 1-15, Williams and Wilkins Co., Baltimore.

Majno, G., Lagattuta, M., and Thompson, T. E. (1960), Cellular death and necrosis: chemical, physical, and morphologic changes in rat liver, Vir. Arch. Path. Anat., *333*:421.

Mueller, G. C. (1969), Biochemical events in the animal cell cycle, Fed. Proc., *28*:1780-1789.

Murayama, M. (1966), Molecular mechanism of red cell "sickling," *Science, 153*:145.

Parsons, D. F. (1965), Recent advances correlating structure and function in mitochondria, Adv. Exp. Path., *5*:1.

Recknagel, R. O. (1967), Carbon tetrachloride hepatotoxicity, Pharmacological Rev., *19*:145.

Reynolds, E. S. (1965), Liver parenchymal cell injury. III. The nature of calcium-associated electron-opaque masses in rat liver mitochondria following poisoning with carbon tetrachloride, J. Cell Biol., *25*:53.

Shinozuka, H., Goldblatt, P. J., and Farber, E. (1968), The disorganization of hepatic cell nucleoli induced by ethione and its reversal by adenine, J. Cell Biol., *36*:313.

Smuckler, E. A., and Arcasoy, M. (1969), Structural and functional changes of the endoplasmic reticulum of hepatic parenchymal cells, *in* Inter. Rev. Exper. Path., Vol. 7, pp. 305-418, G. W. Richter and M. A. Epstein, Eds., Academic Press, New York and London.

Scarpelli, D. G. (in press), Experimental alteration of mitochondrial membrane biogenesis and function, *in* Cell Membranes: Biological and Pathological Aspects, G. W. Richter and D. G. Scarpelli, Eds., Williams and Wilkins Co., Baltimore.

Tosteson, D. C. (1964), Regulation of cell volume by sodium and potassium transport, *in* The Cellular Functions of Membrane Transport, pp. 3-22, J. F. Hoffman, Ed., Prentice-Hall, Inc., Englewood Cliffs, New Jersey.

Trump, B. F., and Ericsson, J. L. E. (1965), Some ultrastructural and biochemical consequences of cell injury, *in* The Inflammatory Process, pp. 35-120, B. W. Zweifach, and L. Grant, Eds., Academic Press, New York.

Trump, B. F., and Ginn, F. L. (1969), The pathogenesis of subcellular reaction to lethal injury, *in* Methods and Achievements in Experimental Pathology, Vol. IV, pp. 1-29, E. Bajusz, and G. Jasmin, Eds., Yearbook Medical Publishers, Chicago.

Trump, B. F., Duttera, S. M., Byrne, W. L., and Arstila, A. U. (1970), Membrane structure: Lipid-protein interactions in microsomal membranes, Proc. Natl. Acad. Sci., *66*:433.

Trump, B. F., Croker, B. P., Jr., and Mergner, W. J. (in press), The role of cell membrane alterations, ion and water movements in the pathogenesis of cell injury, *in* Cell Membranes: Biological and Pathological Aspects, G. W. Richter and D. G. Scarpelli, Eds., Williams and Wilkins Co., Baltimore.

3

INFLAMMATION

Peter A. Ward, M.D.

A. General Description

As one of the most common and visible responses of the vertebrate body to injury, the inflammatory process has occupied the attention of physicians since the time of the early Greeks. It was recognized many years ago that without the inflammatory process a microbe would be free to enter a wound or mucosal surface, establish residence in the warm, well-nourished environment, proliferate, spread, and eventually kill the host. In quite another way, the benefits derived from the body's ability to marshal an inflammatory response have been evident in wound healing, since not only are microbial agents kept in check and infection thus prevented but, concomitantly, events of the inflammatory response set into motion a complex series of reactions that result in healing and repair of the damaged tissue. Without inflammatory responses, then, we would go through life bearing all the open wounds of the past, a body unable to heal itself, quite like a machine that functions until a part wears out or breaks. In all these respects because it swiftly and dramatically copes with sudden changes in the body, the inflammatory response is important to the maintenance of life. But inflammation itself may also be destructive. The loss of homeostatic control in the inflammatory response can lead to self-mutilation or even death. The many hundreds of thousands of victims of rheumatoid arthritis, the thousands of patients dying yearly with glomerulonephritis, the increasing numbers of patients threatened by rejection of a vital homograft, all give testimony to the serious consequences of the inflammatory process that goes, for whatever reason, unchecked.

The constitutional signs and symptoms of an inflammatory process are well known. Who has not experienced the lassitude, the weakness, and the fever that are so prominent when an inflammatory response is in progress, as in the throat, the middle ear, the lungs, or anywhere else in the body? Precisely why a localized process should lead to such profound systemic changes is far from clear. Are substances released from the local area resulting in an effect elsewhere in the body and, if so, how is the inflammatory process involved in such a mechanism? Perhaps the best answers to these questions come from the work of many groups who have defined a mechanism of fever that depends upon the role of granulocytes. It is now well known that a substance termed *endogenous pyrogen* is elaborated from granulocytes as a result of contact of these cells with antigen-antibody complexes, bacterial endotoxin, or soluble substances present in inflammatory foci. Endogenous pyrogen is also elaborated during the phagocytic process of granulocytes. The pyrogen apparently has an action on the central nervous system where the thermal regulatory mechanism is upset and the body's "thermostat" is set higher. In view of the variety of mechanisms for releasing endogenous pyrogen, it is not difficult to see why fever develops once granulocytes have accumulated in an inflammatory focus.

The classical local signs of inflammation—namely, heat, redness, swelling, and pain—are the result of functional changes in the vasculature of tissue in response to an injurious agent or altered state. Water-dissolved electrolytes and macromolecules, and cells, especially leukocytes, escape from the usual intravascular confines. When these substances appear outside the walls of vessels, provided this is not due to a simple physical destruction of the vessel wall, the inflammatory process is, by definition present. Without intact blood vessels and without circulating elements within them, the inflammatory process could not occur, but once the functional integrity of the blood vessels is lost, these substances quickly begin their exodus from the bloodstream. The redness caused by the inflammatory process is attributable to dilatation of vessels, the heat is due to the increased blood flow to the area, the swelling is due to the escape of liquids and cells into the extravascular spaces, and the pain is due to the pressure on nerve endings, and/or the action of mediators such as bradykinin (see below) on these structures. Such changes usually lead to healing, but on occasion they may seriously interfere with the function of the involved organ; this is well represented in post-streptococcal glomerulonephritis, rheumatic carditis, or pneumococcal pneumonia, where the inflammatory process itself leads to a condition that is more life-threatening than the initial insult to the tissue.

B. Histology of the Inflammatory Response

The inflammatory response can be classified according to the types of cells that predominate in the inflamed tissue.

Acute inflammation is the common type that one might see when a wood splinter has penetrated the skin. Within hours redness appears, heralding the vascular dilatation and the accelerated blood flow through the area. Fluid (edema) accumulates in the tissues. Shortly thereafter, neutrophilic granulocytes can be seen clustering along the endothelial margins of blood vessels, the phenomenon of margination or peripheralization, and soon these leukocytes can be seen making their way into the adjacent connective tissue. These events accelerate over the period of several hours so that soon the entire area contains vast numbers of extravascular granulocytes which effectively wall off the foreign body. Much the same sort of response is seen whenever any acute injury to tissue occurs, such as a burn, a mechanical injury like an abrasion, or an infection.

Precisely what accounts for these changes in the functional behavior of the blood vessels is quite unclear. Many years ago Lewis (1927) emphasized the role of the autonomic nervous system in bringing about changes in the caliber of blood vessels. He emphasized that this occurs autonomously, in the nature of a reflex: that is to say, peripheral nerves are involved, the higher center of the central nervous system being by-passed. Why the granulocytes accumulate along the endothelial surfaces just prior to their movement out of the blood vessel has been a point of great controversy. It has been suggested that the endothelium has been modified, becoming "sticky" for leukocytes, but there is no convincing evidence for this conclusion. However, this does not exclude a chemical or physical basis for the adherence of these leukocytes to endothelial surfaces. Precisely why granulocytes would move beyond the confines of the vessel at this point could be explained by the role of chemotactic factors, that is, attractants which are present in the surrounding area and which cause the unidirectional movement of leukocytes toward a concentration gradient of attractant. In the acute inflammatory response very few lymphocytes or monocytes accumulate in the extravascular sites. Possible reasons for this could be either a lack of specific mediators such as chemotactic agents causing extravascular migration of monocytes and lymphocytes, or the much slower responsiveness of lymphocytes and monocytes to stimuli such as chemotactic factors.

Ordinarily within one to three days the character of the cells in the acute inflamatory process has changed: this altered morphology defines the *subacute inflammatory response.* In the place of neutrophilic granulocytes, lymphocytes and monocytes can be seen scattered in the extravascular area. The most striking manifestation of the subacute inflammatory response, however, is the appearance of lush sprouts of very actively growing, tiny, fragile blood vessels and connective tissue cells. This angioblastic and fibroblastic proliferation, in aggregate referred to as *granulation tissue,* indicates that a stimulus to cell growth has occurred. It is because of the profusion of vascular sprouts and fibroblasts which begin to lay down collagen that the stage is set for the formation of a scar.

If the inflammatory process does not subside, particularly if the agent responsible for inducing the inflammatory process remains, the granulation tissue will continue to form, and dense collagenous connective tissue may be found. In addition, the population of leukocytes begins to change, almost exclusively, to lymphocytes, monocytes, and plasma cells. The persistence of these cells in areas where they ordinarily exist in small numbers, if at all, the continued laying-down of ever increasing amounts of dense collagenous connective tissue, the continued influx of cells from the circulation and the accelerating disintegration of leukocytes (and also cells native to the area of injury) leads to a *chronic inflammatory process* which may present serious problems to the functional capacity of tissue, particularly if a critical area such as the central nervous system or the myocardium is involved.

As just indicated, the staging of the inflammatory process is usually based upon histologic criteria, that is, the nature of the inflammatory cells (leukocytes) present. While the type of leukocyte in the inflammatory response can usually be predicted according to duration of the process, the clinical terms *acute* or *chronic inflammation* may also be based solely upon temporal considerations. Accordingly, acute inflammation usually implies a process of fairly short duration (days). It is usually characterized by an exudate of neutrophils, although in some cases, for instance viral hepatitis, mononuclear cells predominate. On the other hand, persistent osteomyelitis would be termed a *chronic* inflammatory process because of its long duration, although histologically the inflammatory cells might consist almost exclusively of neutrophilic leukocytes. In this chapter the terms *acute, subacute,* and *chronic* are used according to established histologic criteria.

C. Phases of the Acute Inflammatory Response

In order to understand these very complex events, it is important to examine the various phases of the inflammatory process. It is possible to consider separately the permeability changes and the accumulation of leukocytes; these are independent events which may occur simultaneously or in sequence.

1. Permeability changes

Wilhelm and Mason (1960) and subsequently several other workers have now shown that the acute inflammatory process, which can conveniently be induced by thermal injury in rat skin, is characterized by two phases of altered per-

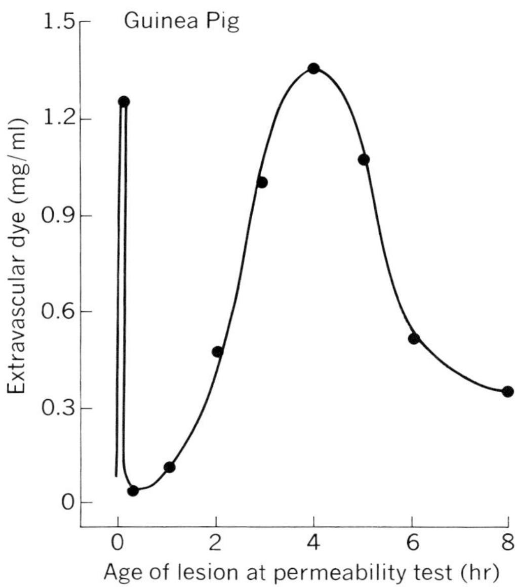

Figure 3-1. The two phases of capillary permeability (in rat skin) induced by thermal injury. The initial phase is transient and histamine dependent, whereas the secondary (delayed) or prolonged phase is independent of histamine. Extravascular leukocyte accumulation in tissue occurs during the secondary phase of permeability. (Courtesy of Wilhelm and Mason, 1960).

meability (Fig. 3-1) (see review of Wilhelm, 1962). The first phase appears to be mediated by histamine since suitable chemical antagonists of histamine will completely ablate the change in permeability. As several groups have pointed out, this histamine-dependent phase is transient, lasting little more than a few minutes. Within two to four hours a prolonged and quite different phase occurs. In contrast to the histamine-dependent phase, the secondary phase is prolonged, lasting over the next three to four hours. It is during this period that leukocytes begin to migrate out of blood vessels (Hurley, 1964). The mediator of this secondary phase has not been identified, but it clearly is not histamine or serotonin.

Both the histamine-dependent and the histamine-independent phases of permeability are associated with the migration of fluids, not through endothelial cells, but between endothelial cells—that is, a percolation of proteins, electrolytes, and water through the junctional zones between endothelial cells, through the basement membrane of the vessel, and into the area around the blood vessel (Fig. 3-2).

Several classes of mediators affecting permeability of blood vessels have been described, and most appear to affect the postcapillary venules rather than the capillaries themselves (Table 3-1). *Vasoactive amines* consist of histamine and serotonin, which ordinarily do not exist free in the circulation but are stored in cells such as basophils, mast cells, and platelets. Intricate mechanisms account for the release of these amines, and when they are released in the vicinity of endothelium, permeability changes in the vessels occur. The natural antagonists to these permeability factors include the catecholamines such as epinephrine and norepinephrine (Spector and Willoughby, 1964), which do not exist in local stores but must be released from secretory granules in cells at a distant site (in the adrenal medulla), which then make their way via the circulation to the site of altered permeability. The *kinins* are a group of peptides derived from $\alpha 2$ globulin in the plasma. They are generated by the action of *kallikrein* which exists as a precursor enzyme (prokallikrein or prokininogenase) and is converted to the active enzyme form by triggering of the Hageman factor (Factor 12, which also exists as a profactor) in plasma. It is likely that between these two steps (active Hageman factor and prokallikrein) another agent (see below) is also required. Upon conversion to its active form, kallikrein cleaves the plasma substrate, resulting in the release of peptides consisting of 9, 10, or 11 amino acids. These bioactive products are known as bradykinin, lysylbradykinin, and methionyl-lysylbradykinin, respectively. Each peptide increases the permeability of vessels and

Table 3-1 Permeability Factors

FACTOR	SPECIAL CHARACTERISTICS
Amines (histamine, serotonin)	Stored in active form in cell (platelets, mast cells, basophils).
Kinins	Generated by plasma kallikrein acting on $\alpha 2$ globulin substrate in plasma
PF/dil	Present as inactive plasma enzyme, active product not defined.
Lymph node permeability factor	Extractable from sensitized lymph node cell; not defined.
SRS-A	Fatty acid; production somehow related to neutrophils.

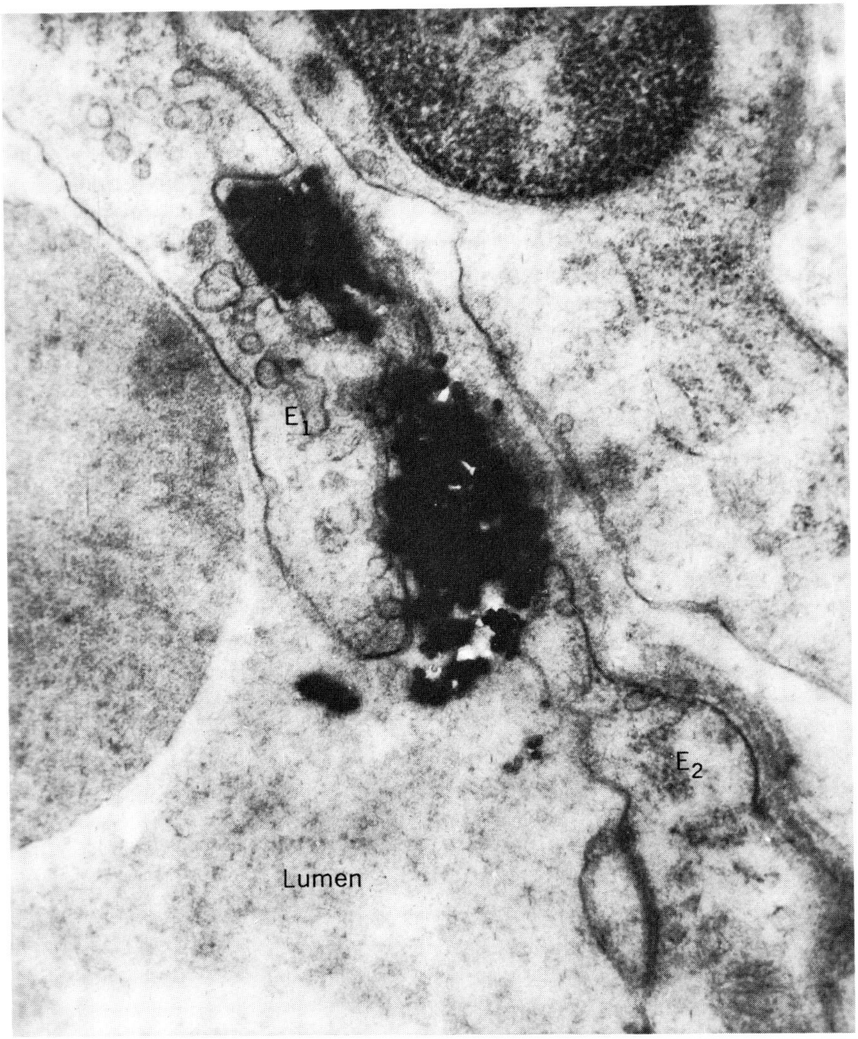

Figure 3-2. Movement of carbon particles through an interendothelial junction (between endothelial cells E1 and E2). The capillary lumen is indicated, with a red blood cell adjacent to the endothelial surface. (Courtesy of Marchesi, 1962).

also causes contraction of smooth muscle. The contraction of venular smooth muscle results in increased hydrostatic pressure, accentuating the permeability change. The kinin system has been the subject of an excellent recent review (Kellermeyer and Graham, 1968). The *anaphylatoxins* constitute a completely separate class of vasoactive peptides and are derived from the third or the fifth components of complement (reviewed by Muller-Eberhard, 1968). Each of these peptides has an approximate molecular weight of 10,000 and apparently alters vessel permeability indirectly by causing the release of histamine from tissue mast cells. In addition, the anaphylatoxins contract smooth muscle, and this contraction may, in critical areas, lead to increased hydrostatic pressure and subsequent increased permeability. The substance termed by Miles (1961) *PF/dil* (permeability factor in diluted serum) appears to be a plasma enzyme which can act on a plasma substrate to produce a material that increases vascular permeability. The nature of this bioactive agent is not known. It is pertinent to emphasize that PF/dil may be an intermediate in the reaction between Hageman factor and prokallikrein, the latter being the most important substrate of PF/dil (see review of Becker, 1968). A substance termed *lymph node permeability factor* has been extracted from lymph nodes of animals exhibiting delayed hypersensitivity to various antigens. This material appears after sensitization and induces increased vascular permeability following intradermal injection. It has not been characterized but Willoughby and Spector (1964) suggest a role for this factor in chronic inflammatory processes where immunologic mechanisms come into play. Finally, a substance termed *slow reacting substance* (SRS-A) is released when sensitized lung tissue is perfused with antigen (Brocklehurst, 1960). SRS-A, which requires neutrophils for its elaboration and may be a product of them (Orange, Valentine, and Austen, 1968), induces increased vascular permeability as well as characteristic contraction of smooth muscle, and it may be that this substance is important in certain allergic reactions where vascular permeability changes are prominent.

2. Transmigration of leukocytes

It is quite clear that permeability change in vessels leading to the escape of proteins is not synonymous with the escape of granulocytes. Indeed, change in permeability may very well occur in the virtual absence of leukocyte emigration, and vice versa. The transmigration of cells across vascular barriers is of central importance in inflammation.

There is no evidence that red blood cells escape by other than passive means, specifically by transit through interendothelial cell junctions (Fig. 3-3). Unless

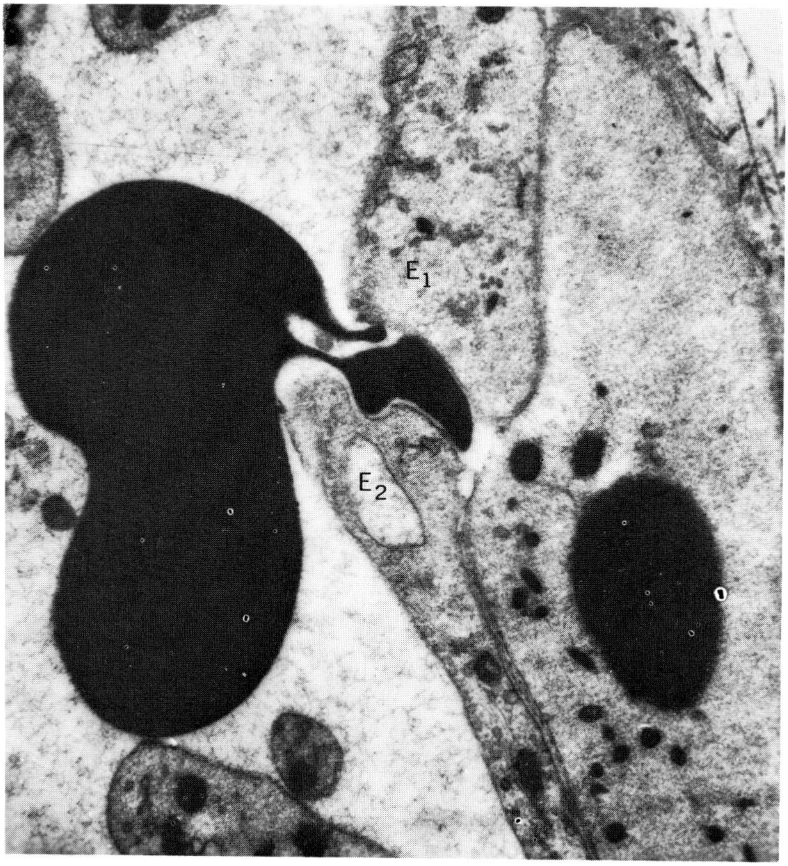

Figure 3-3. Movement of a red blood cell through an interendothelial junction, similar to the escape of carbon particles during inflammation. Plasticity of the red cell is evident. (Courtesy of Marchesi, 1964).

initial injury to the blood vessels results in their physical disruption, the extravasation of red cells appears to be a late event in the inflammatory process which, when it occurs, usually reflects grave injury to the blood vessel wall. By definition, hemorrhage reflects the severity of the vascular damage and should not be considered an integral part of the inflammatory process, even though a "hemorrhagic exudate" is sometimes described.

Granulocytes escape from the vessel in quite a different manner than red cells. The very elegant electron microscopic observations of Marchesi and Florey (1960) have defined morphologically the process of granulocyte emigration. These authors describe how granulocytes approximate the endothelial surface of the vessel and protrude pseudopods into the interendothelial junction, following which the pseudopod then squeezes along and arrives at the base (outer aspect) of the endothelial cell (Figs. 3-4, 3-5). Once there, the rest of the cell squeezes along this channel and is soon outside the endothelial cell, where it moves through the basement membrane of the vessel and into the extravascular connective tissue space.

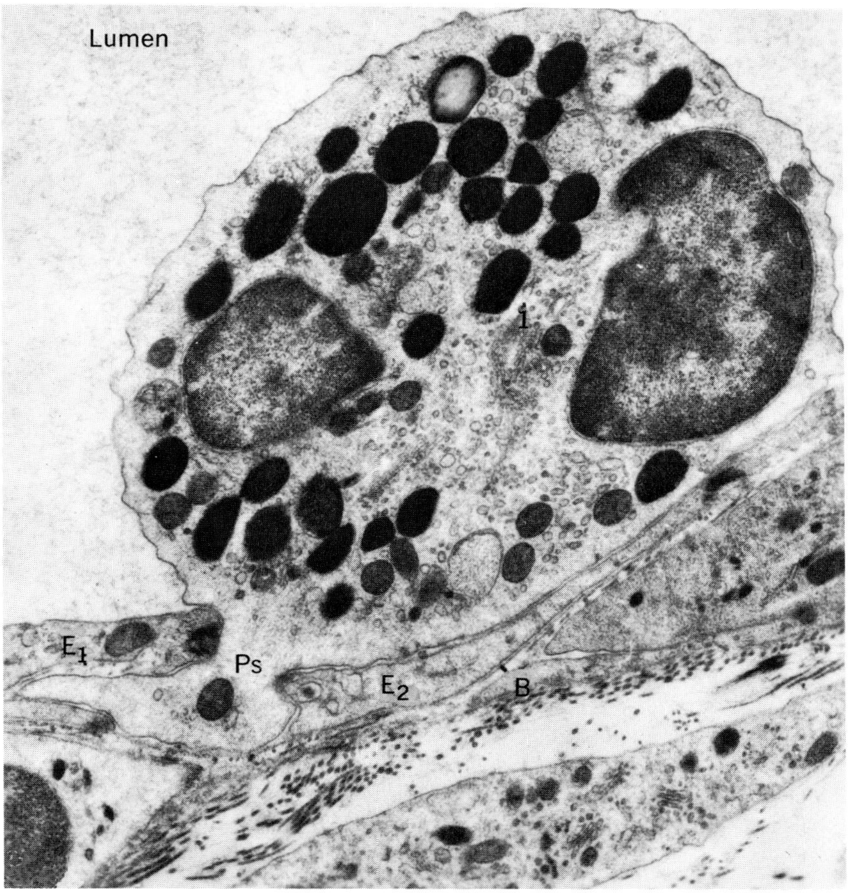

Figure 3-4. Intrusion of a pseudopod (Ps) from a neutrophil (1) through an interendothelial junction (defined by cytoplasmic processes of endothelial cells E_1 and E_2) as the cell moves through the capillary wall. (B represents basement membrane). Collagen fibers are in evidence outside the vessel wall. (Courtesy of Marchesi, 1961).

The movement of leukocytes from the bloodstream into areas beyond the endothelial barrier has been explained at least in part by chemotactic mechanisms. For years, it has been known that leukocytes on surfaces of glass slides will move toward certain substances, such as bacterial clusters, and time-lapse photography has revealed that this is a unidirectional linear movement rather than an aimless random migration (Harris, 1960). The possibility that such mechanisms apply *in vivo* has appealed to many although the evidence for this has not been convincing. Nevertheless, it has been possible to demonstrate that neutrophilic granulocytes respond chemotactically to specific factors *in vitro*.

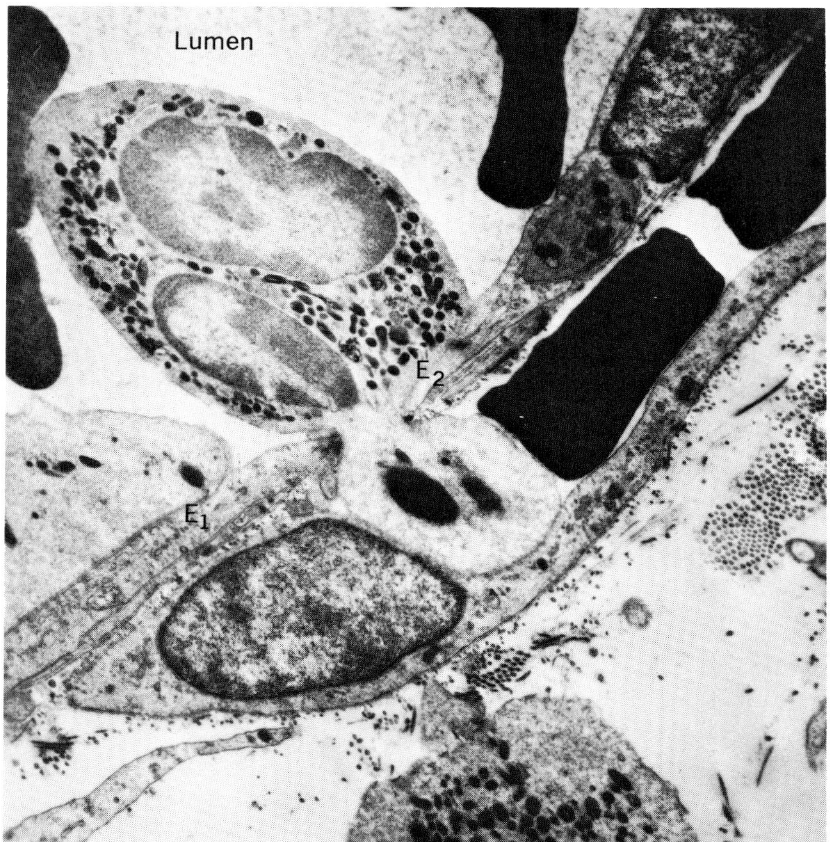

Figure 3-5. Movement of a neutrophil through a venular wall with intrusion of a pseudopod into the periendothelial space. Several red cells have escaped beyond the point through the same channel. (Courtesy of Marchesi and Florey, 1960).

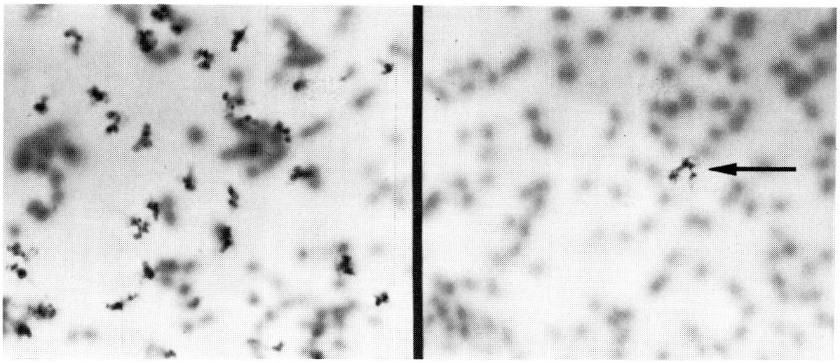

Figure 3-6. Chemotaxis of neutrophilic leukocytes, micropore filter technique. Micropore filters are from two chemotaxis chambers. The left frame from negative control chamber contains a single cell (arrow) that has migrated into the filter, while the right frame shows numerous neutrophils that have moved into channels of the filter in response to a complement-dependent chemotactic stimulus. (Courtesy of Ward, Cochrane, and Muller-Eberhard, 1965).

The latest era in the study of chemotaxis began in 1962 when Stephen Boyden popularized a new method for studying leukocyte chemotaxis, namely, by the use of a micropore filter which would separate leukocytes on the one side from the chemotactic substance on the other side of the membrane. It has now been rather convincingly shown that granulocytes will migrate only if the chemotactic factor is present at a distance from the cell (i.e. in the opposite compartment). Using various concentrations of the chemotactic factor on the two sides of the membrane, it was found that the cells were responding to a gradient of concentration of the factor (Fig. 3-6) (Ward, Cochrane and Muller-Eberhard, 1965, 1966; Keller and Sorkin, 1968). With this system it became possible to obtain precise quantitative data for leukocyte responsiveness, and the micropore filter technique has now become the most popular method for studying chemotaxis.

Neutrophilic granulocytes respond over a short interval of time, which is reminiscent of the behavior of leukocytes *in vivo*. Specifically, these cells require only ninety minutes to complete their response in the chemotactic chamber, in sharp contrast with the time course of response for mononuclear cells (Fig. 3-7). Several different factors which are chemotactic for neutrophils have been isolated. Curiously, many of these are derived from the nine-component complement system either as products of complement or as substrate products produced by an enzyme extrinsic to the complement system but acting as a single complement

Table 3-2 Products of the Complement System with Chemotactic Activity for Neutrophils

FACTOR	METHOD OF PRODUCING FACTOR
High molecular factor	
$C\overline{567}$	Sequential interaction of first 7 components of complement
Low-molecular-weight factors	
C3a	Complement enzyme ($\overline{C4,2}$ or "C3 convertase") trypsin plasmin cobra venom factor –β globulin complex
C5a	Sequential interaction of first five components of complement trypsin

component (Table 3-2). Sequential interaction of the complement system results in the activation of the macromolecular complex consisting of the fifth, sixth, and seventh components of complement. This factor with a relatively high molecular weight thereupon acquires chemotactic activity. Additionally, two fragmentation products of low molecular weight also possess similar biologic activity. The first, cleaved from the third component, is produced by sequential interaction of the complement system, by the direct action on C3 of the enzymes plasmin or trypsin, or by a complex containing a cobra venom factor and serum cofactor. A fragmentation product of the fifth component of complement (C5) also contains chemotactic activity and is generated by interaction of the first five complement components or by the direct action of trypsin on C5. In addition to all these chemotactic agents, most bacteria produce a variety of soluble factors which, in their own right, are chemotactic for neutrophils (see review by Ward, 1970). It is tempting to conclude that the production of such substances in tissues accounts for the ability of most bacteria to induce an acute inflammatory response which is characterized by the massive accumulation of granulocytes. The fact that the complement system appears to be closely involved in the generation of chemotactic factors suggests that the complement system consists of a series of substrates involved in the production of mediators capable of initiating the acute

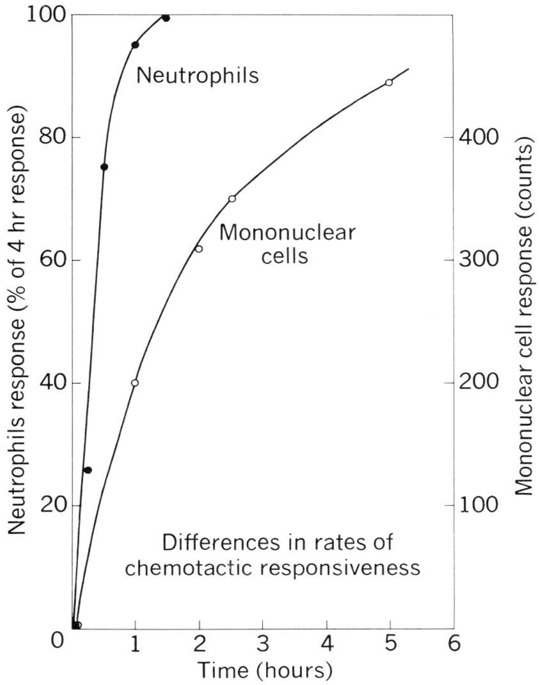

Figure 3-7. Differences in rates of responsiveness of neutrophilic and mononuclear leukocytes as measured by chemotactic migration. Neutrophils respond rapidly within 90 minutes, whereas mononuclear cells respond much more slowly. (Drawn from data of Ward and Becker, 1967; Ward, 1968).

inflammatory response. It should be pointed out that in addition to the chemotactic factors, the *anaphylatoxins* are also generated by sequential interaction of the complement system or by direct action of enzymes on C3 or C5 (see above). These factors increase the permeability of blood vessels. It is now well substantiated that many bioactive products can be derived from the complement system; one set of factors causes the soluble contents of plasma to leak out while the other set of factors affects the escape of circulating leukocytes. As a result of all these actions, the stage is set for the acute inflammatory response. Precisely which factors are involved in a given inflammatory reaction is a very difficult question because of the very short life span of these mediators.

Some information is available concerning the nature of the interaction of one of the complement-derived chemotactic factors with the neutrophil. It is now recognized that at least two different enzymes in the neutrophil are necessary if

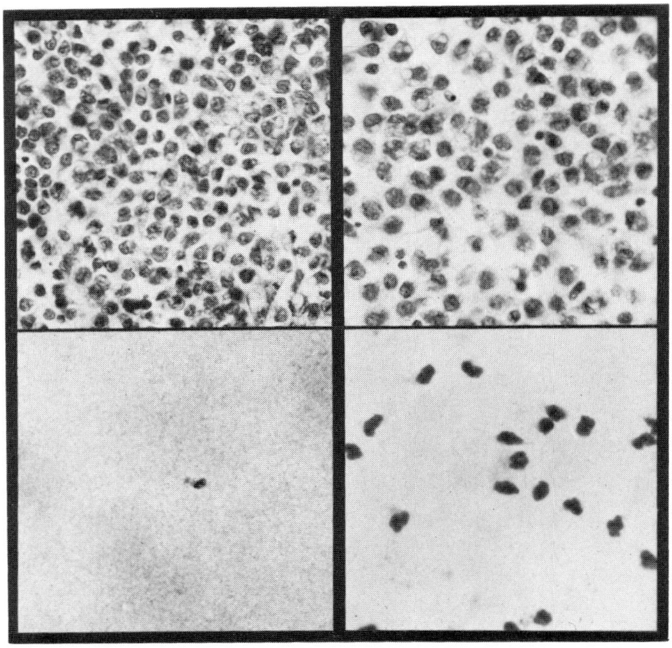

Figure 3-8. Chemotactic response of mononuclear cells. Two micropore filters are included showing non-responding cells (upper frames) and those which have moved completely through the filter to the opposite side (lower frames). In the lower right frame, cells have responded to a chemotactic stimulus, whereas the negative control (with a single migrated cell) is seen in the left lower frame. (From Ward, 1968).

the cell is to respond to the chemotactic factor of high molecular weight. One of these enzymes exists as an inert precursor which, upon contact of the cell with the chemotactic factor, is triggered to an active enzyme (Ward and Becker, 1967). This enzyme or esterase has some features suggestive of chymotrypsin (Ward and Becker, 1968). The second exists naturally in the granulocyte in an active form and appears to be similar to an acetylase (Becker and Ward, 1967). Undoubtedly, a large series of enzymes is involved in the interaction of chemotactic factor with the leukocyte. The net result is that the cell eventually begins to move in a specific and unidirectional manner, probably by an expenditure of energy through glycolytic pathways. It will be important to understand those biochemical events if novel non-empirical approaches to anti-inflammatory therapy are to be developed.

Mononuclear cells also respond to chemotactic stimuli in a manner which is much more sluggish than that of neutrophils; the migrational response requires up to five hours, whereas neutrophils have completed their migration within a ninety-minute period (Fig. 3-7). Such differences might account for the fact that mononuclear cells are rarely seen in inflammatory exudates in the first few hours but appear in significant numbers by the fifth or sixth hours. Chemotactic behavior of mononuclear cells can also be studied by the micropore filter technique

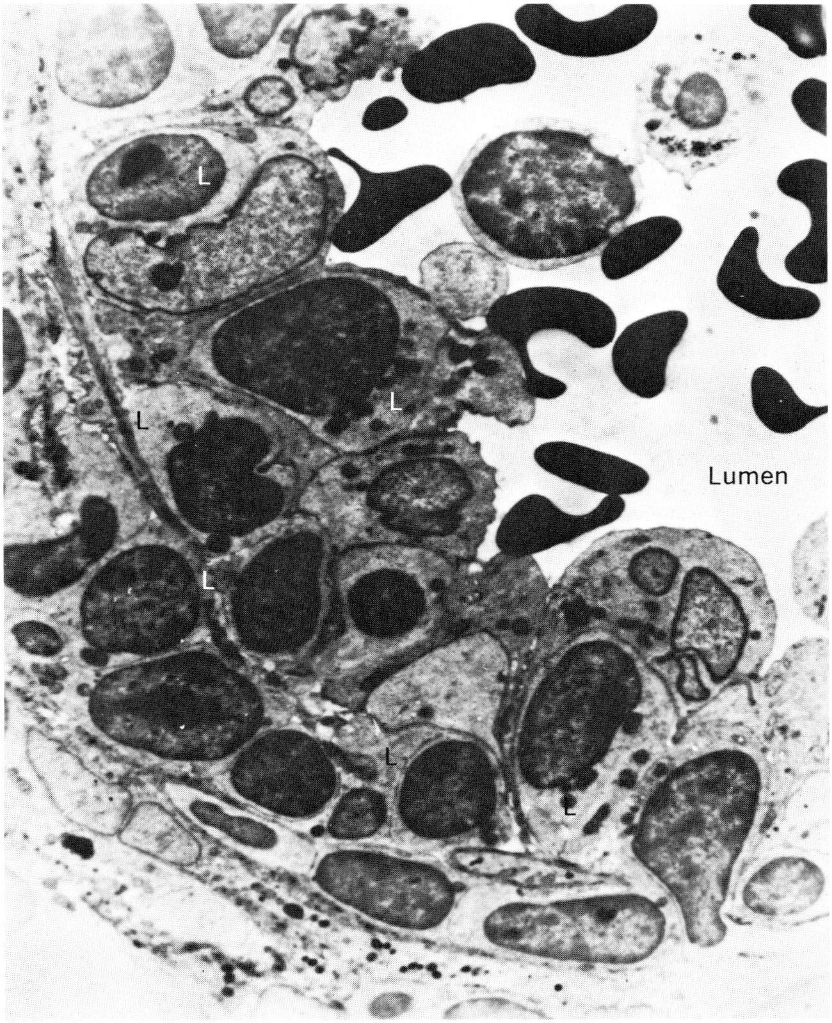

Figure 3-9. Postcapillary venule in a lymph node of a normal rat. Red blood cells are present in the lumen. Endothelial cells contain lymphocytes (L) characterized by their electron-dense nuclei. (Courtesy of Marchesi and Gowans, 1964).

(Fig. 3-8). Mononuclear cells respond to the following chemotactic factors: a factor generated in serum by interaction with antigen-antibody complexes which is apparently not related to the complement system, fragmentation products of the third and fifth components of complement, soluble bacterial factors, a factor produced by the interaction of sensitized lymphocytes with specific antigen, and a factor present in lysates of neutrophils (Ward, 1968; Ward, Remold, and David, 1969; Ward, unpublished observations). It is obvious that both complement-associated and non-complement-associated systems are important in the generation of factors which are chemotactic for mononuclear cells. The fact that sensitized lymphoid cells produce upon contact with antigen a chemotactic factor for mononuclear cells could explain the presence of these cells in reactions of delayed hypersensitivity. The neutrophil-contained factor which is chemotactic for mononuclear cells could explain the sequential appearance of mononuclear cells after the arrival of neutrophils in an exudate. It has been shown in cyclic neutrophenia of human beings that monocytes do not appear in inflammatory exudates unless there is an adequate supply of circulating neutrophils (Page and Good, 1958).

Concerning enzyme mechanisms involved in the chemotactic response of mononuclear cells, all that can be said is that mononuclear cells contain at least one enzyme, a serine esterase, which is required for the chemotactic response of the cell but which is distinct from either of the two enzymes required for the chemotactic response of the neutrophil (Ward, 1968).

How *lymphocytes* traverse blood vessels has been a mystery for a long time. It has been known for many years that lymphocytes are relatively slow moving and there is no convincing evidence for their chemotactic responsiveness to any factor. Marchesi and Gowans (1964) and subsequently others have provided evidence that lymphocytes migrate out of blood vessels by at least one mechanism which is totally different from the emigration of neutrophils and mononuclear cells. By the process of *emperipolesis,* lymphocytes in contact with endothelial cell surfaces become surrounded and engulfed by the cytoplasmic processes of the endothelial cells (Figs. 3-9 to 3-11). The lymphocytes are then transported intact across the endothelial cell to be deposited on the basement membrane side. At this point, the lymphocytes are effectively outside the blood vessel. The phenomenon of emperiopolesis has been observed in post-capillary venules of lymph nodes, in choroidal vessels of the eye, and in vessels of nerves involved with experimental allergic neuritis. The fact that the emigration of lymphocytes from blood vessels involves an interaction (which may be passive on the part of the lymphocyte) with endothelial cells implies a mechanism of migration totally different from that for granulocytic leukocytes.

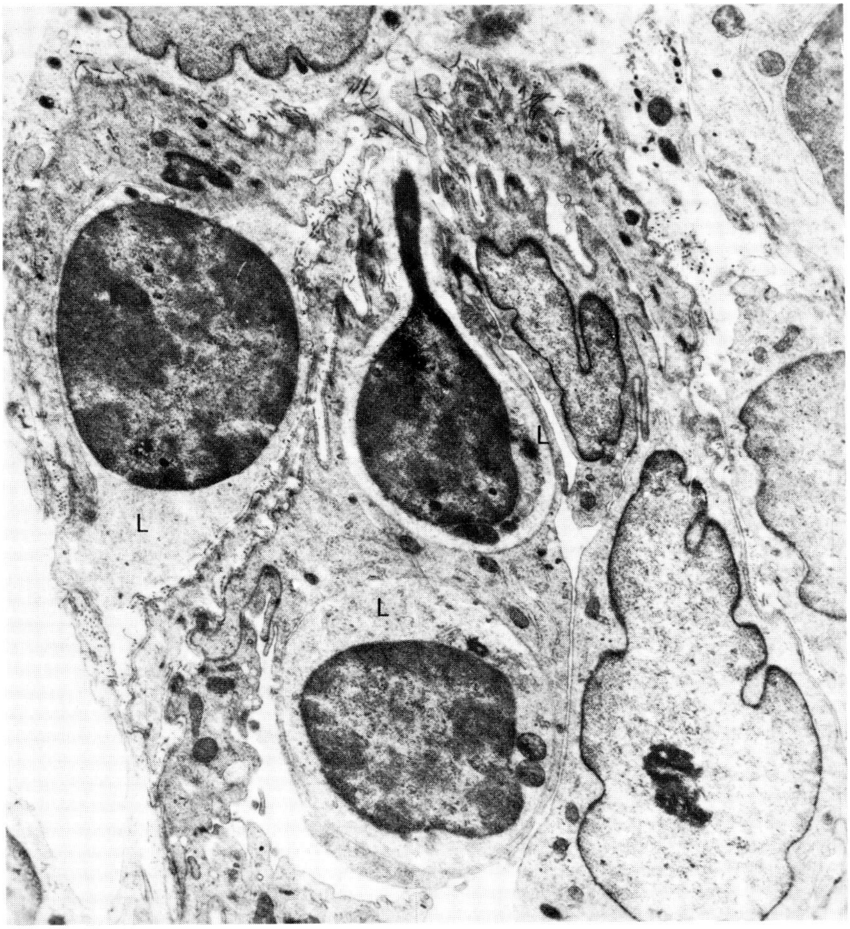

Figure 3-10. From the same vessel as Fig. 3-9. Three lymphocytes (L) with electron-dense nuclei are enclosed within endothelial cells. One lymphocyte has a pseudopod extending through an interendothelial junction. (Courtesy of Marchesi and Gowans, 1964).

D. Reticuloendothelial System

At an inflamed site, phagocytic uptake and metabolic degradation of foreign material is readily accomplished by the macrophages (derived from blood monocytes) and the granulocytes that have arrived from the circulation. If the injurious agent is quickly contained, these cells are functionally adequate and no other clearance mechanism is required. However, there also exists an auxilliary system of phagocytosis which has as its main purpose the clearance of foreign matter

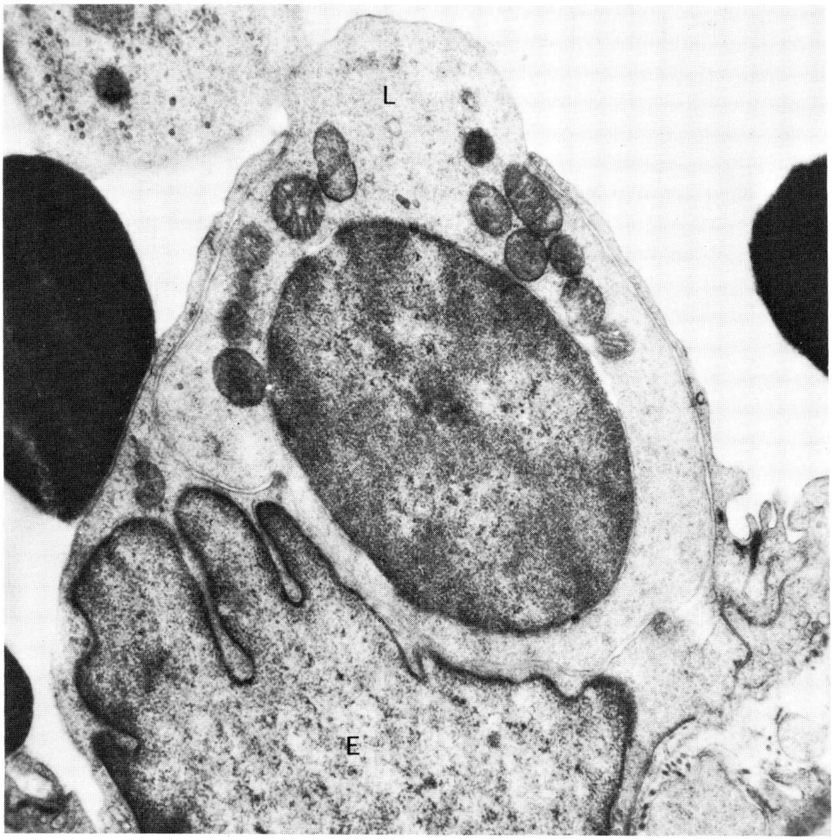

Figure 3-11. Additional area of the vessel pictured in Fig. 3-9, showing the intimate relationship between a lymphocyte (L) and an endothelial cell (E). Cytoplasmic processes of the endothelial cell almost completely enclose the lymphocyte. (Courtesy of Marchesi and Gowans, 1964).

from blood or lymphatic channels. The material being phagocytosed may be particulate, as in the case of a microbe or protozoan, or soluble as in the case of an aggregated protein (autologous, homologous, or heterologous) or an antigen-antibody complex. All of these substances will disappear from the circulation within hours. The clearance mechanism can be ascribed to the fact that the body has a highly specialized system, termed the *reticuloendothelial system* (RES), that acts as an effective back-up system of phagocytosis for the inflammatory cells. In some instances the RES may be the sole means for phagocytic removal of foreign material, as in the case of erythrocytes that become coated with antibodies rendering them "foreign." The actively phagocytic cells of the RES lie along vascular channels of the liver and spleen. There are occasional, scattered cells in vascular channels of various other organs that, under the proper stimulus engage in phagocytic function. The lymphatic channels and especially the peripheral sinuses of the lmyph nodes contain macrophages that are very avidly phagocytic. These cells may completely remove microbes that have escaped from a wound site and have begun to percolate into the interior of the body. The RES even includes phagocytic cells (histiocytes) that are scattered throughout the connective tissue of the body. In a special sense, the RES is the reserve system that takes over protective, phagocytic functions when leukocytes that have been mobilized during an inflammatory response have failed in their efforts to contain an invading microbial agent.

E. Fate of Inflammatory Cells

Because both mononuclear cells and neutrophils carry stores of enzymes potentially destructive of tissue proteins, the function and the fate of these cells once outside blood vessels is of considerable importance. Both types of leukocytes are actively phagocytic and possess numerous lysosomal enzymes such as lysozyme, which is ideally suited for destruction of bacteria by hydrolysis of sugar groups in the cell wall.

The engulfment and ingestion by the neutrophil of particulate material, such as bacteria, has been expertly documented by Hirsch (1962) among many others. The discharge of lysosomal contents into phagocytic vacuoles in the leukocyte cytoplasm, a necessary step in the destruction and digestion of phagocytosed particles, is a well-known phenomenon. Following phagocytosis, there is within the neutrophil a burst of metabolic activity associated with glycolysis, increased oxygen consumption, oxidation of glucose via the hexose monophosphate shunt, and formation of hydrogen peroxide (see review of Karnovsky, 1962). As will be seen in Chapter 4, when these mechanisms fail, bacterial invaders remain viable and can cause serious disease.

Much less is known about mononuclear cells except that, while their enzyme content differs from that of neutrophils, the mechanism for phagocytosis is probably similar to that of the neutrophil.

The fate of neutrophils and mononuclear cells once outside the blood vessel is not clear. Neutrophils have little proliferative potential and probably have a life span of only a few days. If their accumulation is rapid and emigration from the area fails to occur, they may begin to break down, as occurs in an *abscess* (see Fig. 4-1), with the discharge of enzymes potentially destructive to the tissue

Table 3-3 Enzymes and Other Substances Associated with Lysosomes[a]

Acid phosphatase	Hyaluronidase
Acid ribonuclease	Lysozyme
Acid deoxyribonuclease	Collagenase
Cathepsins B, C, D, E	Aryl sulfatases A and B
Phosphoprotein phosphatase	Phospholipase
Phosphatidic acid phosphatase	Acid lipase
Organophosphate-resistant esterases	Phagocytin and related bactericidal proteins
β-Glucuronidase	Endogenous pyrogen
β-Galactosidase	Plasminogen activator (? urokinase)
β-N-acetylglucosaminidase	Hemolysin(s)
α-L-fucosidase	Mucopolysaccharides and glycoproteins
α-1,4-glucosidase	Basic proteins: (a) Mast-cell-active; (b) Permeability-inducing, independent of mast cells
α-mannosidase	Kininase
α-N-acetylglucosaminidase	Elastase
Kininogenase	
Collagenase	

[a] Adapted from Cochrane (1968).

of the host. Neutrophils contain an elastase which is capable of breaking down the internal elastic lamina of arteries and a collagenase which may disrupt connective tissue fibers. There exist numerous other hydrolases which are capable of acting upon a variety of substances in tissue (Table 3-3). There are even enzymes in the neutrophil that produce kinins and phlogist factors from the complement system. The breakdown of neutrophils also releases cationic (basic) peptides which cause disruption of mast cells with the release of histamine, and thus increased permeability. The sum of these actions is destruction of tissue, intensification of the inflammatory reaction, and accelerated tissue damage.

Mononuclear cells apparently contain many enzymes similar to those in neutrophils, but they behave differently in several respects. Mononuclear cells are derived from precursor cells in the bone marrow and are undergoing continuous, rapid division (Volkman and Gowans, 1965). It appears quite possible that mononuclear cells may continue to proliferate once in the extravascular site, accounting for a rapid increase in numbers of these cells in exudates. Under certain influences mononuclear cells merge one with the other to acquire a common cytoplasm, while at the same time maintaining their distinct nuclei, and form the so-called giant cells (Fig. 3-12). Often the giant cell appears when a vigorous

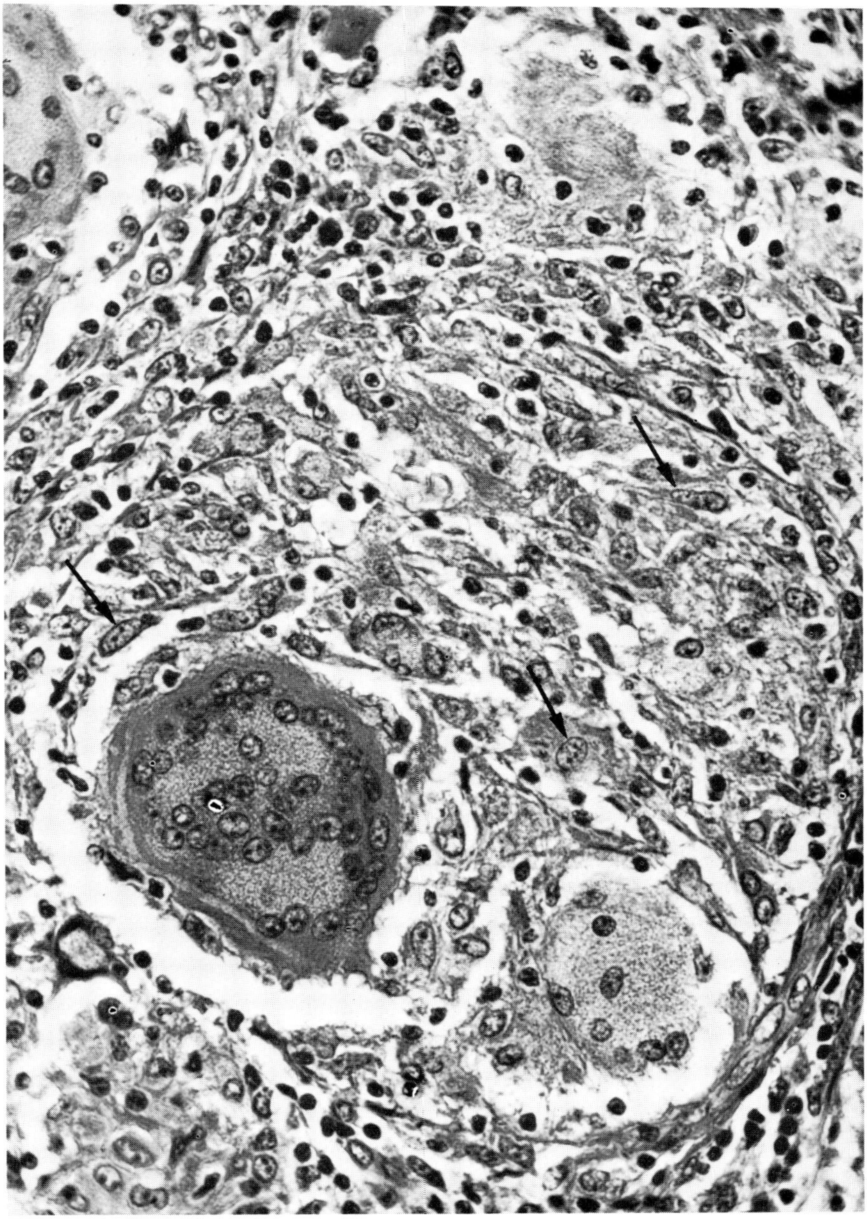

Figure 3-12. Granulomatous inflammation (sarcoidosis) in a human lymph node. A giant cell is present and loosely arranged epithelioid cells (arrow) contain clear, elliptical nuclei and abundant cytoplasm.

attempt by the mononuclear cells to remove foreign material by phagocytosis has failed. Tuberculous inflammation, fungal infection, a wood splinter, or silk suture often exemplify this reaction.

The fate of lymphocytes in exudates is slightly clearer. These cells carry immunologic memory (see Chapter 5), and if they come into contact with the appropriate antigen, they may undergo a curious *transformation* process. The nucleus enlarges, the cytoplasm acquires new lysosomal structures, and the cells simultaneously begin mitotic division. In transformation such soluble substances as the so-called migration inhibitory factor which causes cessation of random movement of mononuclear cells, a factor chemotactic for mononuclear cells, a substance cytotoxic for virtually any cell type, and a broad spectrum anti-viral agent (*interferon*) may be elaborated. In addition, several serum proteins are synthesized (see review of David, 1970). The arrival at extravascular sites of specifically sensitized lymphocytes which then come in contact with the appropriate antigen can lead to the production of a mediator which will lead directly or indirectly to tissue damage. There is very little proof, however, that all lymphocytes which make up a chronic inflammatory exudate are specifically sensitized to an antigen present at the site of inflammation. In fact, it has been shown that in a skin reaction of delayed hypersensitivity, more than 90 per cent of the lymphoid cells are not specifically sensitized (Hamilton and Chase, 1967; Turk, 1962; McCluskey *et al.,* 1963). If there are factors present, however, that can transfer "naïve" lymphocytes, they can be recruited in the inflammatory response to produce injury of tissue. It might be noted that no one has yet described a function for lymphocytes unrelated to an immunologic mechanism.

The fact that lymphocytes continually recirculate in a shuttle between the bloodstream and lymphoid tissues is firmly documented by the studies of Gowans (1959). This phenomenon allows for a conservation of immunocompetent cells in the body, while providing a mechanism for the return of lymphocytes to lymphoid tissues and to the bloodstream once the cells have passed beyond the endothelial barrier. Thus, lymphoid cells can be cleared from an exudate, provided lymphoid channels are intact.

F. Exudates

Most inflammatory responses are morphologically identified by the presence of protein and cells outside blood vessels, giving rise to the so-called exudate. The cellular character of the exudate, as implied above, defines the morphologic stage of the inflammatory response as acute, subacute or chronic. The exudate may be water-rich (serous) exudate, protein-rich, fibrin-rich (fibrinous), and so forth. An exudate consisting primarily of neutrophils is termed a *purulent* exudate. One in which numerous neutrophils are associated with tissue destruction would be a *suppurative* exudate, as in the case of an abscess. The presence of fibrin in an inflammatory exudate has been described as a mechanism for walling off organisms which might otherwise spread to distant parts of the body. Again, the accumulation of proteins and leukocytes presents the problem of removing all of the inflammatory products of the exudate (leukocytes, fibrin, water, protein) and restoring the tissue to its original form. Perhaps the most important factor is whether the agent responsible for the induction of the inflammatory response is neutralized, removed, or destroyed. If the responsible agent consists of bacteria, successful phagocytic destruction of the organisms will result in the disappearance of leukocytes, a reduction in permeability, and a return of the tissue to its original state. However, if for some reason, the inciting agent is not successfully dealt with, the continued accumulation of leukocytes may lead to the release of tissue-destructive enzymes from leukocytes and the subsequent liquefaction of host tissue. When this happens, an *abscess* appears. Nowhere is this complication more serious than in the central nervous system, as in the case of bacterial meningitis. The acute inflammatory response may also progress into the subacute phase at which point granulation tissue, lymphocytes, and monocytes predominate. This becomes an important defense mechanism in the case of myocardial necrosis where heart muscle, having very limited regenerative capability is replaced by very young, angioblastic and fibroblastic tissue. In this type of inflammation the laying down of dense, collagenous connective tissue is followed by formation of a scar. As the scar matures, all evidence of the inflammatory episode disappears. As will be discussed in more detail below, the inflammatory response by this progression may be very important in the healing process.

The persistence of an inflammatory exudate ("nonresolution") is a serious hazard to the functional integrity of the involved tissue. In the lung, progressive accumulation of inflammatory cells, fibrin, and granulation tissue may result in a chronic inflammatory focus. If the margin of this zone becomes sufficiently walled off with inflammatory cells, and fibrin or fibrous scar tissue, a chronic festering wound develops. In the pleural cavity, the consequence may be serious compression of adjacent lung tissue and/or erosion into the underlying lung parenchyma or the overlying chest wall with discharge of debris. Rarely will the persistence of an inflammatory response over a long period of time lead to any beneficial results for the individual.

G. Consequences of Inflammation

During the development and resolution or progression of the inflammatory process, it may happen that instead of healing or repair, damage to the host occurs. It has already been shown that when an inflammatory exudate persists too long, destruction of host tissue may result. In the rejection of a homografted tissue, it is the lymphocytes and monocytes of the inflammatory exudate that mediate the destruction of the grafted tissue. The presence of leukocytes along glomerular capillary loops may lead to hydrolysis of the underlying basement membrane and functional aberrations in glomerular filtration (see review of Cochrane, 1969). Along the articular surface of a joint, the presence of granulation tissue with its lysosomal-rich cells may lead to enzymatic destruction of articular cartilage. A great deal of effort in clinical medicine is expended in attempts to suppress these harmful effects of the inflammatory process.

1. Host reactions

The reaction of the stromal and parenchymal elements in a tissue which has been the site of the inflammatory response varies according to the tissue and the circumstances of the inflammatory episode. Both parenchymatous and stromal connective tissue elements may be involved in a proliferative response. In the dermis, the proliferation of fibroblastic and angioblastic elements occurs during the formation of granulation tissue. This results in the appearance of new blood vessels as well as increased numbers of fibroblastic elements which are capable of laying down ground substance and collagen fibers. When inflammation in renal glomeruli takes the form of acute exudative glomerulonephritis following streptococcal infection, numerous neutrophils appear along glomerular capillary loops, and a marked proliferation of endothelial and epithelial cells frequently follows (Figs. 3-13, 3-14). Precisely what purpose, if any, this type of response serves is unclear. It may represent an attempt by the kidney to replace damaged cells. These changes may, however, be detrimental if extensive proliferation of endothelial elements leads to an occlusion of glomerular capillaries, or if rapid proliferation of epithelial cells lining glomerular loops and Bowman's capsule lead to the formation of continuous sheets of epithelial cells which obliterate the urinary space. The advantageous element of such proliferative activity is seen in convoluted tubules or renal tubules where the epithelium has been destroyed by a poison such as ethylene glycol; here the only hope for recovery of renal function is the regenerative proliferation of tubular epithelial cells.

A frequent accompaniment to the acute or chronic inflammatory response in the central nervous system is the proliferation of intrinsic supporting tissue cells or glial elements. This accumulation of glial cells accompanied by a limited angioblastic response is the only way the central nervous system can respond to injury,

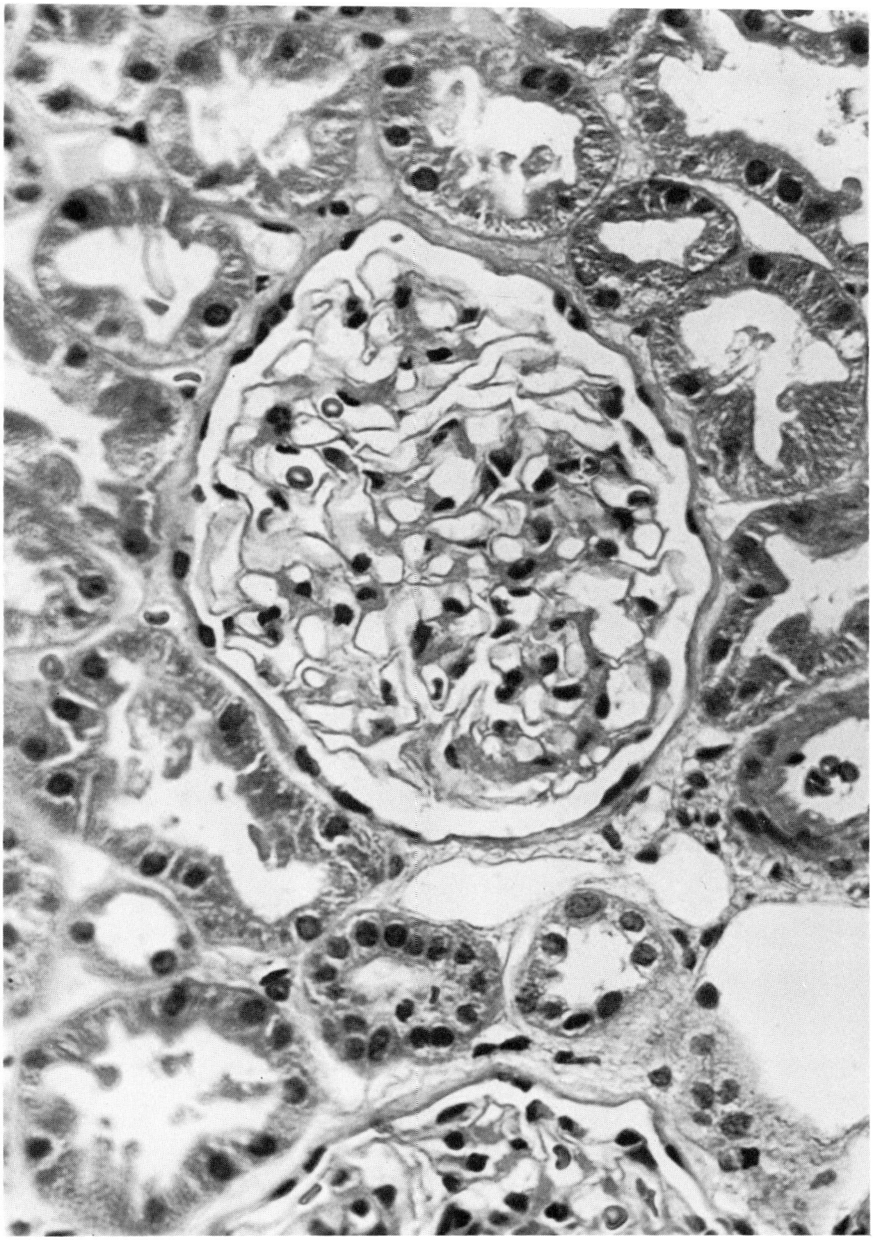

Figure 3-13. Normal glomerulus for comparison with that in Fig. 3-14. Capillary loops are widely patent.

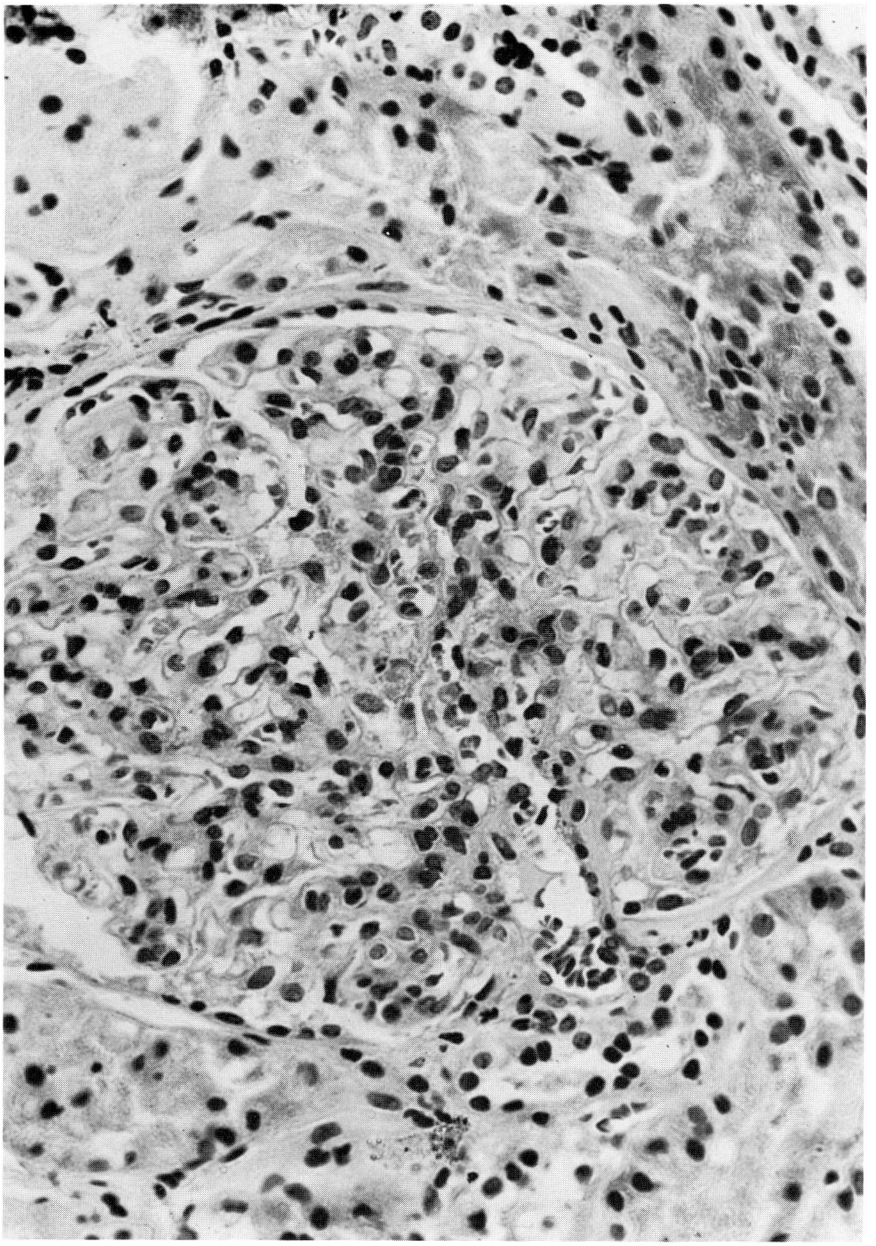

Figure 3-14. Glomerulus from a case of acute post-streptococcal glomerulonephritis. The glomerulus is enlarged due to the proliferation of endothelial and epithelial cells within capillary loops, causing partial occlusion of blood flow.

since it lacks regenerative potential. If excessive, this accumulation of glial cells may interfere with neural function.

2. Repair—healing and regeneration

This reaction of tissue to inflammation is the basis of the phenomenon of repair, which includes healing and regeneration. In the repair of tissue, the area either becomes replaced with a scar, or the tissue is restored to its original state by the regenerative capacities of that tissue (see review of Schilling, 1968). The outcome of the reparative processes in injured skin at the site of a laceration may be either a tissue that is indistinguishable from the original one, or there may result an ugly scar which must be considered less than optimal repair of damaged tissue. In a laceration of the skin where there has been the release of blood cells, protein, and fibrin by mechanically ruptured vessels, the acute inflammatory response results in a profusion of polymorphonuclear leukocytes surrounding the zone of damage. In a few days the angioblastic and fibroblastic proliferation ensues, and these elements bridge the gap where disruption of tissue has occurred. Fibrin which has formed in the exudate will be invaded by the granulation tissue. Shortly thereafter, epithelial cells begin rapid proliferation and proceed to overgrow the wounded area. If all goes well, within a week or so the area is completely covered by epithelial cells which have regenerated from the margins of the wounds or from retained hair follicles in the area of the injury; the tiny blood vessels which have grown into the area of the wound begin to disappear. In some circumstances, fibroblasts begin to lay down an inordinate amount of connective tissue, which may result in the formation of a scar. The continued presence of bacteria predisposes an area to this undesirable end. In the case of the liver which has been damaged by hepatitis virus, the region being repaired is often the site of competition between fibroblastic proliferation and regeneration of hepatocellular elements and bile ducts (Figs. 3-15, 3-16). The presence of fibrous scar tissue in so vital an organ is detrimental not only because it effectively precludes the expansion and regeneration of hepatic lobules, but also because it may seriously interfere with blood flow, resulting in portal hypertension. There is no clear indication as to why, in certain individuals with hepatitis, the inflammatory process persists in the liver. Nevertheless, as long as it continues, there is grave danger that the process will be resolved by the laying down of fibrous scar tissue. It may well be the local persistence of the virus that results in continued inflammation, although many have postulated the role of an auto-immune process. Whatever the cause, it is vital that the inflammatory reaction subside if the liver is to return to normal function.

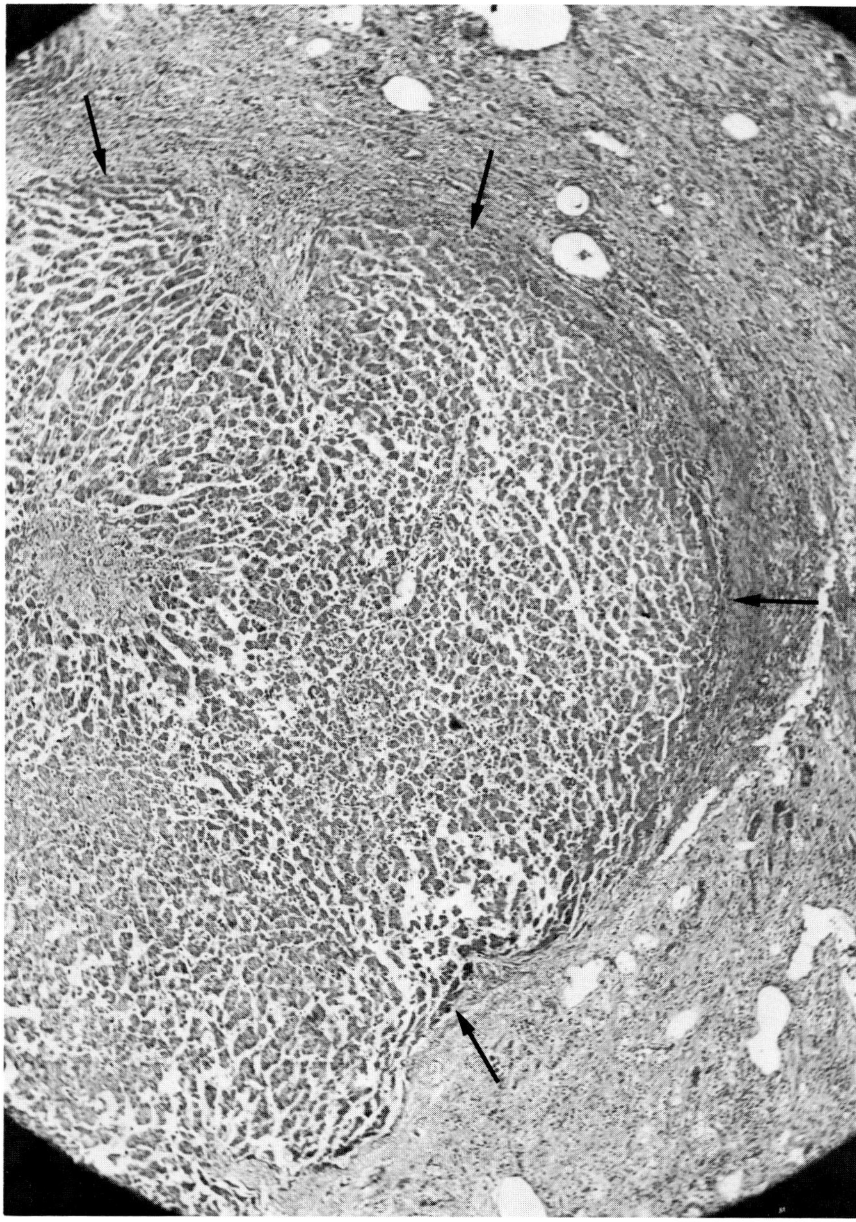

Figure 3-15. "Pseudolobule" (arrows) in the liver from a case of postnecrotic cirrhosis in a human being. The nodule contains irregular collections of liver cord cells that have undergone proliferation in an attempt to replace other destroyed liver tissue. Fibrous scar compresses periphery of lobule.

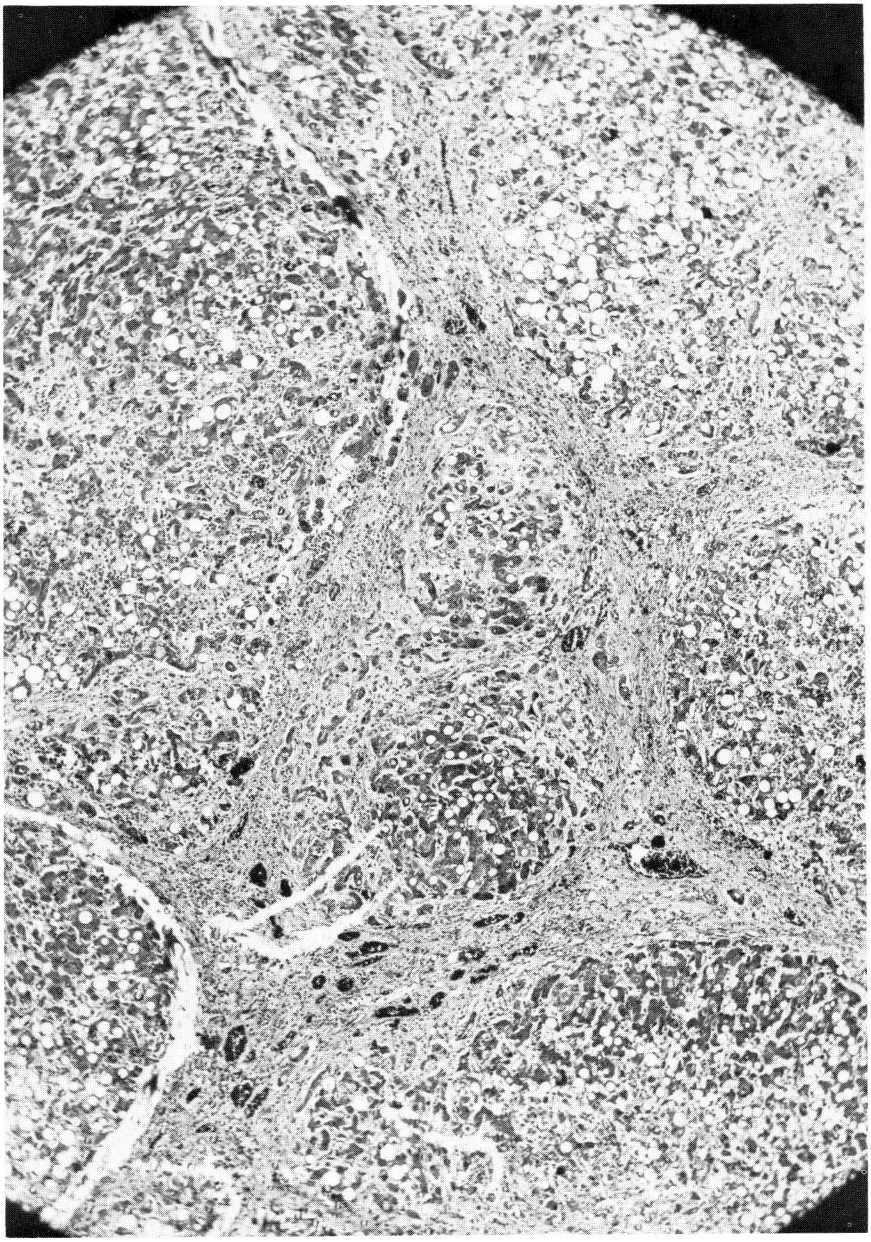

Figure 3-16. Postalcoholic cirrhosis of the liver in a human being, with residual nodules of parenchymal cells. The extensive amount of connective tissue (with interspersed bile ducts) has caused irreversible interruption of hepatic lobules. Fatty (vacuolar) changes can be seen in liver cord cells.

Table 3-4 Examples of Regenerative Capacities of Various Tissues and Organs

UNLIMITED OR MODERATE CAPACITY	LIMITED OR NO CAPACITY
epithelium of skin, gastrointestinal and genitourinary tracts	skeletal, cardiac and smooth muscle
formed elements of bone marrow (red cells, white cells, platelets)	lung parenchyma
renal tubular epithelium	renal glomeruli
liver parenchyma	neurons of central nervous system
lymphoid tissues	retinal tissue and all sense organs
endothelium	endocrine glands
bone	gonadal parenchyma
peripheral nerves	dental structures
ductal epithelium of exocrine glands	

Repair in the central nervous system is seen primarily as scar tissue formation because neuronal elements have little or no capacity to regenerate. As indicated above, the inflammatory process, if unchecked, may lead to the formation of large amounts of glial scar, resulting in serious functional disturbances in the central nervous system. In the peripheral nervous system, Schwann cells, which function as nutritive and supporting tissue elements around axons of peripheral nerves, participate in the laying down of new myelin sheaths after a nerve has been damaged or destroyed. Table 3-4 lists the various regenerative capacities of tissues in the body. It is obvious that if an injured tissue is unable to regenerate, repair can only be accomplished by the formation of a scar.

H. Granulomatous Inflammation

Granulomatous inflammation is almost impossible to define. Originally the term *granuloma* descriptively defined the tiny granular, white bodies which could be seen in tissues such as the peritoneum, where they appeared as a result of systemic (hematogenous) spread of the tuberculous organism and the peculiar local inflammatory reaction to the mycobacterium. The term was later redefined according to certain microscopic criteria. At the present time, granulomatous inflammation usually refers to an inflammatory response which is characterized by the presence of lymphocytes, monocytes, and plasma cells. The monocytes or histiocytes may be clustered in a characteristic elliptical formation around the causative agent or around a central necrotic area. Large histiocytic cells with abundant cytoplasm are usually referred to as *epithelioid cells,* and it seems more than likely that they are derived from circulating monocytes. It is not unusual for multiple histiocytes to unite to form giant, multinucleated cells with common cell membranes (Fig. 3-12).

Recently it has become evident that in at least one experimental model, granulomatous inflammation may be dependent upon an intact immunologic responsiveness of the individual, but it is equally clear that in other situations granulomatous inflammation can occur in the face of severe immunologic suppression. Using experimental schistosomiasis in the mouse, it has been found that immunosuppressive agents, which preclude the development of a state of delayed hypersensitivity, will prevent the formation of granulomas in response to the infective agent (Domingo, Cowan, and Warren, 1967). Considering the multiplicity of mediators produced by contact of sensitized lymphocytes with antigen, it is not difficult to visualize the accumulation of monocytes in clusters that might define a granuloma and, by the action of enzymes released from the leukocytes as well as the elaboration of a cytotoxic factor (Perlmann *et al.,* 1968; Kolb and Granger, 1968), the subsequent death of cells in the central areas of the granuloma. This central necrosis is very characteristic of granulomas in tuberculosis and syphilis. For a long time it has been assumed that the granulomatous inflammation of pulmonary tuberculosis represents an immunologic response with allergic manifestations, although at present there is no firm evidence for this conclusion. Nevertheless, the association between granulomatous inflammation and immunocompetence suggests that this assumption may be correct.

Situations also exist in which immunologic responsiveness is apparently not required for the development of granulomatous inflammatory responses. The condition of "blue velvet disease" seen in addicts who inject themselves with substances containing talc crystals, results in the formation of diffuse pulmonary granulomas. However, evidence suggests that no immunologic mechanism is involved in this type of cellular response. Warren and Kellermeyer (1968) have demonstrated that, in mice, talc granulomas form in the face of severe suppression of immunocompetence, and it has been suggested that kinin formation may be necessary for the production of talc granulomas.

Most granulomatous inflammatory response will fade as the inciting agent is removed. In the case of tuberculosis or syphilis, however, extensive destruction of cells within the central portions of the granulomas occurs. The reasons for such cellular destruction are not clear (see above), but once necrotic tissue forms there will be a continuing inflammatory response unless this tissue is removed. If extensive necrosis of granulomas develops in peripheral lymph nodes, rupture through the skin surface may occur with discharge of contents. Similarly, in the lung necrotic granulomas may rupture into pulmonary vessels or into the bronchial tract. Occasionally, if the area of necrosis is not extensive, calcification and even bone formation can ensue and the end result will be a fibrocalcific or osseous nodule.

I. Defective Inflammatory Responsiveness

Among clinical aberrations of the inflammatory response, the most obvious is that cells may be defective in numbers. In conditions such as severe bone-marrow depression due to drugs or radiation, neutrophils, having one of the shortest life spans of any cellular element in the marrow, are the first cells to disappear from the circulation. Under such circumstances, a typical acute inflammatory response is not possible, at least in so far as the cellular elements are concerned. The inability to mobilize neutrophils renders the individual susceptible to infections which may become life-threatening. As in cases of lymphopenic agammaglobulinemia (Swiss type) or thymic aplasia, the absence or severe reduction in the number of circulating lymphocytes results in this same susceptibility to infectious agents. It is presumed that lymphocyte precursors are absent from the bone marrow or that they lack the thymic environment which allows them to undergo "maturation" and thus provide the individual with immunocompetent cells.

An individual whose leukocytes are functionally defective is immunologically vulnerable. It is well known that in chronic granulocytic leukemia, neutrophils are unable to cope with infectious agents, especially bacteria, although the basis of this defect has not been discovered. In the "stem-cell" leukemias, precursor cells are ineffective against bacterial agents and appear to crowd out the functionally (and morphologically) mature cells. It is common in autopsy specimens from leukemic patients to see colonies of bacteria in lung tissue without any significant mobilization of neutrophils in the area.

In chronic granulomatous disease of childhood, neutrophils phagocytose bacteria but fail to kill and digest them. This is especially true with *Staphyloccus* and *Serratia sp.* In this disease, the customary burst of respiratory oxidative activity and production of hydrogen peroxide following phagocytosis are both lacking (Holmes, Page, and Good, 1967), and an oxidase for reduced nicotinamide adenine dinucleotide (NADH) is apparently lacking. Precisely how these metabolic aberrations are related to defective killing of bacteria after the ingestion phase of phagocytosis is not clear, but seems to be related to defective lysosomal function (see Chapter 2). The persistence of bacteria in various tissues of these patients leads to the progressive accumulation of mononuclear cells and lymphocytes: thus the term *chronic granulomatous disease.* This defect is a sex-linked recessive character appearing only in males with the carrier female having somewhat decreased leukocytic activity.

The Chediak-Higashi syndrome is another condition in which neutrophilic granulocytes are defective. Morphologically the cells are recognizable by large cytoplasmic granules. For reasons that are not clear, these cells do not effectively phagocytose and kill bacteria, and the affected individuals frequently die after a series of bacterial infections. Acquired failure of leukocytes to deal with infectious agents occurs in renal and in diabetic acidosis, although the nature of this defect is not known.

The inflammatory response may be abnormal because of a functional or structural defect in blood vessels. The most common example of this defect is sunburn, which actually represents a first degree burn. Persistent vasodilatation is caused by the actinic damage to vessels which, if severe, can result in increased capillary permeability with accumulation of water, protein, and electrolytes in extravascular areas. Ionizing radiation, especially that associated with gamma irradiation, can produce endothelial damage resulting in persistent vasodilatation.

Defects in plasma constituents may result in aberrations of the inflammatory response. At least two different types of impaired phagocytosis have been reported, each dependent on deficiency of a plasma opsonin. Individuals with sickle cell disease have been found lacking in a heat-labile opsonin that promotes phagocytosis of pneumococci (Winkelstein and Drachman, 1968). Miller *et al.* (1968) have reported the case of a child in whom deficiency of a plasma factor impairs the ability of leukocytes to phagocytize yeast cells and *Staphylococcus aureus.* This defect is corrected by the addition of highly purified fifth component of human complement.

There has also been a study made on a child who has an *inhibitor* in his serum that renders neutrophils unresponsive to chemotactic stimuli (Ward and Schlegel, 1969). The child fails to show an accumulation of neutrophils in inflammatory sites, presumably due to the presence in plasma of this inhibitor. As a result, neutrophils are not efficiently mobilized and bacterial infections are common.

The loss of *homeostatic factors* in plasma may lead to uncontrolled, acute inflammatory episodes. This is especially well documented in patients who lack the natural inhibitor of the esterase of the first component (C1) of human complement (Landermann, 1962; Donaldson and Evans, 1963). The C1 esterase inhibitor may be totally lacking, or it may be present in normal quantity but in a non-functional form. In either case, the individual is subjected to episodes of angioedema which may be life-threatening. It is now recognized that the C1 esterase inhibitor also acts on plasmin and kallikrein, but it is not known which mediators (products of enzymes) are most important in the associated clinical disorder.

A report has been published about a man in whom both autologous and passively injected homologous C3 are rapidly destroyed (Alper *et al.,* 1968). It is thought that this patient possesses a large quantity of a natural C3 inactivator in his plasma. The rapid destruction of C3 has left him susceptible to frequent and serious infections, which might be explained by the reduction in uptake of C3 onto surfaces of sensitized cells (including bacteria), thus diminishing the threshold of phagocytosis.

"Experiments of nature" provide an array of clinical patterns, pointing out aspects of exaggerated or impaired inflammatory responses. The variety of mediators which participate in the inflammatory response is formidable, but it is from such material so generously provided by nature that an understanding of the role of these mediators will eventually emerge.

References

Alpers, C. A., Abramson, N., Johnston, R. B., Jr., McCall, C. E., Jandl, J. H., and Rosen, F. S. (1968), Increased susceptibility to infection associated with a defect of complement metabolism, J. Clin. Invest., *48*:1a (abst.).

Becker, E. L., and Ward, P. A. (1967), Partial biochemical characterization of the activated esterase required in the complement-dependent chemotaxis of rabbit polymorphonuclear leukocytes, J. Exp. Med., *125*:1021.

Becker, E. L. (1969), The relation of complement to the other systems, Proc. Roy. Soc., Ser. B., *173*:188.

Boyden, S. (1962), The chemotactic effect of mixtures of antibody and antigen on polymorphonuclear leukocytes, J. Exp. Med., *115*:453.

Brocklehurst, W. E. (1960), The release of histamine and formation of a slow-reacting substance (SRS-A) during anaphylactic shock, J. Physiol. (London), *151*:416.

Cochrane, C. G. (1968), Immunologic tissue injury mediated by neutrophilic leukocytes, *in* Advances in Immunology, 9:97, F. J. Dixon and H. G. Kunkel, Eds., Academic Press, New York.

David, J., Mediators produced by lymphoid cells, Fed. Proc. (in press).

Domingo, E. O., Cowan, R. T., and Warren, K. S. (1967), The inhibition of granuloma formation around *Schistosoma mansoni* eggs. I. Immunosuppressive drugs, Amer. J. Trop. Med., *16*:284.

Donaldson, V. H., and Evans, R. R. (1963), A biochemical abnormality in hereditary angioneurotic edema. Absence of serum inhibitor of C'l-esterase, Amer. J. Med., *35*:37.

Harris, H. (1960), Mobilization of defensive cells in inflammatory tissue, Bact. Rev., *24*:3.

Hirsch, J. G. (1962), Cinemicrophotographic observations on granule lysis in polymorphonuclear leukocytes during phagocytosis, J. Exp. Med., *116*:827.

Holmes, B., Page, A. R., and Good, R. A. (1967), Studies of the metabolic activity of leukocytes from patients with a genetic abnormality of phagocytic functions, J. Clin. Invest., *46*:1422.

Hurley, J. V. (1964), Substances promoting leukocyte emigration, Ann. N. Y. Acad. Sci., *116*:918.

Karnovsky, M. L. (1962), Metabolic basis of phagocytic activity, Physiol. Rev., *42*: 143.

Keller, H. U., and Sorkin, E. (1968), Chemotaxis of leucocytes, Experientia, *24*:641.

Kellermeyer, R. W., and Graham, R. C., Jr. (1968), Kinins– possible physiologic and pathologic roles in man, New Eng. J. Med., *279*:754, 802, 859.

Kolb, W. P., and Granger, G. A. (1968), Lymphocyte *in vitro* cytotoxicity: characterization of human lymphotoxin, Proc. Natl. Acad. Sci., *61*:1250.

Landerman, N. S. (1962), Hereditary angioneurotic edema. I. Case reports and review of the literature, J. Allergy, *33*:316.

Lewis, T. (1927), The blood vessels of the human skin and their responses, Shaw, London.

Marchesi, V. T. (1961), The site of leukocyte emigration during inflammation, Quart. J. Exp. Physiol., *46*:115.

Marchesi, V. T. (1962), The passage of colloidal carbon through inflamed endothelium, Proc. Roy. Soc., Ser. B., *156*:550.

Marchesi, V. T. (1964), Some electron microscopic observations on interactions between leukocytes, platelets, and endothelial cells in acute inflammation, Ann. N. Y. Acad. Sci., *116*:774.

Marchesi, V. T., and Florey, H. W. (1960), Electron micrographic observations on the emigration of leukocytes, Quart. J. Exp. Physiol., *45*:343.

Marchesi, V. T., and Gowans, J. L. (1964), The migration of lymphocytes through the endothelium of venules in lymph nodes: an electron microscope study, Proc. Roy. Soc., Ser. B., *159*:283.

Miles, A. A. (1961), Local and systemic factors of shock, Fed. Proc., Suppl. #9, *20*:141.

Miller, M. E., Seals, J., Kaye, R., and Levitsky, L. C. (1968), A familial, plasma-associated defect of phagocytosis, Lancet *ii*:60.

Muller-Eberhard, E. J. (1968), Chemistry and reaction mechanisms of complement, *in* Advances in Immunology, *8*:1, F. J. Dixon and H. G. Kunkel, Eds., Academic Press, New York.

Orange, R. P., Valentine, M., and Austen, K. F. (1968), Antigen-induced release of slow reacting substance of anaphylaxis (SRS-A^{rat}) in rats prepared with homologous antibody, J. Exp. Med., *127*:767.

Page, A. R., and Good, R. A. (1968), A clinical and experimental study of the function of neutrophils in the inflammatory response, Amer. J. Path., *43*:645.

Perlmann, P., Perlmann, H., and Holm, G. (1968), Cytoxic action of stimulated lymphocytes in allogenic and autologous erythrocytes, Science, *160*:306.

Pickles, V. R. (1969), Prostaglandins, Nature, *224*:221.

Schilling, J. A. (1968), Wound healing, Physiol. Rev., *48*:374.

Spector, W. G., and Willoughby, D. A. (1964), Vasoactive amines in acute inflammation, Ann. N. Y. Acad. Sci., *116*:839.

Volkman, A., and Gowans, J. L. (1965), The production of macrophages in the rat, Brit. J. Exp. Path., *46*:50.

Ward, P. A., Cochrane, C. G., and Muller-Eberhard, H. J. (1965), The role of serum complement in chemotaxis of leukocytes *in vitro*, J. Exp. Med., *122*:327.

Ward, P. A., Cochrane, C. G., and Muller-Eberhard, H. J. (1966), Further studies on the chemotactic factor of complement and its formation *in vivo*, Immunol., *11*:141.

Ward, P. A., and Becker, E. L. (1967), Mechanisms of the inhibition of chemotaxis by phosphonate esters, J. Exp. Med., *125*:1001.

Ward, P. A. (1968), Chemotaxis of mononuclear cells, J. Exp. Med., *128*:1201.

Ward, P. A., and Becker, E. L. (1968), The deactivation of rabbit neutrophils by chemotactic factor and the nature of the activatable esterase, J. Exp. Med., *127*: 693.

Ward, P. A., and Schlegel, R. J. (1969), Defective leukotaxis in a child with recurrent infections, Lancet, *ii*:344.

Ward, P. A., Remold, H. G., and David, J. R. (1969), Leukotactic factor produced by sensitized lymphocytes, Science, *163*:1079.

Ward, P. A. (1970), Neutrophil chemotactic factors and related clinical disorders, Arth. and Rheum., *13*:181.

Warren, K. S., and Kellermeyer, R. W. (1968), Foreign body granuloma as a response to chemical mediators of inflammation, J. Clin. Invest., *47*:99a.

Wilhelm, D. L., and Mason, B. (1960), Vascular permeability changes in inflammation: the role of endogenous permeability factors in mild thermal injury, Brit. J. Exp. Path., *41*:487.

Wilhelm, D. L. (1962), The mediation of increased vascular permeability in inflammation, Pharmacol. Rev., *14*:251.

Willoughby, D. A., and Spector, W. G. (1964), The lymph node permeability factor: a possible mediator of the delayed hypersensitivity reaction, Ann. N. Y. Acad. Sci., *116*:874.

Winkelstein, J. A., and Drachman, R. H. (1968), Deficiency of pneumococcal serum opsonizing activity in sickle-cell disease, New Eng. J. Med., *279*:459.

4

HOST-PARASITE INTERACTION

Charles E. McCall, M.D.

A. Introduction—Parasitism

Within the evolutionary process there has always existed a constant interplay between both the offensive and the defensive forces of all forms of life. Underlying these reactions within the biologic world are the quests of all forms of life for food and a suitable environment for self-preservation and replication. Theobald Smith (1934) in his classic discussion of parasitism has suggested that two universal habits have evolved from these biologic necessities: the predatory and the parasitic.

Parasitism does not necessarily evoke a pathobiologic reaction, for it has its foundation in the interdependence of all life. Indeed, most of man's parasites do not harm him. An inoffensive relationship between host and parasite is called *commensalism*. Occasionally, mutual benefits result from host-parasite interaction (*mutualism*), as demonstrated by the production of vitamin K by the indigenous intestinal bacterial flora of man.

It is beyond the scope of this discussion to describe uneventful parasitism in any detail. Instead, the determinants which transform the host-parasite interaction in man into an abnormal or diseased state will be emphasized. These determinants do not emanate solely from properties of the parasite. They include the genotypic and phenotypic constitution of both host and parasite interacting within a specific biologic ecology. Parasitism resulting in disease is aberrant; commensalism is usually a better biologic habit for the parasite as well as the host.

Host-parasite pathobiology has itself been an evolutionary phenomenon. The contemporary state of parasitic diseases of man reflects a fascinating natural history which has been comprehensively reviewed (Burnet, 1966). In man, a relatively constant population of parasites, which usually reside in a balanced relationship with their hosts, has developed through the selection and mutation forces of evolution. Soon after birth man encounters a large number of microbes which then colonize his skin, mucous membranes, and gastrointestinal tract, establishing a pattern which, with intermittent alterations, persists throughout life. Members of this indigenous microbiota are *endogenous parasites*. Within recent years alterations of the equilibrium between these endogenous parasites and man have allowed expressions of endogenous microbial disease with increasing frequency.

The most rapidly fatal host-parasite reactions occur in unnatural hosts who are ill-prepared for the invasion, and the microbes producing such disease cannot be considered members of the normal human flora. Many of the great plagues of human history fall within this category of exogenous infection: smallpox, yellow fever, typhus, diphtheria, typhoid fever, malaria, bubonic plague, and cholera. This truly infectious kind of microbial disease caused by *exogenous parasites* is still immensely important throughout the world, although medical and socioeconomic advances have decreased the incidence in more developed countries.

The evolutionary development of host-parasite relationships and the advances of civilization have not resulted in the so-called perfect parasitic state in which parasitism exists without disease, for many endogenous as well as exogeenous parasitic diseases still plague man. Thus, we are led to the questions which are fundamental to this chapter: What are the specific and nonspecific mechanisms of host response to aberrant parasitism which produce disease? What are the assailants and how do they attack? Why are peaceful parasites, which normally can be held so easily in check, sometimes able to invade host tissue without hindrance?

B. Host Determinants of the Pathobiology of Parasitism

It is axiomatic that host-parasite pathobiology will depend upon both the microorganism and the host. At the present stage in the evolution of the infectious diseases, except for cases of extremely aberrant parasitism, the state of the host is of greater importance in determining the reaction than the parasite itself. The local and systemic host determinants of disease, therefore, will be discussed first.

1. Local interactions

a. Inflammatory injury

Although inflammation is described extensively in Chapter 3, certain aspects merit repetition because of their fundamental importance in infectious disease.

Indeed, the inflammatory process is undoubtedly the most basic of the pathobiologic host-parasite reactions. It involves the primary mechanisms by which the anti-parasitic properties of the host, particularly the phagocytic cells, are mobilized at the site of parasite invasion in an attempt to erect a defense barrier, sequester, and then destroy the parasite. Although an effective defense mechanism, inflammation is a host-parasite reaction which may harm the host as well as the parasite, thus producing disease.

The types of inflammation which follow parasitic invasion are nonspecific responses to parasites, which are adapted either to an extracellular or intracellular existence within host tissues. *Extracellular parasites* primarily evoke an acute inflammatory response in which the neutrophilic phagocyte is the predominating cell. Through the sequence of altered microcirculation, transudation of serum factors, and active transmigration of neutrophils toward the invader, the parasite encounters this first line of defense (Spector and Willoughby, 1963). The neutrophil attempts to phagocytose and then to destroy intracellularly the invading microorganism. These ingestion and killing phases are controlled by separate metabolic and biochemical events. Intracellular bactericidal activity also probably involves at least two mechanisms: the production of hydrogen peroxide via the hexose monophosphate shunt (Klebanoff, 1967) and the release of bactericidal substances from lysosomes into the phagocytic vacuole (Zeya and Spitznagel, 1963).

Other mechanisms participate in the acute inflammatory reaction to parasites. These include interactions of: (1) specific antibody with parasite antigen which

Table 4-1a Microorganisms Adapted to Extracellular Parasitism of Man

GRAM-POSITIVE BACTERIA	GRAM-NEGATIVE BACTERIA
Streptococcus	Meningococcus*
Staphylococcus	Gonococcus*
Pneumococcus	Hemophilus
Clostridia	Enteric bacilli
Diphtheria	Bordetella
Anthrax	Pasteurella
	Bacteroides
	Shigella
	Cholera vibrio

* May also be facultative intracellular parasites.

prepares the invader for ingestion by neutrophils (opsonization), (2) components of complement, together with specific antibody, which may lyse Gram-negative bacteria, (3) substances such as lysozyme and beta lysin which may destroy some microorganisms extracellularly (Myrvik and Leake, 1960).

Most extracellular parasites to which the host responds with acute inflammation are bacteria. Those which man commonly encounters are listed in Table 4-1a.

It is not surprising that acute inflammation results in cell injury and cell death that is harmful to the host as well as to the parasite. Constituents of the

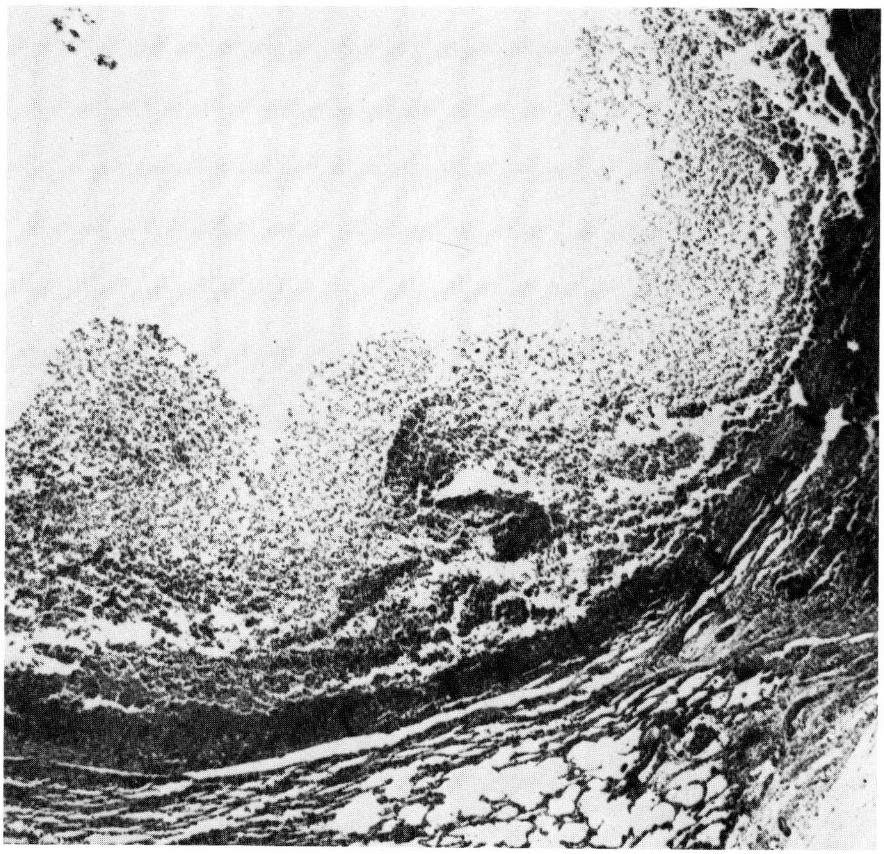

Figure 4-1. Microscopic view of an abscess in the skin due to infection with the extracellular parasite Staph. aureus. The subcutaneous tissue seen at bottom right is replaced elsewhere by pus, a mixture of dead and dying neutrophils and products of tissue digestion. Some of this pus has fallen out of the section, leaving an empty space.

cytoplasm of cells participating in the inflammatory process are released into the environment. Included are vasoactive polypeptides such as bradykinin, and vasoactive amines such as histamine and 5-hydroxytryptamine (Wilhelm *et al.,* 1965). In addition, a sequence of steps following the activation of the complement system results in elaboration of anaphylatoxin which increases capillary permeability and causes constriction of smooth muscle (Nelson, 1965). Enzymes which are capable of causing tissue necrosis and which are ordinarily held in an inactive state within the granules (lysosomes) of neutrophils, may be released into the immediate environment (Weissmann, 1965). These enzymes display powerful proteolytic, lipolytic, and collagenolytic properties which may operate in the immediate vicinity of inflammation.

The host-parasite interaction following invasion by pyogenic bacteria such as *Staphylococcus aureus* is typical of acute inflammatory injury caused by extracellular parasites. An example of this type of infection, which is characterized by abscess formation (liquefaction necrosis containing the cellular and tissue debris of inflammation), is given in Figure 4-1.

Another type of local tissue inflammation is characterized by the host's attempt to sequester and completely destroy a parasite which is partially or totally adapted to an intracellular existence. These *intracellular parasites,* which include certain bacteria (*Mycobacterium tuberculosis,* Brucellae, *Listeria monocytogenes,* and Salmonellae), most fungi, protozoa, and all viruses (Table 4-1b), will be

Table 4-1b Microorganisms Adapted to Intracellular Parasitism of Man

FACULTATIVE INTRACELLULAR PARASITES		
BACTERIA	FUNGI	PROTOZOA
Mycobacteria	Histoplasma	Pneumocystis
Brucella	Blastomyces	Toxoplasma
Salmonella	Coccidiomyces	Leishmania
Listeria	Cryptococcus	Trypanosoma
Streptobacillus	Candida	
	Nocardia	
OBLIGATE INTRACELLULAR PARASITES		
VIRUSES	RICKETTSIAE	PROTOZOA
All	All	Plasmodia (malaria)

discussed in greater detail later. The reaction to these parasites is somewhat delayed compared with the response of the acute inflammatory process, which may at times precede it, and it is characterized by the predominance of lymphocytes, monocytes, and fibrocytes, rather than neutrophils.

The sequence of events which brings the activated lymphocytes and mononuclear phagocytes to the intracellular parasite is similar to the dynamics of acute inflammation. It includes changes in microcirculation, chemotaxis, transmigration, phagocytosis, and intracellular killing. The pathologic lesion which develops, particularly if the phagocyte is unable to destroy all of the invaders quickly, is fre-

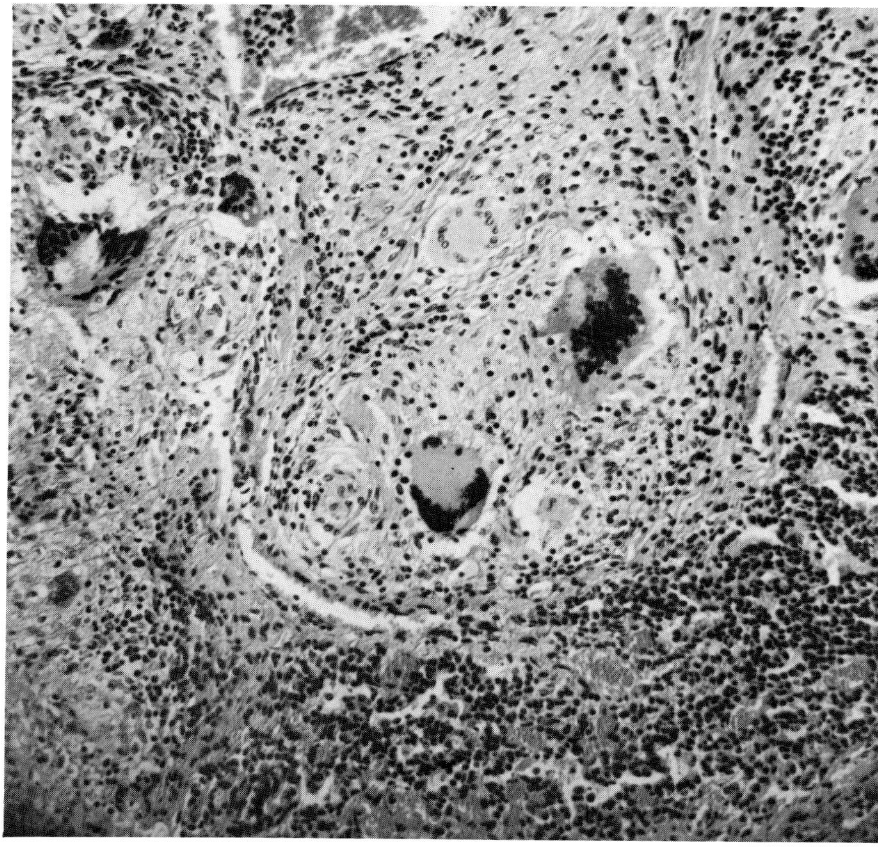

Figure 4-2. Granulomatous inflammation in the lung, caused by reaction to the facultative intracellular parasite, M. tuberculosis. A bronchiole is seen at right, but most of the tissue is replaced by epithelioid cells, giant cells, and lymphocytes. For a higher power view, see also Figure 3-12.

quently characterized by the formation of granulomata (Fig. 4-2). As in acute inflammation, the defense process becomes an expression of disease.

In some granulomatous inflammation, particularly that due to tuberculosis, necrosis develops within the center of the granuloma. Secondary enzymatic injury from the lysosome constituents of monocytes and lymphocytes may be responsible.

The cellular picture of the delayed inflammatory reaction may at times be equated with delayed hypersensitivity. Thus one may also categorize delayed inflammation as a form of immunologic injury.

b. Allergic injury

The mechanisms of immunologic (allergic) injury are described in detail in Chapter 5. The expression of allergic injury, at least in part, involves elements of the types of inflammation just discussed, but these hypersensitivity reactions should be considered separately, for in parasitism they are secondary rather than primary responses. Presensitization, usually with the formation of antibody, is a prerequisite.

Since parasites, either alive or dead, are fertile sources of antigen, one might expect the antigen-antibody interaction, which is based upon the specific antigenic nature of the parasite, to be frequent. At times, this interaction activates a train of cellular and biochemical events in which tissues are injured. Our knowledge in this area is incomplete, but it is probable that all major categories of parasites, which include bacteria, fungi, viruses, protozoa, and metazoa, are at times agents of allergic injury.

Following invasion of *Mycobacterium tuberculosis,* the development of delayed hypersensitivity, which in itself is probably an immune response, also becomes a pathologic process. Similar injury may be associated with deep fungal infections such as histoplasmosis, blastomycosis, cryptococcosis, and coccidiomycosis. The tissue damage in postviral encephalitides and polyneuropathies may also involve the delayed hypersensitivity process (Epstein, 1967).

Allergy may play a role in the symptomatology of measles. Whether the rash, which develops about the time antibodies are detectable in the serum, is due to a direct viral effect on epithelium and vascular endothelium or to an immune reaction is not clear. Support for the latter theory is found in the fact that when children acquire fatal giant-cell pneumonia, they do not form neutralizing antibodies and do not develop a rash. Infection with certain rickettsiae is also characterized by a rash. In the case of epidemic typhus, after an incubation period, fever develops and persists until the infection resolves. Between the fourth and seventh day of the disease process, a characteristic rash appears. Since rickettsiae are demonstrable in this lesion, one might assume that it results from a direct toxicity of the localized rickettsiae. It is of interest, however, that the rash occurs about five to seven days after the onset of the fever. Together with the accumulation of cells of the lymphoid series, this observation suggests that an immune reaction may also participate in the pathogenesis of this rash.

The sequelae of Group A streptococcal infections resulting in the syndromes of acute rheumatic fever, acute glomerulonephritis, and vascular (Schönlein-Henoch) purpura have long been a part of the annals of medicine (Cluff and Johnson, 1965). Although the mechanisms underlying these syndromes have not been established with certainty, antigen-antibody reactions are probably operative. The M-protein antigens (see below) of the streptococci have been strongly suspected as possible agents. One possible explanation for tissue damage in these syndromes is that specific antibodies cross-react with antigens of streptococci and similar antigens of target tissue (Kaplan, 1964). The pathobiologic reactions also suggest similarities between these syndromes and experimental serum sickness, in which soluble antigen-antibody complexes are deposited in target tissue, causing damage by an Arthus-like reaction (Dixon *et al.,* 1961).

c. Hyperplasia

Local parasitic invasion frequently results in hyperplasia of neighboring lymphoid tissue, a manifestation of disease. This reaction may extend throughout the entire reticuloendothelial system and causes enlargement of the liver and spleen. The stimulus to such hyperplastic reaction within lymphoid and reticuloendothelial tissue has not been adequately delineated, but it probably involves the recognition and processing of parasite antigens which in turn directly or indirectly stimulate the cells which participate in antibody formation and other immune processes. Virtually all parasites are capable of eliciting such a hyperplastic response. The extracellular parasites more frequently cause local reactions, whereas the intracellular parasites cause hyperplasia, both locally and systemically.

d. Neoplasia

The oncogenic potential of viral host-parasite interaction is described in Chapter 6. The alterations by viruses of the basic replicating mechanisms of human cells immediately suggest that they might have oncogenic potential. Indeed, viruses have been clearly implicated as the cause of animal neoplasia; examples are the polyoma virus of mice and the SV_{40} virus of monkeys. Moreover, human viruses such as adenoviruses have caused neoplasia in animals.

As yet the evidence that viruses cause human neoplasia is at best circumstantial. The possibility that a herpes-like virus causes Burkitt's lymphoma, a neoplasm endemic in Africa, is explored in Chapter 6.

The problems of paramount importance in the theory of the viral etiology of neoplasia are the elucidation of the mechanisms of transformation of supposedly normal cells into neoplastic cells and the determination of the fate of the viral genome in neoplastically transformed cells. A general concept of transformation by polyoma and SV_{40} DNA tumor-producing viruses is that their viral DNA enters the infected cell and activates cellular activities to produce one or more proteins required for the transformation (Eckart, 1969). Viral genetic material becomes a part of the heredity of the transformed host cells, and as transformed cells develop, neoplastic potential emerges.

2. Systemic reactions

It hardly needs to be mentioned that systemic reactions occur in infectious disease as well as local injury at the site of the parasite invasion. These are the cardinal symptoms and signs of advanced host-parasite interaction: malaise, headache, alterations in pulse rate, shock, fever, negative nitrogen balance, electrolyte imbalance, elevated serum glucose, and leukocyte responses. As in the case of local reactions, these phenomena are frequently called non-specific, although such a classification may reflect our ignorance of the specific mechanisms responsible. Indeed, there is much to be learned concerning the mechanisms by which local invasion of parasites precipitates a chain of events leading to systemic symptoms and sometimes to death.

a. Metabolic and hormonal reactions

Host-parasite interaction elicits many metabolic and biochemical events which may be responsible for certain generalized symptoms of infection, for they are qualitatively similar, relatively stereotyped, and apparently not specifically related to the etiology of the infection. For the most part these reactions are systemic, although it is obvious that infections involving particular organ systems, such as hepatitis, myocarditis, and pneumonitis, would cause local metabolic changes and impairment of organ function secondary to tissue invasion.

Protein catabolism with a negative nitrogen balance is a prominent systemic reaction in infection and probably is a result of fever and decreased dietary intake (Beisel *et al.,* 1967). This persistent catabolism during chronic infections such as tuberculosis probably causes the wasting state which characterizes these diseases. In contrast, selective anabolism also occurs during host-parasite interaction as increased synthesis of interferon, alpha globulins, specific enzymes, and antibody proteins indicates. During certain experimental bacterial and viral infections, there is increased synthesis of ribonucleic acid, perhaps reflecting a need to produce proteins utilized in host defense mechanisms.

Through increased aldosterone output, there is renal retention of salt, with secondary depression of serum sodium and chloride during infection. Increased elaboration of the adrenocortical hormones and/or growth hormone during infection may be responsible for the glucose intolerance which sometimes occurs during severe host-parasite interaction. This may be followed by depletions in tissue carbohydrates and a terminal hypoglycemia.

It is likely that specific systemic metabolic events may be associated with specific parasitic infections. One such mechanism has recently been elucidated. During Gram-negative but not Gram-positive bacterial infections, there is an elevation of plasma-free fatty acids, triglyceride, and phospholipid (Gallin *et al.,* 1969). An increase in pre-beta lipoprotein appears to be responsible for this elevation. As a consequence there may be increases in gluconeogenesis, conversion of glucose to lactate, suppression of glycolysis, and activation of clotting processes.

b. Cardiovascular reactions

During severe host-parasite pathobiologic processes, altered cardiovascular reactivity is frequently seen (Weil *et al.,* 1964). The peripheral vascular resistance decreases, the pulse becomes rapid, and the cardiac output increases. Although the blood pressure falls, this generalized reaction, sometimes referred to as *warm shock* because of the peripheral vasodilatation, is usually reversible. At times, however, an irreversible shock-like state (*cool shock*) appears, which in contrast is characterized by a decrease in cardiac output and an increase in peripheral vascular resistance. Occurring distant from the site of host-parasite interaction, these changes still defy simple explanation. It has been postulated that the vasoactive substances released at the site of host-parasite reactions are responsible. It has also been postulated that specific parasite toxins, acting directly on the heart and blood vessels, or mediated through the central nervous system, precipitate these drastic systemic reactions. Recent evidence links disseminated intravascular coagulation with shock caused by infection (Corrigan *et al.,* 1968). Since most fatalities in host-parasite disease are the result of cardio-vascular collapse, the need for a specific explanation is apparent.

c. Fever

Recognition of the elevation of body temperature in most forms of parasitic disease dates back to ancient history. Indeed, this is perhaps the most common and best known manifestation of infectious disease. Yet it is only recently that the pathogenesis of fever has been somewhat clarified. Most evidence suggest that parasites induce fever primarily by stimulating certain cells (usually neutrophils and monocytes) to elaborate a substance which acts on the thermoregulatory centers of the brain (Atkins and Snell, 1965). This *endogenous pyrogen* has not been purified but is probably a lipoprotein. The process of phagocytosis is in many situations associated with and perhaps responsible for the release of endogenous pyrogen, after which there is a latent period before the host increases body temperature by vasoconstriction and increased muscular activity. This chill phase is later followed by vasodilatation and diaphoresis in an attempt by the host to return body temperature to its closely held norm.

The release of endogenous pyrogen is not specific to host-parasite interaction, for allergic fevers are probably generated in a similar fashion. (Furthermore, neither a beneficial nor deleterious effect of fever has been established.) A

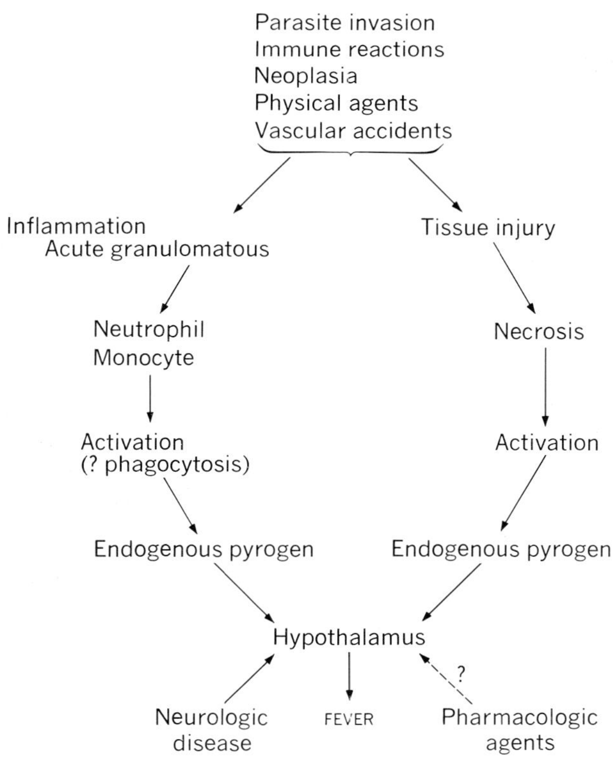

Figure 4-3. Pathways in the pathogenesis of fever.

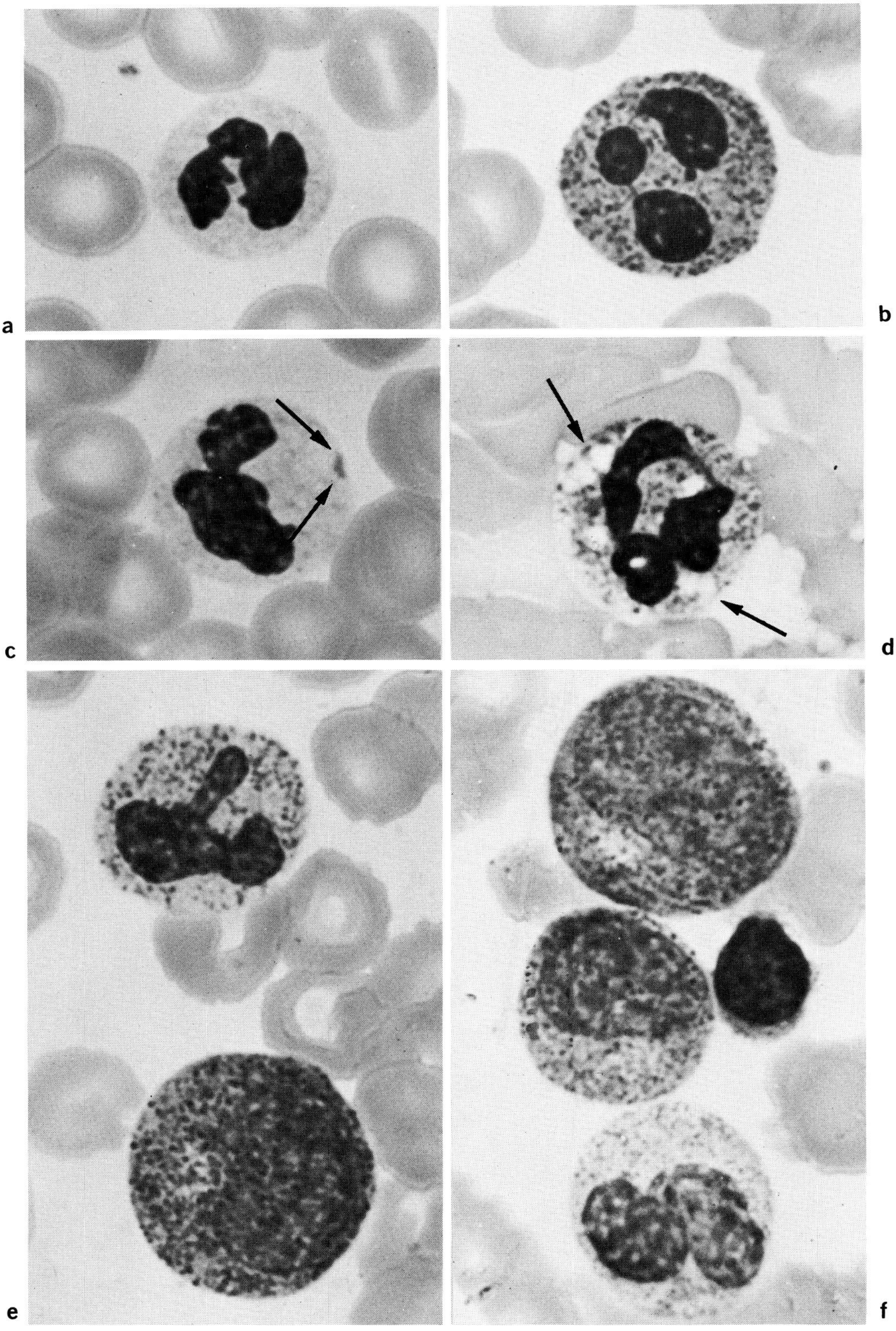
a
b
c
d
e
f

schematic diagram of known and hypothetical mechanisms of the pathogenesis of fever is given in Figure 4-3.

d. Hematologic reactions

Another classic, generalized response to host-parasite interaction is the alteration in the quantity and quality of blood neutrophils which occurs during serious bacterial infection. Although nonspecific to many types of bacterial host-parasite infection, these changes in blood neutrophils occur infrequently in viral, protozoan, and fungal infections. Perhaps the determinant to this response is extracellular parasitism in which the primary inflammatory cell is the neutrophil. It has been suggested that certain leukotactic factors are elaborated at the local inflammatory site and that these substances then act as a stimulus to the production and release of neutrophils from the bone marrow (Menkin, 1956). Teleologically, the reason for an increase in total neutrophils is clear—a need for more phagocytes.

The increase in quantity of neutrophils is also accompanied by an increase in the proportion of immature cells and by specific changes within cell cytoplasm. When observed with a Romanowsky stain, these cytoplasmic changes appear as heavily stained granules called *toxic* granules, vacuoles, and inclusions of rough endoplasmic reticulum called *Dohle bodies* (McCall *et al.,* 1969) (Fig. 4-4). The morphology of these toxic neutrophils reflects alterations in the constituents and activity of lysosomes and in cytoplasmic autophagy. The neutrophils so affected are dysfunctional, having decreased migratory, chemotactic, phagocytic, and bactericidal activities (McCall and Caves, 1970). Collectively, the pathobiology of toxic neutrophilia may reflect cellular immaturity, a reaction to cellular injury, or a stimulus of infection. The phenomenon probably is not specific to bacterial infection, for such changes have been described in other severe inflammatory states.

Hematological changes also occur in intracellular parasitism. As in the case of the neutrophil response, the cells involved are those participating in the specific defense reaction. For example, in tuberculosis there may be an increase in

Figure 4-4. Stained blood films from human blood and bone marrow:
a. Normal blood neutrophil.
b. Blood neutrophil with toxic granulation.
c. Dohle body (arrows).
d. Vacuoles (arrows) in a toxic neutrophil.
e. Toxic granulation in a mature blood leukocyte and metamyelocyte.
f. Toxic neutrophils and precursors in bone marrow. (Courtesy of McCall, Katayama, Cotran, and Finland, 1969)

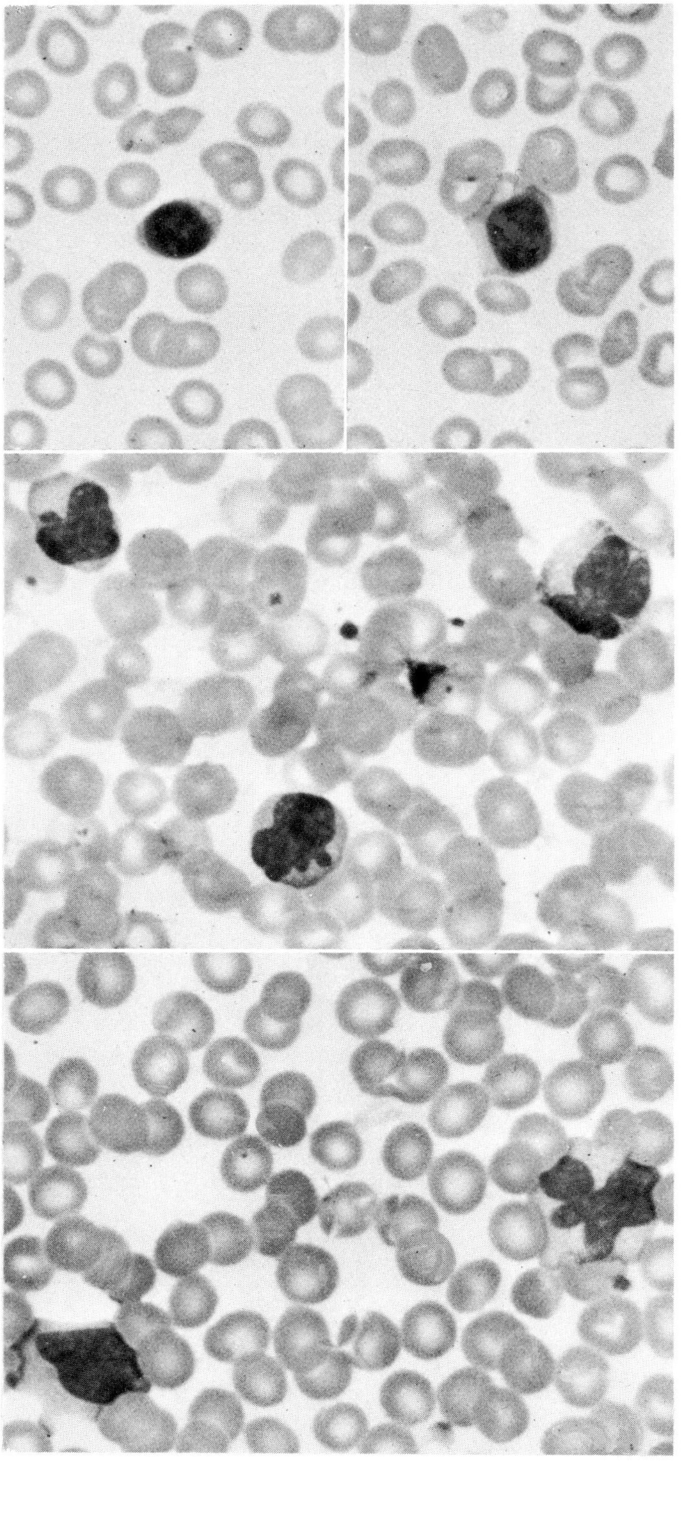

a b c d

the number of circulating monocytes, the cytoplasm of these cells may become vacuolated, and there is an increase in the quantity of certain of their lysosomal enzymes. In infectious mononucleosis, presumably a viral disease, the cytopathologic reactions of the circulating lymphocytes are highly characteristic. These *atypical lymphocytes* are morphologically and metabolically distinct from lymphocytes of uninfected hosts, reflecting an increase in the synthesis of lysosomal enzymes, rough endoplasmic reticulum, and RNA (Wood and Frenkel, 1967) (Fig. 4-5).

Other blood constituents may be altered during host-parasite interaction. An anemia due to decreased red cell production and/or increased red cell destruction is common. There may be destruction or decreased production of blood platelets. At times there is a disorder in the clotting mechanism in which many of the essential clotting factors are consumed (McKay, 1965). The ensuing disseminated intravascular coagulation, which results in both thrombosis and bleeding, has been implicated as a cause of shock and death in a number of severe infections both by extracellular and intracellular parasites. The initiating factors in this injury are unclear, but immunologic interaction of host and parasite may precede the event. The generalized Shwartzman reaction in animals, which is a response to the endotoxin of certain bacteria, has been equated with the same process in humans.

C. Parasite Determinants of the Pathobiology of Parasitism

1. Concepts and definitions

The emphasis in the preceding discussion upon the host's response in aberrant parasitism was not meant to imply that the parasite is a neutral element. Indeed, the popularity of Robert Koch's germ theory of disease, which emphasizes the parasite, has continued to foster extensive research into the specific mechanisms whereby parasites cause disease. Three concepts which permit biologists to understand better the offensive capacity of the parasite have evolved. To satisfy the need for food, self-preservation, and replication, the parasite must: (1) have a natural habitat (reservoir), (2) be able to move to a new reservoir or suscep-

Figure 4-5. Stained blood films from human blood.

a. Normal small lymphocyte.

b. Normal large lymphocyte.

c,d. Atypical lymphocytes from patients with infectious mononucleosis.

tible host by means of spread, and (3) be able to penetrate host tissue and thereafter either subsist or be excreted. Since this discussion is primarily concerned with direct host-parasite interaction, the third category will be stressed.

The pathogenic potential of a parasite, however, cannot be separated from the first two concepts of reservoir and spread to a susceptible host which are epidemiologic features of parasitism. If man is an unnatural host, for example, contracting the disease depends upon his proximity to a natural reservoir and to a vehicle which can transmit the parasite to the susceptible tissues in his body. In Rocky Mountain Spotted Fever, which is caused by a rickettsia, the prevalence of disease in man depends upon the prevalence of parasites in the natural reservoir (e.g. wild animals), the availability and prevalence of carriage within the vector (e.g. tick), and the exposure of the susceptible host to these epidemiologic determinants.

In concert, the forces underlying transmission from a reservoir through a vehicle of spread to a new host constitute *communicability*. Communicability does not mean that after transfer to a new host, the parasite is necessarily capable of eliciting a pathologic interaction. The capacity to cause disease is a separate property called *pathogenicity*. The variability in pathogenicity among strains within a group of parasites reflects individual *virulence*.

The most pathogenic parasites usually cause disease in an unnatural host. In a natural host the pathobiologic reaction depends upon a change in the dynamics of commensalism, which renders the parasite a potential pathogen. The ensuing host-parasite interaction is called *opportunistic infection*. These infections by parasites within natural hosts are of paramount importance, and they will be discussed in greater detail later.

2. Extracellular parasitism

a. Invasive properties

The interactions of pathogenic parasites may be conveniently divided into two categories: those that occur extracellularly and those that occur intracellularly. The extracellular parasites include most pathogenic bacteria (Table 4-1a).

Pathogenic bacteria arrive at the site of host-parasite interaction either by primary penetration, by secondary inoculation from vectors (insects, etc.) or accidental breaks in environmental barriers (skin, mucous membranes, etc.). Unfortunately, the characteristics of primary tissue penetration by pathogenic bacteria have almost completely eluded the researcher. It has been clearly shown, for example, that salmonellae can invade epithelium of the small intestines of man and make their way into the lamina propria where they then elicit the inflammatory response. How they are able to do this is an enigma, but it must reflect an offensive property of the parasite.

Once in an appropriate environment for multiplication, bacteria produce disease by two mechanisms (Davis *et al.*, 1968): invasion of tissue and elaboration of toxins.

The capability of invading tissue usually reflects the pathogen's defensive mechanisms against the host's own defenses. A common defense in bacteria is the formation of a thick capsule of gummy material which effectively repels the phagocyte. This is advantageous for extracellular parasites, most of which are unable to maintain life once they have been ingested.

Capsules are heterogeneous in composition. For example, the capsule of the pneumonococcus is a complex of a high-molecular-weight polymer of glucose and glucuronic acid, while that of the anthrax bacillus contains a polypeptide of glutamic acid. That these capsules are indeed virulence factors is clearly exemplified in the case of pneumococcal infections. The smooth, fully encapsulated strains cause disease, whereas the unencapsulated, rough strains do not (MacLeod and Krauss, 1950). Moreover, specific host antibody against the capsule reduces or abolishes the virulence of the bacteria. In human disease the heavily encapsulated Type 3 pneumococcus is more virulent than the less encapsulated types of pneumococcus. Likewise, the capsule size of *Klebsiella pneumoniae* varies, and strains with thicker capsules are more virulent than those with thin capsules.

Little is known of the molecular mechanisms by which capsules inhibit phagocytosis. One hypothesis has been that the hydrophobic lipid components of neutrophil membranes are prevented from making intimate contact with the hydrophilic capsular gel. Another is that there are repelling electrical forces between capsule and neutrophil.

Not all antiphagocytic substances in microorganisms are capsules. For example, the streptococcus has a virulent antiphagocytic protein which resides in the cell wall. This is called M-protein and is both antiphagocytic and antigenic.

Some bacteria elaborate extracellular enzymes that would appear to directly facilitate invasion and spread in host tissue. Many Gram-positive bacteria produce hyaluronidase which promote diffusion by depolymerization of hyaluronic acid in the tissue ground substance. Staphylococci elaborate coagulases which clot plasma by converting fibrinogen to fibrin. Both streptococci and staphylococci elaborate kinases that catalyze plasminogen to plasmin, which then lyses fibrin. In contrast with the enzymes mentioned above, about whose *in vivo* potential we still speculate, there is some clinical evidence that collagenases facilitate

Table 4-2 Invasive Factors That Influence Pathogenicity of Some Bacterial Parasites of Man

INVASIVE FACTOR	SOURCE	ACTIVITY
Capsules	*Diplococcus pneumoniae* *Hemophilus influenzae* *Klebsiella pneumoniae* *Bacillus anthracis* *Staphylococcus aureus* *Pasturella pestis*	Antiphagocytic
M-protein at cell surface	Streptococci-Group A	Antiphagocytic
Extracellular enzymes*		
hyaluronidases	Streptococci-Group A	Lysis of tissue ground substance
coagulases	*Staphylococcus aureus*	Clots fibrin
kinases	Staphylococci, Streptococci	Lysis of fibrin
collagenase	*Clostridium perfringens*	Lysis of collagen

* The role of extracellular enzymes in the pathogenesis of human infections is uncertain.

the invasion of the Clostridia bacilli which cause gas gangrene. Invasive factors that influence the pathogenicity of some bacteria parasites of man are listed in Table 4-2.

b. Exotoxins

A small but significant group of bacterial pathogens cause pathologic host-parasite interaction by elaborating exotoxins (van Heyningen, 1955). Although one might define bacterial enzymes which act locally as *toxins,* the term is usually confined to substances which act at a distance from the site of invasion. The toxin production may depend upon penetration, invasion, and replication, but it is independent of bacterial autolysis. Bacteria producing exotoxins which cause human disease are listed in Table 4-3. The diseases include diphtheria, tetanus, gas gangrene, botulism, food poisoning, whooping cough, cholera, and scarlet fever.

Exotoxins, which are heat-labile proteins, include the most powerful poison known. One ounce of diphtheria toxin, for example, could kill every inhabitant of New York City. Diphtheria toxin inhibits protein synthesis and thus damages

Table 4-3 Endotoxins That Determine Pathogenicity of Some Bacterial Parasites of Man

DISEASE	SOURCE OF EXOTOXIN	ACTIVITY
Diphtheria	*Corynebacterium diphtheriae*	Inhibits protein synthesis; inhibits oxidative processes
Botulism	*Clostridium botulinum*	Anticholinergic
Tetanus	*Clostridium tetani*	Anticholinergic; ? blocks inhibitory synapses
Gas gangrene	*Clostridium perfringens*	Cytolytic
Staphylococcal food poisoning	*Staphylococcus aureus*	? Stimulates brain or peripheral nerves to produce vomiting
Scarlet fever	Streptococci, Group A	Cytotoxic to blood vessels
Whooping cough	*Bordetella pertussis*	Necrotizing to bronchial epithelium; produces lymphocytosis
Cholera	*Vibrio cholera*	Alters water and electrolyte balance in intestine

many types of cells. A strange phenomenon in the production of diphtheria toxin is that a bacteriophage, which is in itself a viral parasite of the bacteria, determines the synthesis of toxin.

The virulent alpha toxin of *Clostridium perfringens* is a lecithinase, which splits lecithin into diglyceride and phosphorylcholine. Since lecithin is probably important in maintaining the structure of cell membranes, its removal results in collapse of the membrane and lysis of the cell.

The exotoxins responsible for botulism and tetanus are neurotropic. Botulism toxin affects production and/or release of acetylcholine at the preganglionic and postganglionic synapses in the autonomic nervous system, in addition to affecting cholinergic mechanisms in peripheral nerves. In contrast, tetanus toxin appears to act within the central nervous system, probably causing spasm by blocking inhibitory motor neurons.

Staphylococci may produce an enterotoxin which acts on the central nervous system or peripheral nerves to produce severe vomiting. Some streptococci produce an erythrogenic toxin which causes injury of small blood vessels to produce the scarlet fever syndrome. The exotoxin produced by *Bordetella pertussis,* the cause of whooping cough, is necrotizing to the bronchial epithelium and is responsible for the unusual lymphocytosis associated with the disease. The cholera toxin alters fluid and electrolyte balance in the gastrointestinal tract.

c. Endotoxins

In contrast to exotoxins, which are produced primarily by Gram-positive bacteria, most Gram-negative bacteria contain a complex macromolecular phospholipid and polysaccharide moiety within their cell wall which is toxic. In contrast with exotoxins, these endotoxins are released only after bacterial lysis, and the reactions with the host are less potent and less specific than those of exotoxins. Indeed, the role of endotoxins in human host-parasite pathobiology has not been established with certainty. Nevertheless, their implication in human disease has long been suspected and the literature is replete with studies of endotoxins (Westphal *et al.,* 1961).

The biologic effects of bacterial endotoxins are numerous, but we will mention only the two which are most likely to be associated with pathobiology in man. First is the production of fever due to either primary hypothalamic activity or secondary elaboration of endogenous pyrogen, perhaps through the phagocytosis of the macromolecules of endotoxin or from its effect at the cell-tissue interphase. Second, in experiments, endotoxins produce a shock syndrome; the cause of this syndrome is not yet clear. Investigators debate whether the cardiovascular collapse results from direct effects of the toxic lipid moiety on the peripheral vascular system, or whether it is secondary to a generalized Shwartzman reaction in which vasoactive substances are released from cells and the clotting mechanism is activated. The shock and massive bilateral adrenal necrosis which sometimes occur in meningococcal sepsis have been attributed to the Shwartzman-like effects of endotoxin.

3. Intracellular parasitism

In contrast to extracellular parasites which cannot live within cells, certain parasites are adapted to intracellular existence. Within this group are *facultative* intracellular parasites, which can live and replicate either inside or outside cells, and *obligate* intracellular parasites, which can live only inside cells because they require certain cellular events for subsistence and replication (Table 4-1b). Examples of facultative intracellular parasites include the bacilli causing human tuberculosis, salmonellosis, and brucellosis, and many of the pathogenic fungi. The obligate intracellular parasites include all rickettsiae, all viruses, and some protozoa. How these microorganisms are able to maintain intracellular existence is a fundamental question regarding intracellular parasitism.

a. Facultative intracellular parasites

The facultative intracellular parasites are perhaps more puzzling than the obligate. Virulent tubercule bacilli are able to live within cells while avirulent tubercule bacilli cannot. The virulent bacilli may either neutralize the destructive forces within the cell or repress the mechanisms which activate them. Both Brucella and *Mycobacterium tuberculosis* have been subclassified on the basis of catalase production. The virulent strains which multiply freely within host cells produce considerably more catalase than those which are avirulent and cannot multiply intracellularly. The role of catalase is uncertain, but since the peroxides of host cells are probably important in the intracellular bactericidal reaction, the bacterial catalase may control the amount of hydrogen peroxide produced. Whatever the mechanisms, the ability to resist rapid intracellular destruction is a property of all facultative intracellular parasites, which perhaps by this resistance then cause the tissue inflammation characterized by formation of granulomata. Support for this theory can be seen in chronic granulomatous disease of children. In this unusual disease, the neutrophils and the monocytes can ingest but can not intracellularly destroy certain bacteria (Quie *et al.,* 1967). The host-parasite tissue reaction in this disease is characterized by the formation of granulomata. Instead of acute inflammation with abscess formation, granulomatous inflammation follows infections with extracellular parasites such as staphylococci, which because of a defect in host defense have become adapted to intracellular existence.

b. Obligate intracellular parasites

The obligate intracellular parasites require either a host substrate or a host metabolic activity or both, for subsistence and replication (Moulder, 1962). An example of the use of host-cell substrate by an obligate intracellular parasite can be seen in malaria, caused by the protozoan, *Plasmodium vivax.* When within a red cell, malarial sporozoites are capable of completing all the intermediate pathways in carbohydrate, nucleic acid, and lipid metabolism of free living microorganisms. Outside the host cell, the sporozoite is apparently unable to synthesize co-enzymes which are necessary to many metabolic reactions in the organisms. The intracellular environment of the host cells provides these important enzymes for the parasite. Another interesting observation is that the malarial parasites have developed a unique manner of obtaining amino acids for protein synthesis. The plasmodium phagocytoses a portion of the red cell's cytoplasm, secretes hydrolytic enzymes into the vacuole, and absorbs from the vacuole the amino acids provided through the digestion of hemoglobin. The iron pigment remains in the vacuole until the red cell ruptures.

Rickettsiae cannot metabolize glucose or glucose-6-phosphate, apparently because they lack a complete set of glycolytic enzymes. Therefore, instead of using glucose as a primary substrate, rickettsiae utilize glutamate, most likely by oxidative deamination to oxaloacetate. The oxaloacetate then enters the Krebs cycle. Apparently the electrons derived from glutamate oxidation can be carried to oxygen thus providing the energy source for rickettsiae through oxidative phosphorylation. Another weakness of rickettsiae is the instability of their membranes and their transport mechanism. When rickettsiae are removed from host cells, their membranes lose essential substances such as adenosine diphosphate and triphosphate. Thus, rickettsiae seem to depend on the host cell for structural as well as metabolic integrity.

Viruses are the most intriguing of the obligate intracellular parasites. One may still wonder what they represent within the order of biology. Composed of a block of genetic material without metabolic machinery and surrounded by a protective protein envelope (capsid) which serves as a vehicle of transmission, does a virion qualify as a living organism? Indeed, the composition of the envelope may at times contain specific components of the host cell and therefore might be considered a part of the host. Regardless of the position we espouse, we must accept that viruses are probably the most common parasites of man. More than forty different disease syndromes result from the interactions of viruses with their hosts. These reactions are so varied and so many of them depend upon poorly defined mechanisms, that our discussion must be confined to generalizations and examples.

Viruses contain either RNA or DNA which carries into the host cell new genetic information. When functioning, this viral genetic material leads to synthesis of new virus within the nucleus or cytoplasm of the host cell. This cycle of virus synthesis can be divided into a series of steps (Buddingh, 1965). After the virus particle has established contact with the host cell (attachment), the nucleic acid (RNA or DNA) reaches a replicating site (penetration) (see Fig. 2-29). The nucleic acid then "instructs" replication of itself and the protein units which constitute its envelope. These basic units are assembled into virus particles (maturation) and the mature viruses may then be freed from the host cell (release) to repeat the cycle. If the viruses are released it is a *productive infection,* and if they do not complete the cycle of reproduction and release, it is an *abortive infection.*

Not all of these steps necessarily follow a chronological sequence. For example, some viruses may remain latent for a period during which the viral molecules and cellular molecules are in intimate interplay. The individuality of both virus and host cells can be considered as lost, the infected cell constituting a new unit called *virus cell complex.* Activated by various exogenous stimuli, the *latent infection* may complete the viral replication cycle months or years after the original penetration. A classic example of latency in man is herpes simplex infection of the lip. The lesion which we call the fever blister disappears, only to recur at irregular intervals under the conditions (fever, stress, ambient heat) which activate the virus to complete a productive cycle.

If virus replication slowly produces abnormalities in the host over the course of months or years, the term *slow virus infection* is used (Gajdusek, 1967). Such reactions are often localized in a single organ. Kuru, a unique disease confined to New Guinea, is characterized by central nervous system symptomatology which progresses inexorably to death; it is likely to be a slow virus infection. This unusual host-parasite interaction has suggested that slow viruses might cause diseases that have hitherto been considered fundamentally genetic, immunologic, neoplastic, or metabolic disorders.

The cell injury in virus-host interactions usually occurs in the infected tissues and organs. A common by-product of the productive viral infection is a cytotoxic effect upon the infected cell, in which vacuolization, ballooning degeneration, syncytium formation, hypertrophy, and hyperplasia may appear. The products of injured tissue may then evoke an acute inflammatory reaction secondarily. The cytopathic changes in specific organ systems may alter the function of cells in the infected tissue. For example, the agent of infectious hepatitis, presumably a virus, may destroy the host through hepatic failure. This alteration of the host cells' basic function is perhaps the major disease-producing mechanism in viral parasitism. The role of viruses in allergic injury and neoplastic transformation is discussed in other chapters.

4. Organotropism

Many parasites not only select a specific host but may select the tissue which they invade. For example, both meningococci and pneumococci frequently reside in the human nasopharynx; yet of the two only pneumococci consistently invade the lower respiratory tract to cause pneumonia. Whereas the meningococci usually infect the upper respiratory tract of man before they invade the meninges, the closely related species which causes gonorrhea invades the genitourinary tract. This phenomenon of tissue preference is called *organotropism* and is seen with all types of parasites. Examples of this phenomenon in common bacterial, viral, and rickettsial pathogens are listed in Table 4-4.

When *Bordetella pertussis,* the agent of whooping cough, is introduced in chick embryos, the microorganisms, in addition to producing a local lesion on the membrane, frequently invade the embryo and eventually localize on the cili-

Table 4-4 Parasites Which Display Specific Organotropism in Host-Parasite Interactions

PARASITE	ORGANOTROPISM
Bacteria	
Meningococcus	meninges
Pneumococcus	lower respiratory tract
Gonococcus	genitourinary tract
Mycobacteria	lower respiratory tract
Cholera bacillus	gastrointestinal tract
Salmonella and Shigella	gastrointestinal tract
Mycoplasma	
Mycoplasma pneumoniae	lower respiratory tract
Rickettsiae	blood vessels
Metazoa	
Trichinella	muscle
Filaria	blood vessels and lymphatics
Protozoa	
Malarial protozoa	red blood cells
Trypanosomes	blood vessels and brain
Viruses	
Enteroviruses	GI tract, central nervous system
(polio, coxsackie, ECHO)	respiratory tract
Reoviruses, rhinoviruses,	skin
adenoviruses, myxovirus	central nervous system,
(influenza)	liver (yellow fever)
Myxovirus (measles)	skin, nervous system
Arboviruses	skin
	central nervous system
Herpes viruses	liver
Poxviruses	salivary glands
Rabies virus	
Hepatitis viruses	
Mumps	

ated epithelium of the bronchial mucosa. If they are injected into the amniotic cavity, the same localization results. When, on the other hand, inoculation occurs before ciliated cells have appeared, infection of the bronchial epithelium fails to occur. These findings are in keeping with the pathobiology of whooping cough in humans. Similarly, *Neisseria meningitidis,* which causes bacterial meningitis in man, localizes in the meningeal tissues of embryos.

The obligate intracellular parasites also have tissue preferences. Of the examples listed in Table 4-4, the neurotropic viruses have received the greatest attention. Dissemination to the nervous system may occur by transmission along the axial structure of peripheral nerves as well as through the blood (viremia). The centripetal transmission of herpes simplex virus in mice can be followed by making serial sections of nerves. The virus may diffuse within the axon or multiply in endoneural cells. In the case of herpes simplex, there is organotropism of both skin and nervous system. Similarly, some Echo viruses and Coxsackie viruses prefer both respiratory and nervous tissue. Although infections in two tissue sites may reflect dissemination by viremia, this is perhaps not always the case. The nature of tissue preference remains an enigma.

D. Opportunistic Host-Parasite Interactions (Table 4-5)

While great progress in medical therapy has resulted from research on host-parasite pathobiology and while we no longer face with frequency most of the grave, infectious diseases of history, a new challenge has evolved. The forces underlying the equilibrium of uneventful parasitism have been so altered that interactions have developed which favor an aberrant course. These are called *opportunistic* infections, and in the prosperous countries most are caused by invasion of endogenous parasites.

Two primary changes underly opportunistic, aberrant host-parasite interactions which lead to infection by endogenous parasites: altered microbial ecology and compromised host defense.

As previously discussed, man's microbial ecology is composed of indigenous microbiota which develop soon after birth (Rosebury, 1962). These parasites are accepted as natural inhabitants, residing at the interphase between tissue and external environment. Included are many bacteria and fungi, and at times protozoa, metazoa, and viruses. If the number of one of these parasites becomes great enough, the state of commensalism is transformed into pathogenicity. When such an opportunity arrives, one cannot rightly say that the acquired pathogenicity resides only in specific offensive properties of the parasite. A better explana-

Table 4-5 Indigenous Microbiota Which Produce Disease by Opportunistic Host-Parasite Interactions

SKIN	UPPER RESPIRATORY TRACT	LOWER INTESTINE	GENITOURINARY TRACT (VAGINA AND ANTERIOR URETHRA)
Coagulase-negative staphylococci	Coagulase-negative staphylococci	Coagulase-negative staphylococci	Coagulase-negative staphylococci
Coagulase-positive staphylococci	Coagulase-positive staphylococci	Coagulase-positive staphylococci	Coagulase-positive staphylococci
Candida species	Group A Streptococci*	Anaerobic streptococci	Anaerobic streptococci
	Microaerophilic streptococci	Enterococci	Candida species
	Meningococci*	*Clostridium perfringens*	
	Corynebacteria	*Escherichia coli*	
	Hemophilus influenzae	Klebsiella-Enterobacter-Serratia Group	
	Bacteroides	Proteus species	
	Actinomyces	*Pseudomonas aeruginosa*	
	Candida species	Bacteroides	
		Candida species	

* Intermittent carrier states

tion is that an unnatural interaction occurs between a natural parasite and a natural host.

Opportunistic host-parasite interactions became increasingly evident following the introduction of antibiotics. Optimists had prematurely looked upon this group of drugs as a panacea which would rid man of all pathogens, if not all parasites. The medical profession did not readily appreciate that along with suppression of the pathogen the antibiotics induced suppression of many members of the normal indigenous flora. The more resistant organisms thereafter could multiply to the extent that their sheer quantity and the lack of interference by other microorganisms apparently made them pathogenic. The result has been a rising incidence of many Gram-negative infections (coliform, Klebsiella, Proteus, Pseudomonas) and some Gram-positive infections (staphylococcal, enteric, streptococcal) (Finland *et al.,* 1959), usually occurring in the hospitalized patient. At present, the new microbial ecology, consisting of both the altered flora of hospital environs and the altered flora within patients, serves as a constant source of endogenous opportunistic infection.

Compromises in host defense have been as forceful as alterations in indigenous flora in causing endogenous infections. A number of factors associated with depression of host-defense mechanisms can be listed: increased age of the host; frequent use of medical instruments which act as foreign bodies in host tissues (urinary catheters, intravenous catheters, heart valves, etc.); prevalence of chronic disease states such as diabetes, alcoholism, chronic bronchitis, congestive heart failure, cirrhosis of the liver, and neoplasia; and use of immunosuppressive drugs such as adrenocorticosteroids, antimetabolites, and alkylating agents. The mechanisms responsible for the suppression of normal host defense in these states still confuse the investigator. It is clear, however, that drugs such as adrenocorticosteroids, antimetabolites, and alkylating agents do suppress immunity, perhaps by compromising a number of immunologic reactions including acute and delayed inflammation, antibody synthesis, and phagocyte production and function (Schwartz, 1969).

Other examples of opportunistic interactions somewhat different from those listed above can be cited. An infection involving the influenza virus in the lung also predisposes the host tissue to infection by bacteria. In this instance of supra-infection it appears that the influenza virus specifically blocks the metabolism of glucose at the phosphohexose-isomerase level (Fisher and Ginsburg, 1956). Since phagocytosis depends upon glycolysis, the inhibition of the metabolic event depresses this mechanism of host defense.

Another opportunistic infection occurs when certain bacteria acquire a symbiotic pathogenicity. For example, staphylococci and streptococci may together cause a necrotizing skin infection which cannot be produced by either organism alone. Similarly, certain members of the mouth flora (streptococci, bacteroides, fusiforms) may in concert cause a necrotizing, anaerobic infection within the lung or pleural cavity, an effect which cannot be produced by any one of the organisms.

Although in contemporary usage the term *opportunistic infection* usually refers to endogenous infections, it would be unfair to history and disrespectful of the future not to mention the role of opportunism in exogenous infections. The most vigorous and lethal host-parasite reactions occur between an exogenous pathogen and a population of hosts that has neither the acquired nor genetic gift of self-defense against the parasite. History is replete with examples. After the Spanish conquest, the Indians were ravaged by smallpox. Microbial diseases became rampant among South Sea islanders soon after Captain Cook arrived. Albert Schweitzer recorded that when African trypanosomiasis, also known as sleeping sickness, moved from Loango where it was endemic, to Uganda where it was unknown, one village lost most of its inhabitants.

References

Atkins, E., and Snell, E. S. (1965), Fever, *in* The Inflammatory Process, p. 495, B. Zweifach, L. Grant, and R. T. McClusky, Eds., Academic Press, New York.

Beisel, W. R., Sawyer, W. D., Ryll, E. D., and Crozier, D. (1967), Metabolic effects of intracellular infections in man, Ann. Int. Med., *67*:744.

Buddingh, G. J. (1965), Pathogenesis and pathology of viral infections, *in* Viral and Rickettsial Infections of Man, p. 339, F. L. Horsfall and I. Tamm, Eds., J. P. Lippincott Co., Philadelphia.

Burnet, F. (1966), Natural History of Infectious Disease, 3d Ed. Cambridge University Press, New York.

Cluff, L. E., and Johnson, J. E. (1965), Post-streptococcal disease, *in* Immunologic Diseases, p. 418, M. Samter, Ed., Little, Brown and Co., Boston.

Corrigan, J. J., Jr., Ray, W. L., and May, N. (1968), Changes in the blood coagulation system associated with septicemia, New Eng. J. Med., *279*:851.

Davis, B. D., Dulbecco, R., Eisen, H. N., Ginsburg, H. S., and Wood, W. B., Eds. (1968), Pathogenic properties of bacteria, *in* Principles of Microbiology and Immunology, p. 574, Harper and Row, New York.

Dixon, F. J., Feldman, J. D., and Vazquez, J. J. (1961), Experimental glomerulonephritis. The pathogenesis of a laboratory model resembling the spectrum of human glomerulonephritis, J. Exp. Med., *113*:899.

Eckart, W. (1969), Cell transformation by polyoma and S.V.^{40}, Nature, *224*:1065.

Epstein, W. L. (1967), Granulomatous hypersensitivity, Prog. in Allergy, *11*:36.

Finland, M., Jones, W. F., Jr., and Barnes, M. W. (1959), Occurrence of serious bacterial infections since introduction of antibacterial agents, J. Am. Med. Assoc., *170*:2188.

Fisher, T. N., and Ginsburg, H. S. (1956), The reaction of viruses in guinea pig polymorphonuclear leukocytes, Virology, *2*:618, 637, 656.

Gajdusek, D. C. (1967), Slow-virus infections of the nervous system, New Eng. J. Med., *276*:392.

Gallin, J., Kaye, D., and O'Leary, W. M. (1969), Serum lipids in infection, New Eng. J. Med., *281*:1081.

Kaplan, M. H. (1964), Immunologic cross-reaction between Group A streptococcal cells and mammalian tissues–possible relationship to the induction of autoimmunity in rheumatic fever, *in* The Streptococcus, Rheumatic Fever, and Glomerulonephritis, p. 169, J. W. Uhr, Ed., Williams and Wilkins Co., Baltimore.

Klebanoff, S. J. (1967), Iodination of bacteria: a bactericidal mechanism, J. Exp. Med., *126*:1063.

MacLeod, C. M., and Krauss, M. R. (1950), Relation of virulence of pneumococcal strains for mice to the quantity of capsular polysaccharide formed *in vitro,* J. Exp. Med., *92*:1.

McCall, C. E., and Caves, J. (1970), Dysfunction of human neutrophils during severe bacterial infection. Clinical Research, *18*:49.

McCall, C. E., Katayama, I., Cotran, R. S., and Finland, M. (1969), Lysosomal and ultrastructural changes in human toxic neutrophils during bacterial infection, J. Exp. Med., *129*:267.

McKay, D. G. (1965), Disseminated Intravascular Coagulation: An Intermediary Mechanism of Disease, Paul B. Hoeber, Inc., New York.

Menkin, V. (1956), Biochemical Mechanisms, *in* Inflammation, Thomas Pub., Springfield, Illinois.

Moulder, J. W. (1962), The Biochemistry of Intracellular Parasitism, University of Chicago Press, Chicago.

Myrvik, Q. N., and Leake, E. S. (1960), Studies on antibacterial factors in mammalian tissues and fluids. IV. Demonstration of two nondialyzable components in the serum bactericidal system for *Bacillus subtilis,* J. Immunol., *84*:247.

Nelson, R. A. (1965), The role of complement in immune phenomena, *in* The Inflammatory Process, p. 819, B. W. Zweifach, L. Grant, and R. T. McClusky, Eds., Academic Press, New York.

Quie, P. G., White, J. G., Holmes, B., and Good, R. A. (1967), *In vitro* bactericidal capacity of human polymorphonuclear leukocytes: diminished activity in chronic granulomatous disease of childhood, J. Clin. Invest., *46*:668.

Rosebury, T. (1962), Microorganisms Indigenous to Man, McGraw-Hill, New York.

Schwartz, R. S. (1969), Immunosuppression: challenge of selectivity, Hospital Practice (February), p. 42.

Smith, T. (1934), Parasitism and Disease, Princeton University Press, Princeton, New Jersey. Reprinted 1963, Hafner Publishing Co., New York.

Spector, W. G., and Willoughby, D. A. (1963), The inflammatory response, Bact. Rev., *27*:117.

van Heyningen, W. E. (1955), The role of toxins in pathology. Society of General Microbiology, Symposium No. 5, Cambridge University Press, p. 17.

Weil, M. H., Shubin, H., and Biddle, M. (1964), Shock caused by Gram-negative organisms. Analysis of 169 cases, Ann. of Int. Med., *60*:384.

Weissmann, G. (1965), Lysosomes, New Eng. J. Med., *273*:1084.

Westphal, O., Luderitz, O., and Staub, A. M. (1961), Bacterial endotoxins, J. Med. Pharm. Chem., *4*:497.

Wilhelm, D. L., Spector, W. G., and Willoughby, D. A. (1965), Chemical mediators *in* The Inflammatory Process, p. 389, B. W. Zweifach, L. Grant, and R. T. McClusky, Eds., Academic Press, New York.

Wood, T. A., and Frenkel, C. P. (1967), The atypical lymphocyte, Am. J. Med., *42*:923.

Zeya, H. I., and Spitznagel, J. K. (1963), Antibacterial and enzymic basic proteins from leukocyte lysosomes: separation and identification, Science, *142*:1085.

5

IMMUNOLOGIC INJURY

Mariano F. La Via, M.D.

A. The Immune Response

1. Introduction

Administration of antigen to an animal usually leads to the formation of antibody, which is characterized by the capacity to combine specifically with the antigen eliciting its production. This immune response, as we understand it today, is restricted to the vertebrate species and is typical of the integrated cellular responses of higher organisms to external stimuli.

The most obvious function of the immune response is in resistance to infectious disease. Antibodies produced against bacterial capsules facilitate phagocytosis and destruction of many organisms, combine with and neutralize bacterial toxins, and combine with viral protein to prevent entry of viruses into cells (Abramoff and La Via, 1970).

The immune response plays an opposite role in the pathogenesis of disease. *Immunological diseases* encompass a number of reactions injurious to the host. In some of these the antigen is external, while in others the host becomes sensitized to his own tissues or to cross-reacting antigens, and *auto-immune* diseases with widespread pathologic manifestations may result (Medawar, 1957; Shaffer *et al.*, 1959; Gell and Benacerraf, 1961; and Mackay and Burnet, 1965).

This chapter will deal primarily with this second aspect of immune responses. First, however, it will be useful to review briefly the process of immunological responsiveness and some of the damaging consequences of its faulty development.

2. Phylogeny and ontogeny of the immune response

The development of immunological competence parallels the differentiation of the lymphoreticular system; antibody production is a function of this system. Defense mechanisms in invertebrates depend upon phagocytosis, and only in the lower marine vertebrates is a rudimentary adaptive immunity found. The well-defined, adaptive immune response with development of serum immunoglobulins starts in the elasmobranchs (Smith *et al.*, 1966).

Paralleling the phylogenesis of immune responses, no antibody is produced during fetal life until thymic and lymph node lymphocytes are present (Smith *et al.*, 1967). At birth, human infants have a gamma globulin level which is usually at least equal to that of the mother. This immunoglobulin, in fact, is almost entirely maternal antibody which has been transferred to the fetus *in utero* (Koch *et al.*, 1959). For a period of from three to ten weeks after birth, the gamma globulin level declines and then levels off, subsequently rising until adult levels are reached at between one and four years of age. The decline after birth can be ascribed to failure of synthesis by the infant, natural decay of maternally derived protein and growth of the infant with increase in the blood volume. The ability to respond to antigenic stimulation thus develops during fetal life and is completed after birth.

There is considerable variation among different species in the degree of maturation of the immune response at birth. In fetal lambs, for example, an antibody response can be induced against some antigens as early as the sixty-sixth day of gestation (normal gestation period 150 days) (Silverstein *et al.*, 1963). On the other hand, chickens show a lack of response to antigenic stimulation until approximately four to five weeks after birth (Wolfe *et al.*, 1957). In man, although natural antibody synthesis does not normally occur until after birth, there is evidence that under appropriate artificial stimuli immunocompetence can be demonstrated as early as the fourth month of gestation (Koch *et al.*, 1959).

The studies on fetal lambs have suggested that the ability to respond to different antigens develops at different times during gestation. For instance, the capacity to reject homografts appears earlier than other immunologic phenomena, while the ability to exhibit a delayed hypersensitivity reaction develops later (Cannon *et al.*, 1958; Fowler *et al.*, 1960; and Schinckel and Ferguson, 1953).

As already mentioned, development of immunological responsiveness parallels the development of lymphoid organs. The thymus develops first in all species examined except the cat (Ackerman, 1967). Lymph nodes, spleen, bone marrow, and other lymphocytes appear subsequently, probably under the influence of the thymus.

3. Characteristics of the immune response

Specificity, memory, and *self-recognition* are three fundamental characteristics of immune responses.

Immunologic specificity is of a very high order. It is dependent on the recognition mechanism by which an antibody reacts with the antigenic configuration which is most complementary to its combining site. An antibody induced by an antigen *A*, however, will cross-react with a second antigen *B* if antigen *B* contains antigenic determinants very similar to those of antigen *A*.

Immunologic memory, still largely unexplained, accounts for two very important features of the immune response: (1) the more vigorous "anamnestic" reaction elicited by antigen when it is administered to an animal for the second time, even after apparent cessation of antibody synthesis in response to the first stimulation; and (2) the phenomenon of tolerance in which the initial treatment with antigen leads to a state of non-reactivity to subsequent stimulation with the same antigen. This can be considered "negative" memory (Abramoff and La Via, 1970).

Self-recognition is essential to the integrity of the animal. Antibodies are not normally made to one's own proteins although these may be highly antigenic in other individuals. This implies that a mechanism exists by which one is capable of discriminating at a very high level of recognition between one's own and very similar but foreign macromolecules (Medawar, 1957).

4. Antigens and antigenicity

Antigens are substances capable of inducing antibody production and of reacting specifically with the antibody. They may be proteins, polypeptides, polysaccharides, or nucleic acids. Although most antigens are complex macromolecules, a compound need not be extremely complex to be antigenic. Polypeptides composed of only two or three amino acids, and dextran composed only of glucose units are antigenic (Maurer *et al.,* 1963; Mage and Kabat, 1963).

Antigens are characterized by determinant groups, i.e. those parts of the modecule which react with antibody and thus impart specificity to the antigen.

Low-molecular-weight compounds may be antigenic if they are conjugated to a carrier (usually a protein). These compounds are called *haptens.* The hapten is the determinant group when it is coupled to a carrier and acts as the inducer of antibody specificity. Thus, it will be capable of subsequently reacting with antibody even when not coupled to the carrier (Landsteiner, 1936).

5. Antibodies

The term *antibodies* is applied to a family of serum proteins which have been well characterized structurally and functionally and which are important in a number of immunologic phenomena. These antibodies have been shown to migrate electrophoretically in the γ and slow β globulin regions and are also termed *immunoglobulins.* Five types of immunoglobulins are most commonly found: IgM or macroglobulin, IgG, IgA, IgD, and IgE. They are responsible for the neutralization of toxins, for bacterial agglutination, for cell lysis and for some allergic reactions. Their production is therefore primarily a defense mechanism (Edelman and Gall, 1969).

In delayed hypersensitivity, in homograft rejection, and in some autoimmune diseases, specific humoral antibody is either not present or can account only for some of the observed reactions. A striking phenomenon seen in these situations is the accumulation of lymphoid cells in large numbers at the reaction sites. When the accumulation of lymphocytes is prevented, these reactions are inhibited. Attempts to isolate an antibody which could be the mediator of injury in lymphoid cells of hypersensitive reactions have thus far yielded inconclusive results. It must be assumed for the moment that while the phenomena are undoubtedly immunological, the presence of lymphocytes is necessary for injury to occur and for passive transfer of immunity. In referring to lymphocyte-dependent immunological phenomena, however, the term *cell-bound (cellular) antibodies* is sometimes used for convenience (Turk, 1967).

6. Antibody synthesis

The production of antibody in response to antigenic stimulation is a complex response that can be divided into three major phases: (1) afferent, with "processing" of antigen and induction of the immune response; (2) central, with multiplication and differentiation of antibody-producing cells and synthesis of antibody; and (3) efferent, with interaction of antibody or effector cells with antigen.

The mechanism by which antigen can induce the production of specific antibody is still obscure. Antigens are carried to lymphoid organs and rapidly degraded, perhaps to expose antigenic determinants not on the surface of the intact molecules. Some stimulus then passes from the phagocytic cell to the antigen target cell. Active proliferation and differentiation of lymphoid cells ensues, and during this process antibody is synthesized and released into the circulation. In laboratory experiments, antibody can be detected at the cellular level beginning about a few hours to a few days after antigen injection, while the serum titer usually rises to a detectable level by the third day.

If an animal which has received a single immunizing dose of antigen is left to rest for a few weeks or months and is then injected with the same antigen, the response to this second injection is somewhat different from that seen after the first antigen administration. The lag period will be shorter, the rise of antibody titer more rapid and to higher levels, the titer will persist for a longer time, and antibody avidity will increase. This is called an anamnestic response to indicate that the cell "remembers" some event which has taken place in the past and is now capable of repeating the operation with greater speed. It seems logical that if information necessary for antibody synthesis is somehow encoded in a cell, after the first exposure this cell would be better able to respond the second time (Abramoff and La Via, 1970).

7. Antigen-antibody interactions

The hallmark of these interactions is their great specificity. An antibody reacts best with the antigen used to induce the production of the antibody; however, some antibody will cross-react with other antigens that have similar determinant groups. In general, cross-reactions are not as strong as homologous reactions. The specificity of antigen-antibody reactions is exquisite enough to allow use of antibodies as reagents to detect very small chemical differences between antigens (Landsteiner, 1936).

The reaction between antigen and antibody is reversible and can be visualized as a series of bimolecular reactions.

$$Ag + Ab \rightleftharpoons AgAb$$
$$Ag + AgAb \rightleftharpoons Ag_2Ab$$

The equilibrium of the reaction is usually in favor of complex formation. Physical-chemical studies have shown that covalent bonds are not formed when antigen and antibody combine. Instead the reaction probably involves hydrogen bonds, hydrostatic interactions, and van der Waals forces (Talmage and Cann, 1961). The initial reaction between antigen and antibody appears to occur rather quickly. However, secondary events, i.e. precipitation or cell lysis, may take hours to appear.

One class of antigen-antibody reaction which is of great importance in immunologic injury is that involving the fixation of complement (C′). The lysis of erythrocytes by hemolytic antibody is the best example of this process. This occurs according to the following scheme:

$$E + Ab \longrightarrow EA$$
$$EA + C' \longrightarrow E^*$$

EA is an erythrocyte which is now activated by the combination of antibody through the primary interaction of antibody and antigen. E* represents the lysed erythrocytes from which hemoglobin has escaped after the membrane has been damaged by the secondary reaction involving C′. Complement is a complex of nine proteins present in the serum, and the secondary reaction of EA + C′ is a complicated reaction of many stages which finally lead to the disruption of the erythrocytic membrane (Muller-Eberhard, 1968) (see Chapter 2).

B. Deficiencies of the Immune Response

Before considering the mechanisms by which injury can be mediated by immunological phenomena, it seems useful to consider briefly those diseases which appear as a result of a faulty development of immune responses. These are due primarily to the lack of the protective action of immunologic reactions. The development of immunologic responsiveness can be affected by genetic defects which lead to various deficiencies in the natural or acquired immune mechanisms.

There are, on the one hand, pure defects involving the phagocytic function, the immunoglobulin synthetic function, or the appearance of cellular immunity. On the other hand, there are mixed defects in which two or more of these mecha-

Table 5-1 Immunologic Deficiency Defects

1. Defects of the phagocytic system
   - Chronic granulomatous disease
   - Splenic insufficiency
2. Defects of immunoglobulin synthesis
   - Congenital hypogammaglobulinemia
   - Acquired hypogammaglobulinemia
3. Defects of cellular immunity
   - A. With slight immunoglobulin synthesis deficiency
     - Thymic dysplasia
     - Thymic aplasia
   - B. With severe immunoglobulin synthesis deficiency
     - Thymic alymphoplasia
     - Swiss agammaglobulinemia
     - Wiskott-Aldrich syndrome
     - Ataxia-telangiectasia

nisms may be deficient (Table 5-1). Some of these defects also involve deficiencies of complement components or of enzymes needed to activate them.

1. Defects of the phagocytic system

Chronic granulomatous disease is the first example of a defect of phagocytosis. This disease, seen in children, is characterized by microabscesses and granulomas containing plasma cells and macrophages. The polymorphonuclear leukocytes in patients with this disease will ingest bacteria or particulate matter normally, but after ingestion, killing and digestion does not occur. The normal lysosomal process of microbial digestion (see Chapter 2) is deficient in chronic granulomatous disease, apparently because an oxidase for reduced nicotinamide adenine dinucleotide (NADH) is lacking. In this disease the inborn error is thus manifested in normal degranulation of the polymorphonuclear leukocytes with no killing and digestion. This defect is a sex-linked recessive character appearing only in males, with the carrier female having somewhat decreased leukocytic activity.

Another syndrome which fits this category of diseases is splenic insufficiency, manifested as decreased resistance to infection. This is a poorly understood condition which depends on the absence of the spleen but is related to the age at which the spleen is removed and to the disease for which the spleen has been removed. In fact, in some children who have had splenectomy for rupture of the spleen or for hematologic disorders (like idiopathic thrombocytopenia), there is no splenic insufficiency; whereas in children who have had splenectomy for lipid storage diseases, splenic insufficiency results.

2. Defects of immunoglobulin synthesis

These are exemplified by congenital and acquired hypogammaglobulinemias. Congenital hypogammaglobulinemia is very clearly a sex-linked inherited disorder limited to boys and manifested in childhood by multiple infections resistant to therapy, particularly pneumonia, otitis media, sinusitis, and sepsis. There are no plasma cells in the bone marrow, lymph nodes, or any other organs, with a resulting lack of immunoglobulin synthesis manifested in very low IgG and in absent IgM and IgA. Lymphocytes are always present in normal number although lymph nodes may be hypoplastic; the thymus appears to be normal. Acquired hypogammaglobulinemia occurs in association with a variety of diseases, especially those associated with the lymphoreticular system.

3. Defects of cellular immunity

These are disorders of thymic function and lymphocytes, and fall into two classes: those which are purely defects of cellular immunity, with little or no immunoglobulin-synthesis deficiency, and those which have a concomitant immunoglobulin-synthesis deficiency.

The first group comprises thymic dysplasia and thymic aplasia. Patients with thymic dysplasia have either normal or slightly low levels of immunoglobulins. The number of circulating lymphocytes may be normal or low, but there is depletion of the lymphoid tissue. Plasma cells are present in normal quantity. The clinical course of this disease is characterized by a lack of delayed hypersensitivity responses. This is not inherited as a sex-linked recessive disease since both males and females are affected and since there are normal siblings where a male and a female in the same family have been affected. Thymic aplasia is a disorder resulting from lack of embryological development of the thymus and parathyroid glands. The symptoms are similar to those of thymic dysplasia but much more severe. There has been some success in treating this disease with fetal thymus grafts.

The combined defects of cellular immunity and immunoglobulin synthesis are represented primarily by thymic alymphoplasia and Swiss agammaglobulinemia. These diseases manifest as total immunological incompetence: no delayed hypersensitivity, no homograft rejection, and no humoral antibody formation. Although the diseases are similar, they have distinct manners of inheritance, thymic alymphoplasia as a sex-linked recessive defect and Swiss agammaglobulinemia as an autosomal recessive. Some have therefore considered the two diseases as one, with a mixed inheritance pattern. Children with these diseases fail to thrive and have chronic pulmonary infections, moniliasis, vaccinia following vaccination, and *pneumocystis carinii* pneumonia; they die very early. There is an absence of lymphocytes in the lymph nodes which are very small and have a poorly developed architecture. The thymus is small with no lymphocytes and no plasma cells can be demonstrated. Variants exist in which some plasma cells are present and little immunoglobulin is formed. An example of such a variant is Wiskott-Aldrich syndrome in which eczema, thrombocytopenia, and recurrent infection are common. The thymus is hypoplastic, there is depression of delayed hypersensitivity, and peripheral lymphocytes are sparse. IgM may be depressed while the IgA is increased. Ataxia telangiectasia, also a hereditary disease, is another example. The thymus shows lymphopenia; there is no delayed hypersensitivity present; IgA is very low, but IgG is present in secretions to replace IgA; and plasma IgG is essentially normal.

As is apparent from this brief description, understanding of immunologic deficiencies is still quite incomplete. As understanding of developmental immunology becomes more complete, the relation between the various steps which occur during immunological ontogenesis, and the pathologic entities which are seen when this ontogenesis is disturbed will be clarified (Janeway, 1968).

C. Immunologic Injury

Understanding of immunologic injury has progressed greatly in the last few years, thanks particularly to the establishment of experimental models which have clarified many phenomena of importance in the production of immunologic diseases. Nevertheless, because of the complexity of these syndromes which may depend on multiple mechanisms of injury, the pathogenesis of many of these diseases remains unclear.

For the sake of clarity, it seems convenient to present first what is known of the various mechanisms by which immune phenomena may cause pathologic manifestations and then discuss some of the complex diseases which are observed in clinical practice. This will by no means be an exhaustive treatise on immunopathology but will for the main part stress simple pathogenetic mechanisms with the understanding that at times more than one of these may participate to cause disease.

1. Differentiation between cell-mediated and serum-mediated hypersensitivities

Historically, hypersensitive responses to antigens were differentiated on the basis of time elapsed between administration of antigen and the appearance of the allergic response. Some of these reactions appeared in as little as thirty minutes to a few hours, while others took forty-eight hours or longer to become apparent. Thus, the names *immediate* and *delayed hypersensitivity* came into use. A more exact differentiation is now used, based on the mechanism by which the hypersensitivity is mediated. Immediate hypersensitivities, or for the purposes of this discussion, humoral hypersensitivities, are mediated by a serum immunoglobulin (primarily IgE in the case of anaphylaxis, and IgM or IgG in the case of Arthus reactions). If these globulins from a hypersensitive individual are injected into a normal individual, he will become temporarily hypersensitive to the specific agent to which the donor was sensitive (Prausnitz and Kustner, translated 1962). The delayed hypersensitivities, on the other hand, cannot be transferred by serum proteins, but can be transferred by lymphoid cells (Chase, 1946). Thus, delayed hypersensitivity appears to be mediated by a cell-bound or cell-associated "antibody." Obviously, the terms *humoral* and *cellular hypersensitivity* are derived from the method by which transfer can be achieved.

Hypersensitivities may also be differentiated histologically (Turk, 1967). In general, the inflammatory exudate in immediate reactions is composed of polymorphonuclear leukocytes (Fig. 5-1). In contrast, the delayed response is characterized by a perivascular infiltrate rich in mononuclear cells (lymphocytes) (Fig. 5-2). Perhaps these cell types reflect nothing more than the difference between chronic and acute inflammatory reactions.

Another major difference between delayed and immediate hypersensitivities is in the pharmacologic mediators which take part in the reaction. In many immediate reactions the antigen-antibody complex causes host cells to release histamine or other vasoactive substances which affect smooth muscle or the autonomic nervous system. In contrast, these agents have not been found to play a role in delayed hypersensitivity.

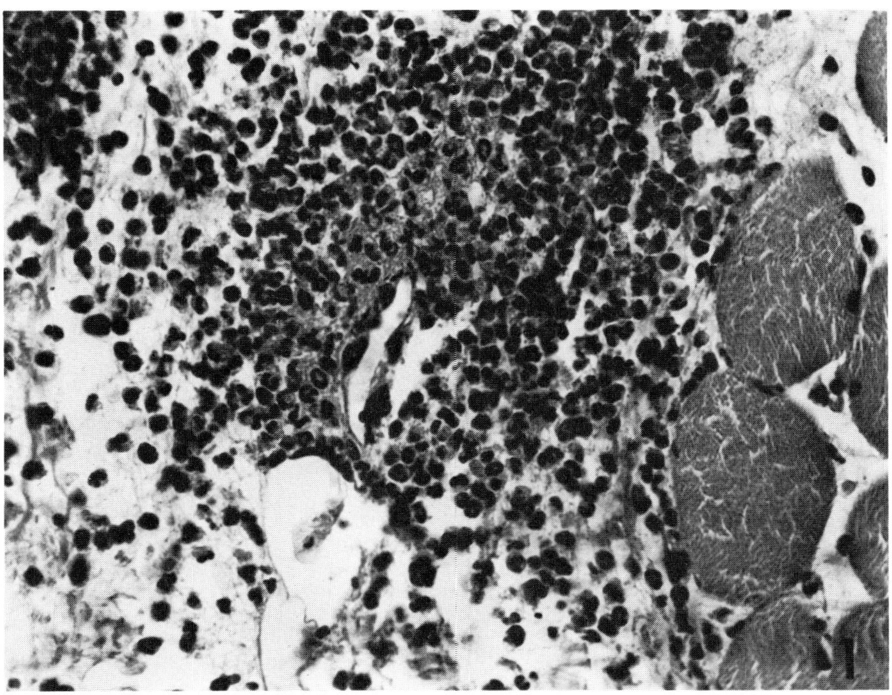

Figure 5-1. Characteristic infiltrate of immediate hypersensitivity consisting of polymorphonuclear leukocytes. (Courtesy of P. Ward)

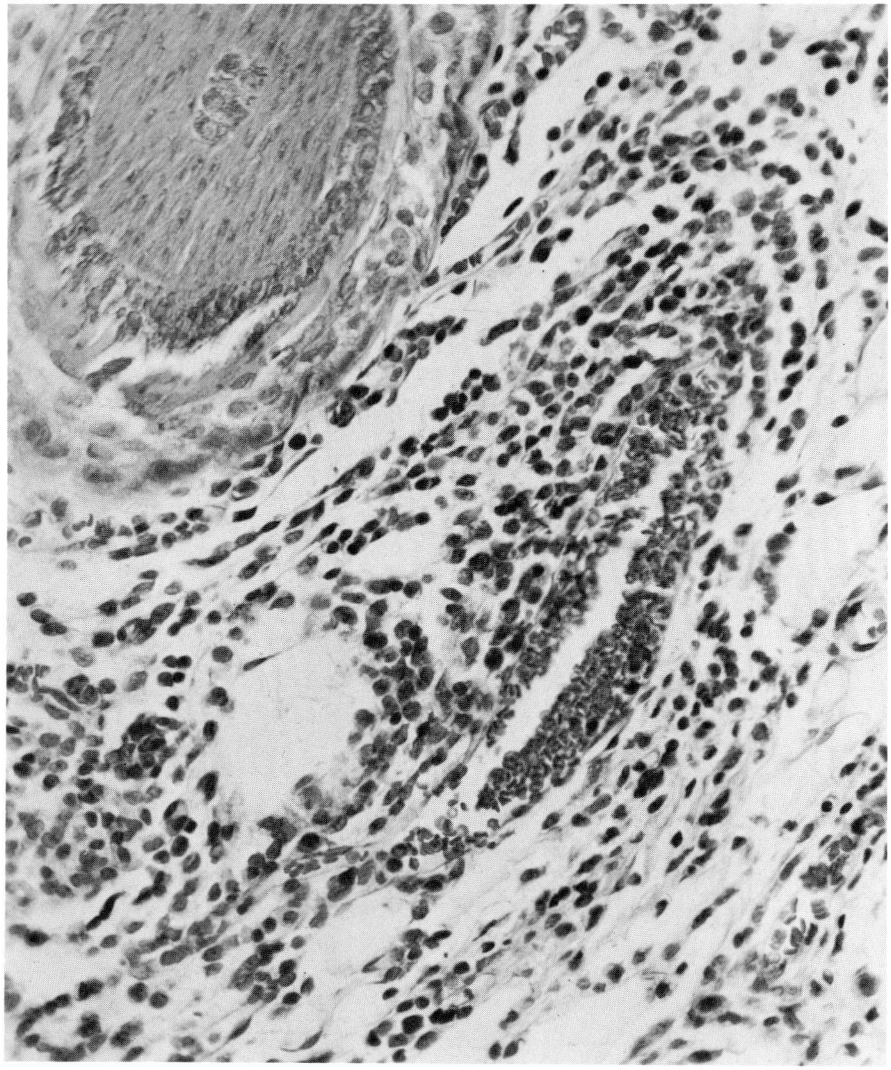

Figure 5-2. Perivascular infiltrate, containing primarily lymphocytes, typical of delayed hypersensitivity responses. (Courtesy of J. Feldman)

2. Classification of mechanisms of immunologic injury

There are four mechanisms by which immunologic injury is mediated. These have been the object of extensive research in the last ten to fifteen years.

On the basis of their characteristics these mechanisms can be divided into the two categories outlined above: humoral or serum-mediated injury in which the antibody is in one of the serum protein fractions; and cellular or cell-mediated injury in which no measurable antibody has been identified thus far, but in which responsibility for the injury can be assigned to cells of the small lymphocyte type (Table 5-2).

Table 5-2 Mechanisms of Immunological Injury

	CELL LYSIS	SERUM-MEDIATED HYPERSENSITIVITY (IMMEDIATE)		CELL-MEDIATED HYPERSENSITIVITY (DELAYED)
		ANAPHYLAXIS—ALLERGY	ARTHUS	
Predominant antibody involved.	IgG, IgM	IgE ($7S\gamma_1$ in guinea pig)	IgG	Cell bound
Predominant cell type involved.	0	Polymorphonuclear leukocyte (eosinophil)	Polymorphonuclear leukocyte	Small lymphocyte
Complement.	+	0	+	0
Mediators.	0	Histamine, serotonin, slow-reacting substance, kinins	Lysosomal enzymes	Not known
Principal type of injury.	Cell destruction	Smooth muscle contraction	Basement membrane damage	Cell destruction (chronic inflammation)

a. Direct injury by circulating antibodies—cell lysis

When an antibody directed against cell surface antigens, usually IgM or IgG, reacts with that antigen and complement, a series of enzymes is activated and the cell wall is punctured with release of intracellular contents (Humphrey and Dourmashkin, 1969).

Lysis of cells after reaction of a cellular antigenic determinant with antibody and complement may be protective in some cases and injurious in others. If the cell lysed is an invading microorganism or a neoplastic cell, lysis is obviously protective to the host. On the other hand, if the cell is the host's erythrocyte, this reaction clearly is harmful.

The mechanism of lysis of erythrocytes by antibody has been carefully studied. For lysis to occur, antibody and complement are necessary; if complement is not present the antibody will agglutinate but will not lyse the cells. The end result of the interaction of antigenic determinants, antibody, and the eleven components of complement is the appearance of small holes, about 80-100 Å in diameter in the cell membrane, which in turn lead to loss of intracellular contents. Red-cell lysis by antibody and complement occurs typically in the case of mismatched transfusions when transfused cells are lysed by the antibodies present in the plasma of the recipient.

b. Indirect injury due to circulating antibodies—immediate hypersensitivity

Certain individuals, on first exposure to an antigen, react by becoming "sensitized" instead of merely immune. When such an individual is exposed a second time to the same antigen, the hypersensitivity reaction between antigen and immunoglobulin leads to release of pharmacologic agents from disrupted basophils and mast cells. These agents cause increased vascular permeability and smooth muscle contraction. Since this occurs within a few minutes after antigen administration to the hypersensitive individual, it has been called an immediate hypersensitivity. When passively transferred, the antibody is capable of sensitizing the tissues of a previously unsensitized individual.

Histamine is the most important pharmacologic agent involved. The symptoms of many types of hypersensitivities can be mimicked by injection of histamine, and in the hypersensitive individual, a reaction can be ablated by antihistaminic drugs. When tissues taken from hypersensitive individuals are exposed to antigen *in vitro,* histamine is released. Recent studies have implicated other pharmacologic agents as well, however. These are: 1) "slow reacting substance," a material of unknown composition which can cause relatively slow contraction of smooth muscle; 2) bradykinin, a basic polypeptide which can cause contraction of smooth muscle, mediates increased vascular permeability, and is leukotaxic (see Chapter 3); and 3) serotonin (5-hydroxytryptamine) which causes broncho-constriction in the guinea pig, cat, and dog (Austen and Humphrey,

1963; Patterson, 1969). Some components of complement are also involved in these reactions.

In some cases of serum-mediated immediate hypersensitivity, the globulins involved ("reagins") are somewhat different from other immunoglobulins and belong to the IgE class. They are heat labile, can not be detected by conventional *in vitro* immunologic techniques, have an unusual affinity for skin and mucous membranes, and tend to become fixed to basophils and mast cells. The lack of a suitable tool for *in vitro* measurement of these antibodies has hampered research in immediate hypersensitivities. It has been suggested that they constitute an "abnormal" class, resulting from splitting of normal immunoglobulins in such a way as to produce a cell-fixing antibody (Ishizaka and Ishizaka, 1968).

The cellular events leading to cell damage by these immunoglobulins are not completely understood. The IgE becomes fixed to specific receptors on the mast-cell surface in a particular conformational state; antigen then appears to bridge two combining sites on two antibody molecules. Degranulation then occurs, with the release of histamine and other pharmacologically active substances, and the complex of symptoms results from the action of these substances. In addition, aggregates of antigen and antibody are sometimes seen obstructing the pulmonary alveolar capillaries.

Anaphylaxis is an important example of immediate hypersensitivity. This occurs when antigen is administered parenterally to a sensitized host; pharmacologic agents are liberated throughout the body with a variety of serious consequences. In the guinea pig, the smooth muscle of the bronchi and bronchioles is the primary shock organ; contraction of these muscles renders the animal unable to exhale and death is caused by suffocation. In the dog, the liver is primarily affected, with pooling of enormous quantities of circulating blood. In man, anaphylaxis is manifested by laryngeal edema, bronchospasm, and pulmonary edema, frequently leading to death.

The atopic hypersensitivities (commonly referred to as *allergies*), restricted almost entirely to man, are another important group of serum-mediated hypersensitivities, exemplified by hay fever. In this case, local administration of the antigen leads to local phenomena, such as edema of the mucosa of the nasal passages.

Not all individuals exposed to antigen develop hypersensitivity. On the other hand, most individuals who are allergic to one antigen are allergic to several antigens. Frequently several members of the same family are atopic. Thus, predisposition to atopic hypersensitivity is thought by some to be hereditary, but the evidence supporting this suggestion is circumstantial and no known genetic mechanism is compatible with the existing data.

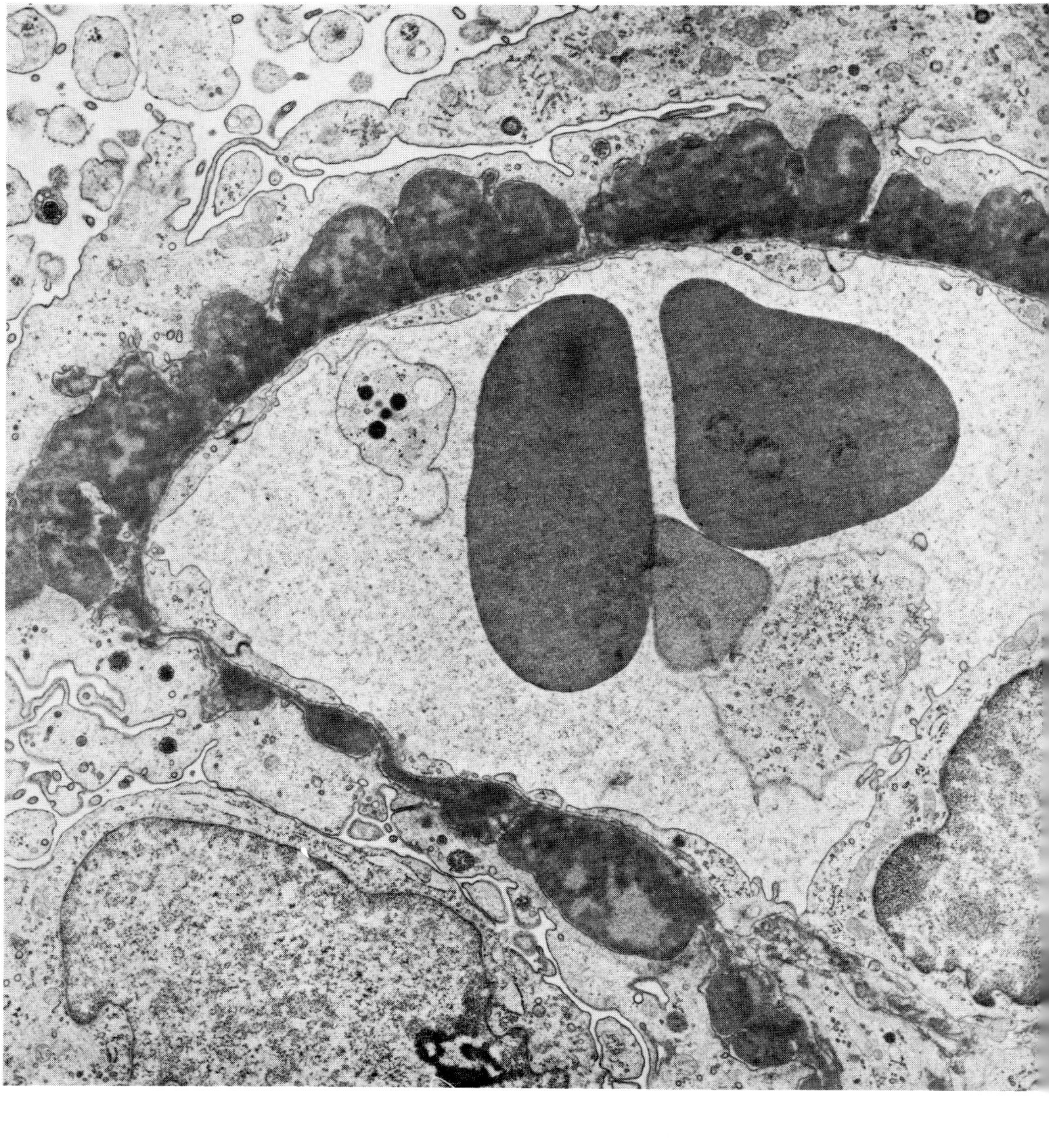

Atopic allergies are often treated by multiple injections of minute quantities of the offending allergen. Antigen administered in this fashion apparently induces a different type of antibody, known as *blocking* antibody, which competes with the reagins upon natural exposure to the allergen. If the titer of blocking antibody is high enough, all antigen will be absorbed, and release of the pharmacologic agents will not occur. This process is not as simple as it seems; circulating antibody titers, for instance, give no clue to an individual's responsiveness or lack of responsiveness to a given allergen (Peterson, 1968).

c. Immune complex formation—Arthus reaction

Antigens and antibodies, usually of the IgG type, may combine in sensitized individuals as antigen-antibody complexes which attach to vascular basement membranes, fix complement, and initiate an acute inflammatory reaction with necrosis (Cochrane, 1968).

The pathogenesis of injury due to immune complex formation is best exemplified by the Arthus phenomenon. Experimentally, the Arthus reaction is produced by injecting an antigen into the skin of an animal previously immunized to that antigen. Within thirty minutes to an hour the injected area becomes hemorrhagic, and if the reaction is severe, necrotic. This reaction is caused by the precipitation of antigen, antibody, and complement (the *immune complex*) in and around capillaries. The complement present in these precipitates acts as a chemotactic agent and attracts polymorphonuclear leukocytes, which are essential to the reaction. A classical, acute inflammatory reaction ensues, the area becomes edematous, and thrombi may form in the vessels; there is destruction of vascular walls and resulting hemorrhage and necrosis. The polymorphonuclear leukocytes contribute to the tissue destruction by releasing cathepsins.

By electron microscopic observation, precipitates of antigen and antibody can be found in the vascular lumen, in the wall of the small vessels between the basement membrane and the endothelium, and in the perivascular spaces (Fig. 5-3). Thus, the Arthus reaction is essentially an acute inflammatory reaction related to deposition of immune complexes and release of enzymes from polymorphonuclear leukocytes.

The mechanism of injury described for the Arthus reaction is not only a laboratory finding but is present in human diseases in the form of serum sickness. This may be encountered in man after therapy involving administration of immune serum from another animal species and is characterized by precipitation of

Figure 5-3. Section of a loop of glomerular capillary showing the heavy deposition of electron opaque material on the basement membrane; this material can be shown to contain antigen and antibody. (Courtesy of J. Feldman)

antigen-antibody complement complexes. The reaction may occur immediately after treatment if the patient was previously sensitive to the antigen, or it may be delayed for a week or more until the patient begins to produce antibodies; enough antigen may persist to form antigen-antibody complexes.

Although serum sickness is not a homogeneous entity, many of the symptoms caused by this mechanism are similar to those seen in the Arthus reaction. Patients with serum sickness develop inflammation associated with immune complex deposits in various organs (joints, lymph node, and kidney). This condition can be reproduced experimentally by injecting foreign protein intravenously into an immune animal. Soluble antigen-antibody complexes circulate in the bloodstream, bind complement, and are deposited in vascular lumina. Ultrastructural studies of the kidneys of rabbits during this time have demonstrated proliferation and swelling of the glomerular endothelium often occluding the lumen.

d. Cell-bound antibodies—delayed hypersensitivity

Administration of certain antigens will lead to a series of cellular reactions resulting in the production of specifically reactive lymphocytes. These in turn will produce injury by means of a yet unknown mechanism which may in part depend on a cell-bound, non-circulating "antibody," when these lymphocytes accumulate at the site of the reaction. The term *delayed hypersensitivity* has been used to identify this type of reaction, since it usually takes several days for it to become apparent (Turk, 1967).

As indicated earlier, delayed hypersensitivity is not dependent on humoral antibodies. It is believed to be an immunological phenomenon because of the following characteristics which are recognized as earmarks of immunological processes: an interval of several days is required between the immunizing injection and the appearance of a positive reaction to the test injection; the reaction is specific for the immunizing antigen; the reaction is mediated by cells of the lymphoid series. The most important consideration, however, for classifying delayed hypersensitivity as an immunological process is that it exhibits an essential characteristic of immune reactions: immunologic memory.

The prototype of delayed hypersensitivity is the tuberculin reaction, a reaction to the proteins of the tubercle bacillus. If one has been sufficiently exposed to *Mycobacterium tuberculosis* and is given an intradermal injection of tuberculin (an extract of the bacterium), the injection site becomes erythematous, indurated, and sometimes necrotic after about twenty-four hours. Histologically, the reaction site is infiltrated first with a small number of polymorphonuclear leukocytes, and later with lymphocytes and histiocytes. The hallmark of this reaction is perivascular accumulation of these mononuclear cells (See Fig. 5-2). The formation of these "granulomas" is typical of many delayed hypersensitivity reactions. A more complete description of granulomatous inflammation can be found in Chapter 3.

In man only, delayed hypersensitivity can be transferred with extracts of peripheral blood leukocytes; intact cells are not needed. Moreover, when delayed hypersensitivity is transferred by means of intact cells, only a small percentage of the transferred cells appear to participate in the reaction (Najarian and Feldman, 1961). Thus, the reaction may be initiated by only a few cells or their products. The cellular component which transfers delayed hypersensitivity in man has been called *transfer factor*. It has not yet been isolated, but has been partially characterized. It is a stable substance unaffected by heating to 37° C for six hours or five months storage at 20° C, and unaffected by treatment with DNase, RNase, or trypsin (Lawrence, 1959a). It is a dialysable material and thus has a molecular weight of less than 10,000 (Lawrence, 1963). When the transfer factor is administered to a normal recipient, he becomes hypersensitive within twenty-four hours. In contrast to the situation in passively transferred humoral or immediate hypersensitivity, the recipient of transfer factor may remain sensitive for as long as two years (Lawrence, 1959b). This long duration of hypersensitivity suggests that the transfer is not merely passive because, if it were, the hypersensitivity in the recipient would decline in a few weeks, the length of time it takes for transferred antibody to be metabolized. Notwithstanding resistance of transfer factor to RNase treatment, these data on duration of transferred hypersensitivity have caused some investigators to suggest that transfer factor is a low-molecular-weight RNA. Possibly the transfer occurs by a mechanism analogous to bacterial transformation. Thus, the host cells would carry the information for the hypersensitivity and the individual would remain sensitive for long periods of time. These studies on transfer factor fail to explain the mechanisms of the delayed response.

In vitro studies have shown that the antigen has marked effects on lymphoid cells taken from a hypersensitive animal. Depending on the concentration of the antigen, either cell death or cell proliferation may be observed. These reactions are specific for the antigen to which the individual is hypersensitive and cannot be elicited in cells derived from a normal person.

Accepting, then, that antigen affects the sensitized cell, how does this antigen-cell interaction cause a lesion? One can only conjecture, but an attractive possibility is that some of the antigen injected into the skin diffuses from the site, retaining hypersensitive lymphocytes which generate mediators. These mediators, in turn, may attract non-specific monocytes and lead to release of toxic products from the monocytes. A substance which increases capillary permeability has recently been described in monocytes of hypersensitive animals (Willoughby and Spector, 1964).

Delayed hypersensitivity has important clinical implications. For example, the pathogenesis of tuberculosis appears to involve this mechanism. The tuberculosis organism itself is innocuous; it does not produce toxins, and it grows slowly. Pathogenicity is related to its ability to induce hypersensitivity in the host which in turn results in an inflammatory lesion around the organism, just as the protein extract of the organism produces a lesion in the skin of the sensitized host. In fact, the lung lesion may be reproduced by placing proteins extracted from *M. tuberculosis* in the lungs of a tuberculin-sensitive animal (Crowle, 1962).

The delayed reaction also is useful in diagnosing the organism responsible for a particular disease. For example, *Mycobacterium tuberculosis* and *Histoplasma capsulatum,* two unrelated organisms, cause diseases which lead to remarkably similar symptoms, both characterized by delayed hypersensitivity. Extracts from each of the possible organisms can be given intradermally; the one corresponding to the infecting organism will produce the total skin reaction of delayed hypersensitivity.

The contact hypersensitivities, induced and elicited by application of the allergen to the skin, are a group of delayed hypersensitivities which are caused by extremely low-molecular-weight antigens. The molecular weight of many contact antigens is so low one would not expect them to be antigens. For example, some individuals become allergic to elemental gold or nickel and others to aniline dyes. Another example is poison ivy. These allergens are not complete antigens, but they do have the capacity to combine as haptens with skin proteins and thus become large enough to be complete antigens. Possibly the hapten-protein interaction changes the tertiary structures of the skin protein making this altered protein antigenic as well. In other respects, contact hypersensitivity is a typical delayed hypersensitivity. It is transferable by cells but not by serum; the reaction takes hours to develop; the inflammatory exudate consists primarily of mononuclear cells.

D. Immunologic Diseases

The processes described in the preceding section illustrate some of the basic mechanisms by which antigen-antibody reactions cause injury, producing pathologic manifestations either by primary action on cells or by the release of pharmacologic agents. Many disease entities have been described in humans and in experimental animals which arise by these mechanisms. These can be subdivided into three main categories: heterologous immunologic diseases if the antigens which cause them are exogenous, auto-immune diseases if there is evidence that the causative antigens are autologous or endogenous, and finally those diseases which are dependent on complex immunological phenomena. These latter include the *collagen diseases,* so designated because of the localization of the secondary inflammatory reactions in the connective tissue.

1. Heterologous immunologic diseases

The allergic diseases, discussed in a previous section, constitute an important group of immunologic diseases due to external antigens. There are other diseases with an immunologic component, poorly understood, which are triggered by an external antigen. Examples are acute post-streptococcal glomerulonephritis and rheumatic fever, in which the kidney and the heart are the primary target organs of immunologic damage, leading to cardiac or renal failure. Other organs may be involved, though less severely.

These diseases occur after an infection with Group A streptococcus, and high titers of antibody to the streptococcus are usually present. The lesions seen in the myocardium of patients with rheumatic fever and in the kidney of those with glomerulonephritis have some similarities to those of serum sickness. Immune complexes, containing complement, are usually present in the glomeruli in acute glomerulonephritis; gamma globulins tend to deposit around vessels in rheumatic fever.

The steps in the development of immunologic tissue injury following streptococcal infection are not known. It has been suggested that the streptococcus is capable of (1) altering host tissue so as to render it antigenic, or (2) inducing the production of antibody which cross-reacts with host tissue (myocardium or glomerular basement membrane). In either case, the presence of antibodies capable of reacting with normal tissue components may lead to tissue injury.

Another group of diseases related to external antigens occurs after the administration of certain drugs. The sedative drug Sedormid, for instance, is capable of sensitizing platelets, which are then susceptible to attack by antibodies which fix complement with lysis of the platelets. This occurs because Sedormid is a hapten; when combined with proteins of the platelet membrane, it is antigenic. The result is that the patient becomes deficient in platelets and may bleed quite severely from minor injuries. Similar mechanisms produce a variety of antibodies directed against other cells of the body.

2. Auto-immune diseases

Antibodies reactive with "self" antigens can arise by several means: (1) Endogenous antigens can be altered in such a way as to be recognized as non-self by the immune mechanism, and the antibody is formed in response to what now appears to be a "foreign" antigen; (2) Endogenous substances such as thyroglobulin, which are inaccessible to the antibody-forming tissue, are normally never recognized as "self," although low levels of antibody to thyroglobulin may be present without injury. If large amounts of such a sequestered antigen reach the immunologically competent tissue, e.g. as a result of injury to the thyroid, antibody production to the antigen is induced; (3) A heritable alteration of the antibody-forming cells may result in abrogation of the property of self-recognition although no data exist in support of this hypothesis. Cells thus altered and their progeny will be capable of producing antibodies to normal self-constituents, and a disease process will result. It is not yet known which of these explanations is correct; in fact, all may be incorrect.

It is important to realize that if one finds antibodies against an organ, this does not necessarily indicate auto-immune disease. In myocardial infarction, for instance, when heart muscle is severely injured, antibodies to heart-muscle protein frequently occur, but it is clear that they are not the cause of myocardial infarction. One must distinguish whether the antibody is a primary cause of the disease or the result of some damage which is not of immunological nature.

For a disease to be defined as auto-immune, the following conditions should be satisfied: (1) the demonstration in the area of injury of antibodies to host tissue, or lymphoid cells capable of reacting with or attaching to host tissue or cells; (2) transfer of the disease with the patient's serum or lymphocytes; and (3) production of the disease experimentally by immunization or sensitization with the specific tissue antigen. These criteria are satisfied infrequently in human pathology.

A group of auto-immune diseases are the so-called auto-immune hematologic disorders, e.g. auto-immune hemolytic anemia. In these, the circulating blood cells and the fixed bone-marrow cells are the target cells of circulating antibodies. The disease can be transferred passively by transferring circulating antibodies. They are detectable on the cells and in the serum. Antibodies can be of two varieties: incomplete (warm) antibodies which react at 37° C and are usually 7S immunoglobulins, and complete (cold) antibodies which react at 2 to 5° C and are found in the 19S macroglobulin fraction. The antibodies are specific and the antigen is usually found in the Rh group of antigens. The sensitization mechanism is not very clear but may involve any of the mechanisms previously mentioned. The destruction of red cells by lysis or hemagglutination and erythrophagocytosis in the spleen leads to chronic insufficiency of circulating red cells, known as *anemia*.

Hashimoto's thyroiditis, or auto-immune thyroiditis, is another example of

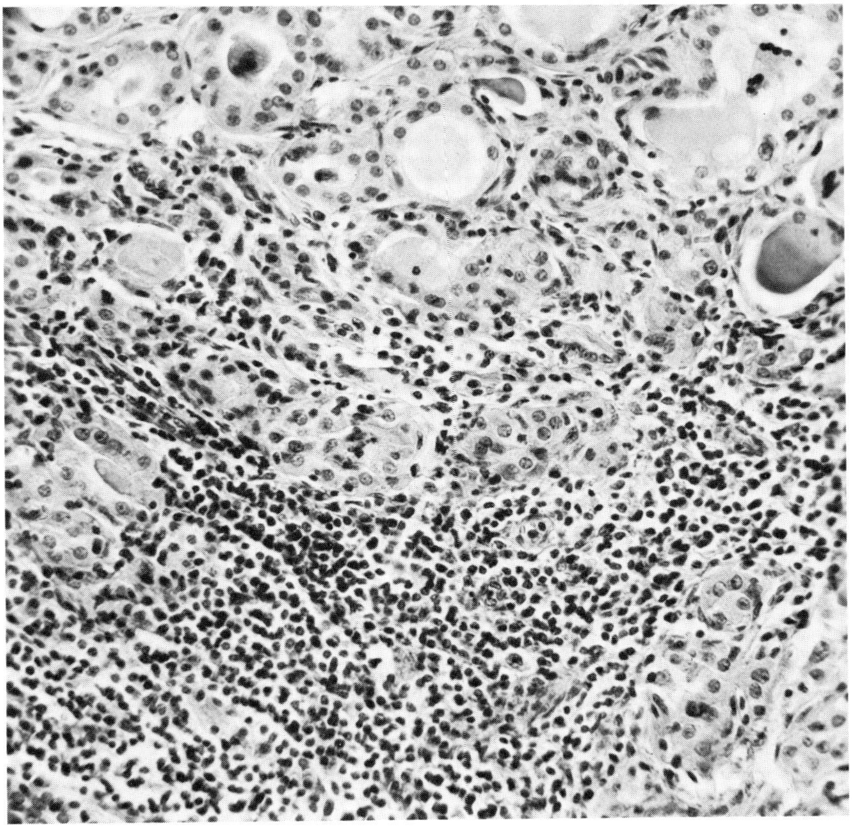

Figure 5-4. A thyroid section from a patient with Hashimoto's thyroiditis showing the typical lymphocytic infiltrate and some still fairly normal thyroid follicles.

auto-immune disease. The antigen appears to be thyroglobulin or another of the constituents of colloid. Patients with this disease have circulating complement which fixes antibodies to thyroid, and lymphoid cells which destroy the thyroid *in vivo* by direct invasion and which attach to thyroid epithelim in tissue culture. Histologically, one observes lymphocytic infiltration of the thyroid with destruction of the epithelium (Fig. 5-4). Eventually, progressive loss of thyroid leads to functional inadequacy or hypothyroidism.

There are many other diseases which may have an auto-immune component. In cases where the cause of a disease is obscure, it is easy to ascribe an auto-immune etiology, particularly if one observes auto-antibodies, elevated levels of circulating immunoglobulins, large numbers of plasma cells in the tissue, and a destructive disease characterized by dense lymphocytic infiltration, or if one demonstrates complement or antibody in the affected tissue by immunofluorescent or other techniques. In most cases, however, rigorous demonstration of an autoimmune etiology is lacking. In the two diseases cited, auto-immunity appears to be clearly implicated.

3. Diseases due to complex immunologic phenomena

These are the diseases which are also known as *collagen diseases,* comprising lupus erythematosus, rheumatoid arthritis, dermatomyositis, polyarteritis, scleroderma, and similar disorders. In these, one can demonstrate affinity of the gamma globulin and lymphocytes of the host for tissue constituents. At least some of the damage is produced by antibodies associated with these constituents. The affinity can be demonstrated by serologic techniques, such as complement fixation, hemagglutination, and antiglobulin consumption, by fluorescent antibody techniques, or by the culturing of lymphocytes in mixed cultures.

An important example of these diseases is lupus erythematosus, characterized by pathologic changes in the vasculature and connective tissue of many organs, leading to a spectrum of symptoms. A wide variety of auto-antibodies to nuclear and cytoplasmic constituents has been identified in the serum of patients with this disease, but the exact relationship of these to the pathogenesis of the disease remains obscure for the most part. In spite of the fact that so many different auto-antigens are present, passive transfer of serum does not cause disease in the recipient. Antigen-antibody complexes also appear to play some role in the pathogenesis of this disease.

One aspect of the disease clearly does have an immunologic pathogenesis and leads to severe disability. This is the deposition of immune complexes in the renal glomeruli, leading to immune complex nephritis which may be progressive and ultimately lethal.

Advantage has been taken of the presence of certain 7S antibodies directed against nuclear components in devising a diagnostic test. When serum from a patient with lupus erythematosus is incubated *in vitro* with white blood cells from his own or other blood, an "L.E. cell" forms (Fig. 5-5). This phenomenon results when a damaged nucleus interacts with antibody and is then phagocytosed by an intact phagocytic cell, usually a neutrophil. This mechanism seems, however, to have little if any relation to the production of disease.

Auto-antibodies can be demonstrated in a number of other collagen diseases. In these other diseases, however, the relation of auto-antibodies to the pathogenesis of the lesions is even less clear. In rheumatoid arthritis, for instance, a

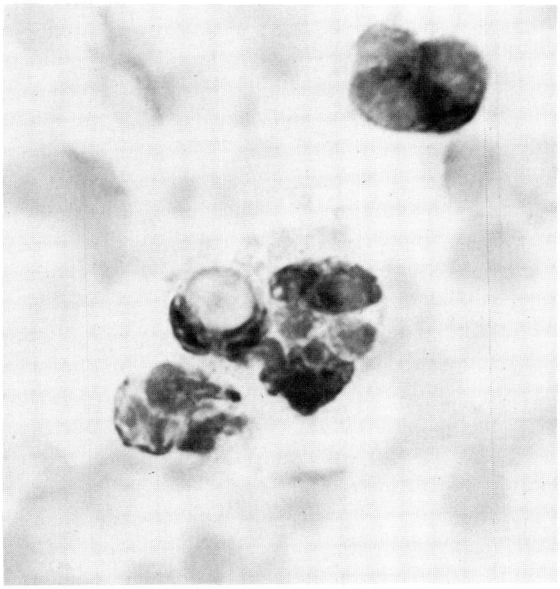

Figure 5-5. Characteristic LE cell in blood smear of a patient with systemic lupus.

complex mechanism for the formation of auto-antibodies exists. Aggregated 7S globulin of indeterminate origin becomes antigenic, and both 19S and 7S antibodies, known as *rheumatoid factor,* are formed to this aggregate and can be demonstrated in the serum of patients with well-developed rheumatoid arthritis. Antibodies similar to but not identical with gamma globulin can be found in the sera of patients with other, unrelated diseases such as bacterial endocarditis, tuberculosis, syphilis—all characterized by prolonged continuous exposure to an external antigen, and in some individuals who are repeatedly immunized to the same antigen.

Manifestations of rheumatoid arthritis cannot be induced by passive transfer of antibodies, however, and there is no other evidence at present that these antibodies are responsible for the chronic progressive destruction of articular surfaces which characterizes rheumatoid arthritis. Some have pointed to the lymphoid aggregates and occasional granulomas seen in this disease as evidence of the role of cellular hypersensitivity in the pathogenesis; proof of this is also lacking.

4. Experimental models

Experimental models exist for the study of auto-immune disease involving either circulating antibodies or cell-bound antibodies. The usual method of production of these diseases is to inject autologous, homologous, or heterologous tissues in conjunction with Freund's adjuvant. Both circulating and cell-bound antibodies will result. For maximal usefulness of the model, the pathologic manifestations should appear in the tissue corresponding to that which is used as antigen, and the damage should be comparable to what is caused by similar diseases in humans. Diseases which have been produced in this fashion are very numerous. Those which have been most thoroughly studied are thyroiditis, glomerulonephritis, and experimental allergic encephalomyelitis. Attempts have been made to produce uveitis, orchitis, adrenalitis, atrophic gastritis, and so on.

Thyroiditis, corresponding to Hashimoto's thyroiditis in humans, has been produced in rats, guinea pigs, rabbits, and dogs by using thyroglobulin and epithelial thyroid antigens as the inducing agent. Cell-bound immunity has been demonstrated, and usually the severity of the disease correlates with this. Circulating antibody has also been shown to exist, however, and the disease can be transferred with serum. The typical mononuclear infiltration and destruction of the thyroid present in the clinical disease is also seen experimentally.

Several animal models for glomerulonephritis have been developed. Models exist for immune-complex nephritis, in which sustained levels of circulating immune complexes are achieved utilizing various antigens. The diseases are very similar to human immune-complex disease, as seen in post-streptococcal glomerulonephritis, or lupus glomerulonephritis. A model for another type of glomerulonephritis with formation of anti-basement-membrane antibody has also been achieved by immunizing animals with basement membranes prepared from other species. This condition, which can be transferred to nonimmunized homologous animals with serum from immunized animals, is similar to that seen in Goodpasture's syndrome in human beings.

The experimental allergic encephalomyelitis produced primarily in monkeys, but also in dogs, rabbits, guinea pigs, rats, and mice, has also been seen in human subjects who have been given rabies vaccine prepared by growing the virus in rabbit spinal cord. The antigen contained in the vaccine is associated with myelin in the white matter of the rabbit central nervous system. Circulating antibodies to myelin are quite prominent, are toxic to the central nervous system cells in tissue cultures, and destroy myelin. Cellular sensitivity has also been shown to exist and the disease can be transferred with lymphocytes. The pathologic changes are characteristic, consisting of demyelination with a concomitant inflammatory process, both acute and chronic, and production of gliosis during repair. The axons are not affected by the pathologic process. It is still not clear what the human counterpart of this experimental auto-immune disease is. The encephalomyelitides, which are seen after viral infections, and multiple sclerosis have been suggested, but no clear-cut evidence can be offered.

The importance of auto-immune reactions in human pathology has been well documented by laboratory experiments. The foregoing discussion has revealed, however, that basic concepts of auto-immune disease are still in need of much clarification. In many cases, the pathogenesis is still in doubt, the antigens are not clearly known, and even the auto-immune nature of the disease may be questionable since the original etiologic agent may be something other than an antigen. Be that as it may, in cases where a reasonably clear endogenous antigenic component, an exogenous cross-reacting antigenic component, or a combination of the two can be demonstrated, and where a reasonable pathogenetic mechanism can be delineated, one is usually justified in calling the pathologic entities auto-immune diseases.

E. Organ Transplantation

The study of tolerance and of its counterpart, rejection, has occupied immunologists for a long time, since it has been hoped that through an understanding of these phenomena, the use of organ transplantation in humans could become feasible. Although great advances have been made toward elucidating the mechanisms regulating histocompatibility, the ultimate goal of transplantation without rejection still eludes the physician. Progress in surgical techniques has essentially eliminated the purely technical obstacles to transplant surgery and has made even more pressing the need for a deeper understanding of histocompatibility and of immunosuppression in order to achieve a very low degree of homograft rejection (Merrill, 1967).

Many of the characteristics of this reaction have been determined by using skin grafts on inbred mouse strains. When a skin graft is placed on a mouse of a strain different from the strain of the skin donor, initially the graft will appear to take. That is, it will begin to heal, become vascularized, and appear to become part of the skin of the recipient. After several days, immunization has been achieved, mononuclear cells invade the graft bed, thrombosis and failure of the blood supply occur, and eventually the graft is sloughed. If a second graft from the same donor is placed on the recipient, the events of graft rejection will be qualitatively unchanged but greatly accelerated. Thus, the first graft immunizes the recipient (Wilson and Billingham, 1967).

Homotransplantation reactions are typically placed in the category of delayed hypersensitivity because passive immunity (accelerated graft rejection) is accomplished by transfer of lymphoid cells, but not, except under unusual circumstances, after transfer of serum. Accelerated graft rejection has also occurred, however, when the transferred lymphoid cells are contained within diffusion chambers. These chambers are built so as to prohibit the movement of cells out of them, but soluble material diffuses freely. Thus, graft rejection appears to be mediated primarily by cellular mechanisms. Nevertheless, it may also be facilitated by humoral mechanisms.

Humoral antibodies are clearly involved in one uncommon type of graft rejection, the "white graft" reaction. The rejection events are different from those described above in that the graft is not vascularized, and sloughing occurs very rapidly. The white graft reaction occurs in animals having humoral antibody to the graft and is transferable by serum. Thus, the white graft reaction is probably mediated by humoral antibodies.

Complete success in homotransplantation is assured only if the donor and recipient are genetically identical. If only those antigens already present in the recipient are administered with the graft, an immune response will not be elicited. Transplantation is therefore possible between identical twins and between experimental animals of the same inbred strain, but in mice a change at only one genetic locus is sufficient to cause rejection. In spite of this, a considerable degree of success has been attained in human homotransplantation with drugs which suppress the immune response. Unfortunately, treatment with these drugs does not completely eliminate the rejection response, and it also decreases the patient's resistance to infectious agents. It is encouraging, however, that the recent development of a variety of methods of suppressing the immune response has allowed the physician more flexibility. One hopes for eventual selective ability to inhibit transplantation rejection with minimal interference with other immune mechanisms.

References

Abramoff, P., and La Via, M. F. (1970), Biology of the Immune Response, McGraw-Hill, New York.

Ackerman, G. A. (1967), Developmental relationship between the appearance of lymphocytes and lymphopoietic activity in the thymus and lymph nodes of the fetal cat, Anat. Rec., *158*:387.

Austen, K. F., and Humphrey, J. H. (1963), *In vitro* studies of the mechanism of anaphylaxis, Adv. Immunol., *3*:3.

Cannon, J. A., Terasaki, P. I., and Longmire, W. P., Jr. (1958), Unexpected manifestations of induced tolerance to skin homografts in the chicken, Ann. N. Y. Acad. Sci., *73*:862.

Chase, M. W. (1946), The cellular transfer of cutaneous hypersensitivity, J. Bact., *51*:643.
Cochrane, C. G. (1968), Immunologic tissue injury mediated by neutrophilic leukocytes, Adv. Immunol., *9*:97.
Crowle, A. J. (1962), Delayed Hypersensitivity in Health and Disease, p. 18, Charles C Thomas Co., Springfield, Ill.
Edelman, G. M., and Gall, W. E. (1969), The antibody problem, Ann. Rev. Biochem., *38*:415.
Fowler, R., Jr., Schubert, W. K., and West, C. D. (1960), Acquired partial tolerance to homologous skin grafts in the human infant at birth, Ann. N. Y. Acad. Sci., *87*:403.
Gell, P. G. H., and Benacerraf, B. (1961), Delayed hypersensitivity to simple protein antigens, Adv. Immunol., *1*:319.
Humphrey, J. H., and Dourmashkin, R. R. (1969), The lesions in cell membranes caused by complement, Adv. Immunol., *11*:75.
Ishizaka, K., and Ishizaka, T. (1968), Human reaginic antibodies and immunoglobulin E., J. Allergy, *42*:330.
Janeway, C. A. (1968), Syndromes of diminished resistance to infection, J. Pediat., *72*:885.
Koch, F., Schultze, H. E., and Schwick, G. (1959), Macroglobulin determination in the blood of healthy children during the first year of life, Arch. Kinderheilk, *3*:199.
Landsteiner, K. (1936), The Specificity of Serological Reactions, Charles C Thomas Co., Springfield, Ill.
Lawrence, H. S. (1959a), Cellular and Humoral Aspects of the Hypersensitive States, p. 279, Harper and Hoeber, Inc., New York.
Lawrence, H. S. (1959b), Homograft sensitivity. An expression of the immunologic origins and consequences of individuality, Physiol. Rev., *39*:811.
Lawrence, H. S. (1963), General perspectives, *in* Cell Bound Antibodies, p. 3. B. Amos and H. Koprowski, Eds., Wistar Inst. Press, Philadelphia.
Mackay, I. R., and Burnett, F. M. (1965), Autoimmunity: experimental and clinical aspects, Ann. N. Y. Acad. Sci., *124*:Parts I and II.
Mage, R. G., and Kabat, E. A. (1963), Immunological studies on dextrans, J. Immunol., *91*:633.
Maurer, P. H., Gerulat, B. F., and Pinchuck, P. (1963), Antigenicity of polypeptides (poly-a-amino acids). V. Studies in rabbits, J. Imunol., *90*:381.
Medawar, P. (1957), The Uniqueness of the Individual, Basic Books, New York.
Merrill, J. P. (1967), Human tissue transplantation, Adv. Immunol., *7*:275.
Muller-Eberhard, H. J. (1968), Chemistry and reaction mechanisms of complement, Adv. Immunol., *8*:1.
Najarian, J. S., and Feldman, J. D. (1961), Passive transfer of tuberculin sensitivity by initiated thymidine labeled lymphoid cells, J. Exp. Med., *114*:779.
Patterson, R. (1969), Laboratory models of reaginic allergy, Progress in Allergy, *13*:332.
Peterson, R. D. A. (1968), Allergy: Status and perspectives, J. Ped., *73*:436.
Prausnitz, C., and Kustner, H. (1962), Studies on hypersensitivity, *in* Clinical As-

pects of Immunology, p. 808, P. G. H. Gell and R. R. A. Coombs, Eds., (translated), F. A. Davis Co., Philadelphia.

Schinckel, P. G., and Ferguson, K. A. (1953), Skin transplantation in the foetal lamb, Aust. J. Biol. Sci., *6*:533.

Shaffer, J. H., Lo Grippo, G. A., and Chase, M. W. (1959), Mechanisms of Hypersensitivity, Little, Brown, and Co., Boston, Mass.

Silverstein, A. M., Uhr, J. W., Kraner, K. L., and Lukes, P. J. (1963), Fetal response to antigenic stimulus. II. Antibody production by the fetal lamb, J. Exp. Med., *117*:799.

Smith, R. T., Good, R. A., Miescher, P. A. (1966), Phylogeny of Immunity, University of Florida Press, Gainesville.

Smith, R. T., Good, R. A., and Miescher, P. A. (1967), Ontogeny of Immunity, University of Florida Press, Gainesville.

Talmage, D. W., and Cann, J. R. (1961), The Chemistry of Immunity in Health and Disease, Charles C. Thomas Co., Springfield, Ill.

Turk, J. L. (1967), Cytology of the induction of hypersensitivity, British Med. Bulletin, *23*:3.

Willoughby, D. A., and Spector, W. G. (1964), The lymph node permeability factor: a possible mediator of the delayed hypersensitivity reaction, Ann. N. Y. Acad. Sci., *116*:874.

Wilson, D. B., and Billingham, R. E. (1967), Lymphocytes and transplantation immunity, Adv. Immunol., *7*:189.

Wolfe, H. R., Mueller, A. P., Neess, J., and Tempelis, C. (1957), Precipitin production in chickens. XVI. The relationship of age to antibody production, J. Immunol., *79*:142.

6

NEOPLASIA

Richmond T. Prehn, M.D.

A. Components of the Physiology of Neoplasia

1. Somatic cell variation

Higher animals are composed of vast numbers of interacting and often highly specialized cells, e.g. liver cells, epidermal cells, myocytes, and nerve cells. Each cell type behaves like a separate species in that each reproduces its own kind. No way has yet been found to induce a liver cell to produce, by mitosis, anything but another liver cell. Nevertheless, it is the present belief that there are no genetic differences among cell types, that they are merely pseudospecies. The nongenetic changes during ontogeny that result in these different pseudospecies of specialized cells are termed *epigenetic* changes. This ontological process of cellular pseudospeciation is called *differentiation* (Harris, 1964).

There is a further aspect of differentiation: namely, the further specializations that occur within each cellular pseudospecies of the adult animal. For example, the epidermal cell population of the skin is not homogeneous but consists of basal cells and cells in various stages of keratinization. The mitotic activity of the epidermal pseudospecies is usually confined to the cells on the basement membrane, the basal cells. Mitosis of these cells produces more basal cells as well as cells which lose the capacity to divide but acquire the specialized capacity to produce keratin. Since the cells cannot divide, no new pseudospecies is formed. Normal differentiation thus may include loss of the capability to divide, as in the case of keratinizing cells of the epidermis, neurons of the adult central nervous system, and the multinucleated contractile cells of striated muscle.

The mechanisms that regulate normal differentiation are largely unknown. It is evident that cell-to-cell interactions often trigger the modifications of gene expression that occur. These interactions may be mediated at the cell surface. Repression of certain nuclear genes may result, i.e. the transcription of particular genic messages to RNA may be halted. Alternatively or additionally, translation of particular messages from RNA into protein may be stopped. In any event, the end result is that in the differentiated cell only a small part of the genome is expressed in the cellular phenotype. What distinguishes a liver cell from a kidney cell is that small, only partially overlapping portions of their common genomes are expressed (Harris, 1964).

Differentiation ordinarily is quite stable. It is heritable through many cell generations. However, most differentiated cells do retain a restricted range of variability, being able to undergo certain changes of phenotype in response to environmental stimuli. A common example is *squamous metaplasia* in the bronchus, in which basal cells differentiate into squamous cells instead of the usual columnar cells. It is commonly observed as a consequence of cigarette smoking or vitamin A deficiency. Since it is apparently a reversible condition, it is not usually considered a new differentiation but is termed a *modulation*. It is probably more dependent upon a continued environmental stimulus than upon a change in cellular heredity (Harris, 1964).

In mammalian systems differentiation usually implies an increased specialization accompanied by a restriction of the cell's potentialities to perform other functions or to give rise to other cell types. However, increased specialization does not necessarily and inevitably imply a restriction of totipotency. This is illustrated in its most extreme form in plant materials. Here a highly specialized cell from a mature plant can sometimes regenerate the entire organism–it has retained all of the totipotency of the seed itself. Thus, the term *differentiation* is used somewhat ambiguously in mammalian systems to refer to either or both of two properties that are not necessarily correlated (Harris, 1964).

Although epigenetic mechanisms probably account for most and perhaps all of normal differentiation, there is another form of somatic cell variation. This is somatic mutation. It is not known if any normal processes are dependent upon it.

Neoplasia, as we shall see, comprises two separate alterations in cell physiology: (1) a form of abnormal somatic cell variation that represents somatic mutation and/or aberrant and defective differentiation; and (2) a pathologic form of hyperplasia.

2. Hyperplasia

Not only do cellular interactions play important and poorly understood roles in regulating differentiation, but they are also vital to the regulation of tissue and organ mass. An increase in the size of an adult tissue or organ due to an increase in the number of cells is termed *hyperplasia.* Hyperplasia can be arbitrarily divided into two different but often overlapping types: (1) physiologic; and (2) pathologic or neoplastic. Physiologic hyperplasia is a normal reaction of a tissue to a variety of environmental stimuli. Perhaps the most commonly observed example is the thickening of the epidermis that occurs in response to trauma. This particular example has been analyzed in greater detail than most and deserves discussion as a general prototype.

It has been observed that any circumstance that kills and/or removes cells in the superficial epidermal layers results in an increase in mitotic activity in the basal layer. In the rat an increase of cell production in the basal layer leads to a restitution of the superficial layers which more than restores the original state. This restitution and overshoot is termed *compensatory hyperplasia.* If the stimulus that originally initiated the process is not recurrent, the mitotic activity in the basal layer eventually subsides and the hyperplasia disappears. Physiologic hyperplasia is thus dependent upon continued application of the external stimulus.

It is, of course, axiomatic that in any tissue at mass equilibrium the rate of formation of new cells must be exactly balanced by the rate of cell death. In a tissue like the epidermis this means that, on the average, exactly half the progeny resulting from mitosis in the basal layer must follow the pathway of cellular differentiation that leads to keratin formation and to eventual cell death. Hyperplasia will be self-limiting only when this ratio is maintained or restored.

The observation that removal of the superficial layers results in mitotic activity in the basal layer led to the hypothesis that the superficial layers were inhibitory to the basal. It has now been demonstrated that the keratinizing layers produce a mitotic inhibitor. The inhibitor has been partially purified and called a *chalone* (Bullough *et al.,* 1967). It does not appear to be specific to the animal species. However, one can anticipate that different chalones probably occur in different tissues.

Chalones are chemical inhibitors that operate at short range, i.e. near their points of origin. Longer range regulatory substances, both stimulatory and inhibitory, have been identified in some tissues. The hormones, somatotropin, gonadotrophin, and estrogen are good examples. Also, there are very short range regulatory effects at the level of cell-to-cell contact, called *contact inhibition of mitosis* (Harris, 1964). Thus it is clear that there are many interacting mechanisms and controls of cell growth and division.

Neoplastic hyperplasia differs from the physiologic type just described, in that it involves a change in the intrinsic cellular heredity. This intrinsic cellular change produces a race of cells less subject to the normal tissue regulatory mechanisms. In the skin, for example, this may mean that neoplastic cells either produce less chalone and/or are less sensitive to the inhibitory effects of chalone. In this race of cells, cellular maturation or differentiation is defective; somewhat less than 50 per cent of the daughter-cells in the basal layer are set on the pathway to keratinization. Of course, a fall in the proportion of differentiated cells implies a fall in the level of the chalone, though this may not always be the case. Some neoplastic hyperplasias have a lower than normal mitotic rate, but the tissue continues to expand because of the imbalance in the ratio between stem-cell renewal and differentiation. The molecular reasons for this imbalance are unknown.

B. Characteristics of Tumors

1. Definition

Neoplasia can be defined as *that form of hyperplasia which is caused, at least in part, by an intrinsic heritable abnormality in the involved cells.* Although it is difficult to define a condition before it is fully understood, this definition successfully excludes those conditions not usually regarded as neoplastic while it encompasses all that are.

It is apparent that this definition includes two portions. The first, that neoplasia is a form of pathological hyperplasia, needs no justification. The second, relating to a heritable cell variation, requires evidence which is derived from experiments of the following kind in animals. Animal neoplasms can be transplanted from animal to animal by the inoculation of living neoplastic cells. This can be done serially ad infinitum provided that immunity to the foreign neoplastic cells is eliminated by some technique. It can be shown with the aid of chromosomal or antigenic markers that the cells of the new neoplasms which arise in the recipient animals are usually the progeny of the transplanted cells rather than of cells of the recipient. In man the process of metastasis supplies somewhat similar evidence; neoplastic cells are carried by the bloodstream or by lymphatics to sites distant from their place of origin. Here they set up neoplasms of the parental cell type. Recently, the inadvertant transplantation of neoplasia during kidney transplantations has also provided evidence of the heritable nature of the disease at the cell level.

From what has been said, it is obvious that neoplasia is a disease characterized by abnormal cell behavior and abnormal interactions among cells. The cells of a neoplasm do not behave in the highly integrated, interdependent manner of normal metazoan cell populations. Thus, neoplasia can perhaps be looked upon as an imperfect cellular reversion to a more primitive, ancestral cell type, in which some of the regulatory mechanisms that normally operate among metazoan cells are defective or absent. This seeming atavism results in abnormalities of function, growth, and territorial behavior. Before going on to discuss in greater detail the characteristics of neoplastic cells, however, it is necessary to consider briefly the conditions of pseudoneoplasia that may closely mimic actual neoplasia.

2. Mimicry of neoplasia

It is not sufficient that a definition of neoplastic hyperplasia specify a change in cellular heredity; it must further specify that this change is present in those cells directly involved in the hyperplasia. Otherwise, some diseases closely related to neoplasia, but not usually regarded as true neoplasms, would not be definitionally excluded. An excellent example of such a disease that mimics neoplasia is pernicious or Addisonian anemia. This disease is characterized by a massive hyperplasia of immature erythroid cells in the bone marrow. Anemia, seen in the peripheral blood, results from the failure of these cells to mature. The ratio of proliferating stem cells to maturing non-reproductive cells has been altered. However, although the condition is due to an alteration in cellular heredity, the lesion exists, not in the cells of the hematopoietic system that are undergoing the hyperplasia, but rather in cells of the stomach which normally provide a factor necessary for the absorption of vitamin B-12. This vitamin in turn is required for the maturation or differentiation of erythrocytes. Pernicious anemia is thus a disease very similar in most characteristics to a true neoplasm. It is furthermore a disease that can be corrected by the injection of a cell-maturing factor.

Chronic physiologic hyperplasia may stimulate neoplasia in almost all its histologic features. The distinction may be difficult even for an experienced pathologist. The two types of hyperplasia, neoplastic and physiologic, are often present simultaneously in varying degree in one and the same lesion. Cells with a heritable abnormality are often capable of responding to some extent to an environmental stimulus.

3. The growth curve

It is often thought that tumor growth is simply exponential. However, there is considerable evidence that this is not strictly the case. With most experimental tumors it can be demonstrated that the rate of tumor growth decreases with time (Laird, 1965). Complex mathematical functions have been presented by several workers to describe this relationship. These curves imply that even the most malignant and fast-growing tumors would eventually reach plateaus of little further

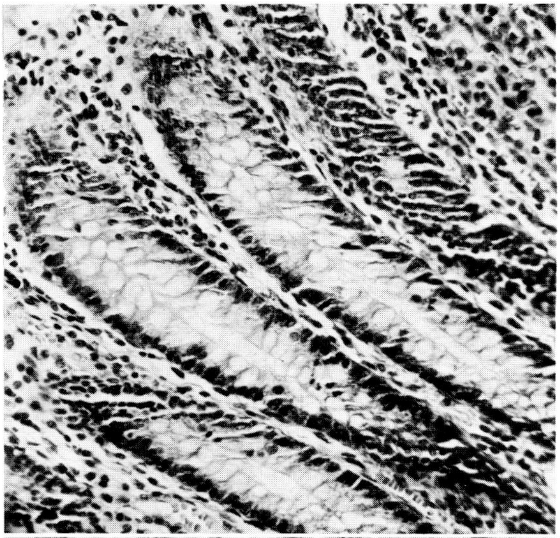

a

Figure 6-1. Photomicrographs of tumors of the colon.

a. This tissue from a benign adenomatous polyp is virtually indistinguishable from normal colonic mucosa. The lamina propria consists of appropriate quantities of connective tissue and various mononuclear cells, and the epithelium of the crypt is regular with normal mucous production in the apical portion of the cells. A few mitoses are seen.

b. In this section from a moderately well differentiated adenocarcinoma, the epithelium is lined up to form glandular spaces with the stroma approximating the appearance of lamina propria. The nuclei of the cancerous epithelium are very

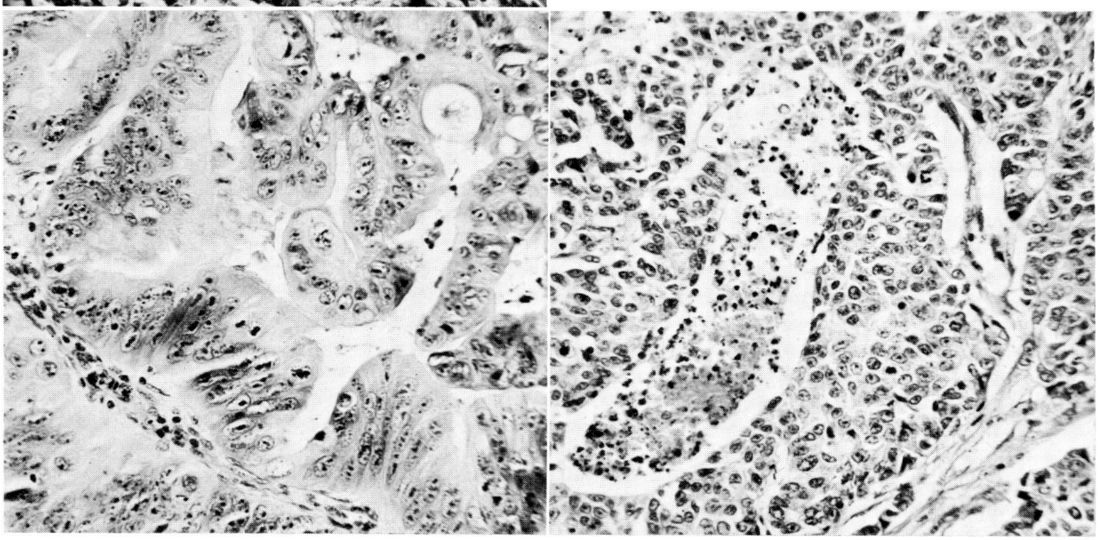

b

irregular in size and shape, and staining qualities. Mitoses are quite numerous. The amount of mucus production is greatly decreased, and the cells are in a considerable degree of disarray with respect to the stroma and the lumen of the "gland."

c. In this example of a rather poorly differentiated adenocarcinoma of the colon, it is difficult to identify a glandular lumen, and the cancerous epithelium does not line up at all but tends to form masses of cancer cells. Some fibrous stroma is still present. In the center the cancerous tissue has become necrotic, presumably because of lack of blood supply, and a mass of dead cells can be seen.

growth if the animals lived long enough. Unfortunately, death usually occurs while the tumors are still in the almost purely exponential portions of their growth curves. With more benign tumors, a plateau is often reached within the lifespan of the animal, and unless further neoplastic progression occurs, the lesion may remain virtually stationary in size. The reasons for this type of behavior are not known.

The fact that immunity may alter tumor growth rates will be discussed in a subsequent section. Nevertheless, it may be appropriate, in connection with tumor growth curves, to point out at this time that in one experimental tumor system, two populations of tumor cells have been demonstrated. One of these was non-replicating. If immunity was blocked, part of the non-replicating subpopulation of cells underwent mitosis (DeCosse and Gelfant, 1968). It would seem that an immune reaction, at least in the systems studied, was capable of reversibly blocking mitosis in a small but variable percentage of the tumor-cell population. It may be that a mechanism such as this can contribute to the complexity of tumor growth curves.

4. Benign and malignant

Neoplasia may involve any vertebrate tissue or organ whose cells are capable of division. The cellular defect may be very mild, the cells hardly varying from their normal counterpart, or it may be so severe that the normal differentiated counterpart is utterly unrecognizable in the distorted cells of the neoplasm. This continuum of differing degrees of aberration is customarily divided into two or sometimes three categories.

Those neoplasms that are highly differentiated and thus differ only minimally in morphology and behavior from their tissue of origin are generally termed *benign,* even though they may rarely prove fatal (Fig. 6-1a). These lesions are usually relatively slow-growing, and the individual cells may in extreme cases be morphologically indistinguishable from the corresponding normal cells. They remain localized and inflict damage by spatial encroachment on normal tissues.

At the other extreme, those neoplasms which show marked cellular atypia and marked deficiency of differentiation (anaplasia) are termed *malignant,* even though cures may sometimes be effected (Fig. 6-1b, c). A *cancer* is a malignant neoplasm. Cancers of ectodermal or endodermal derivation are usually called *carcinomas,* while those of mesodermal origin are, with few exceptions, termed *sarcomas.* The cells of a malignant lesion are usually aneuploid and have a variety of chromosomal abnormalities. There is often much pleomorphism (variation from cell to cell in morphology). Multiple nucleoli are common and the cells are usually larger than normal with large nuclei and large nuclear-cytoplasmic size ratios. There is often a deficiency of rough endoplasmic reticulum with an increase in the number of free ribosomes. Mitoses are often numerous in tissue sections and are frequently abnormal. However, the malignant cell's most important characteristic is a tendency to lose to a variable extent its normal adhesiveness to its neighbors. Cell-to-cell contact is decreased and ionic communication between cells is diminished. The cells acquire an increased propensity for ameboid migration away from their site of origin. This tendency is seen in the entry of neoplastic cells into lymphatics, blood vessels, or the pleural or peritoneal cavities. In this manner, they may be widely disseminated and may establish new and distant secondary sites of neoplastic growth. It is this process, called *metastasis,* that so often defeats attempts at curative surgical excision. Because of its overriding clinical importance, it is the capacity to metastasize, whether it is realized or potential, that is the hallmark of malignancy.

Between these two extremes is a group of lesions that exhibit the cytologic and morphologic characteristics of malignancy but which lack any evidence of invasive tendencies. Such a lesion is commonly called a *carcinoma in situ* (Fig. 6-2).

The existence of carcinoma *in situ* demonstrates dramatically that there is no certain correspondence between the cytologic features usually associated with malignancy and the actual propensity to metastasize. However, the experienced pathologist can usually arrive at a reasonable estimate of malignant potential by studying cytologic and especially histologic evidence. There is no single criterion for this difficult judgment.

It has been a useful practice in the evaluation of malignant neoplasia to assign histologic grades. For this purpose the grading system introduced by Broders is most commonly used. In this system, the lesions are rated on a scale of 1 to 4, according to the percentage of undifferentiated cells—the most differentiated type of lesion is rated 1 and the completely anaplastic is lesion 4. These grades have been shown to have a statistically significant relation to prognosis in a variety of types of malignancies.

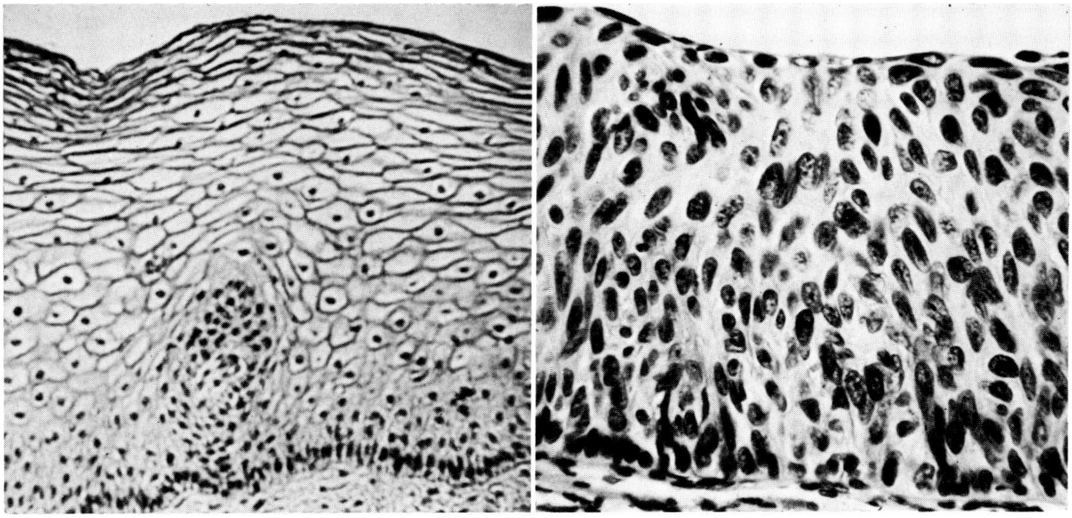

b

Figure 6-2. **a.** Normal cervical epithelium. The basal cells are lined up regularly against the lamina propria, and orderly maturation of cells with formation of parakeratin is apparent. As the cells mature they become flattened and the cytoplasmic contents stain poorly.

b. Carcinoma in situ of the uterine cervix. The cells are in considerable disarray. The basal layer is uneven. No maturation of cells is apparent and there is a great deal of nuclear variability.

Smears of fixed and stained, exfoliated epithelial cells are useful diagnostic tools, especially in assessing the uterine cervix. In the system of Papanicolaou, the smears are rated on a scale of O to V, acording to the cell or clump of cells which appears most malignant. Class V is considered certain carcinoma and class O is completely normal (Papanicolaou, 1958).

5. Metastasis

Despite the fact that the pathologist is often asked, as a matter of grave urgency, to identify neoplasms on the basis of histologic or cytologic criteria as benign or malignant, it must be emphasized that these categories are arbitrary, that there is no sharp biological dividing line between them. The tendency to metastasize like so many biological functions, is a probability function and not an absolute quality.

The process of metastasis, which is so important in prognosis, is not well understood. Before metastasis can occur, however, the neoplastic cells must invade the surrounding normal tissues. Initially at least, the normal tissues are apparently inhibitory to both the growth and migration of small foci of neoplastic cells. With time the characteristics of the cells change so that this inhibition breaks down and the focus can grow and/or spread. The nature of this inhibition is not understood but is undoubtedly complex. It is known to involve cell-to-cell contact processes as well as inhibitors capable of acting over short distances.

Characteristically, the cells of the malignant lesion are less adhesive, one to another, than are normal cells. This is associated with a decreased calcium content in the plasma membrane. Some malignant cells produce hyaluronidase, which may assist the process of invasion. Also, the cells acquire a more negative surface charge which may help to reduce aggregation.

Most individual neoplastic cells that enter the bloodstream die without forming a new nidus of malignant disease (Ziedman, 1965). In order for a metastasis to be established, circulating neoplastic cells must adhere to the vascular endothelium, a process determined by a number of factors such as cell or clump size, diameter of the capillary, and "stickiness" of the capillary wall. The latter property is dependent in part on clotting factors in the blood.

Metastases do not arise with a random distribution throughout the body (Fig. 6-3). Each type and location of malignant lesion has characteristic patterns and routes of most probable metastasis. These patterns are in part determined by purely mechanical factors such as the location of the primary lesion and the extent of the capillary bed in various organs. Many neoplasms have a tendency to lung metastasis because the pulmonary capillary bed serves as the first capillary filter through which the neoplastic cells pass after entering the circulation (Southam *et al.*, 1967).

In addition to these purely mechanical considerations, some patterns are explicable only on the basis of a more receptive "soil" at certain sites for a particular neoplasm (Southam *et al.*, 1967). Since the chemical and physical environment varies from organ to organ, it would indeed be surprising if this were not the case.

It has been pointed out that many neoplasms spread by direct extension or metastasis through the lymphatic channels. The role of the lymph nodes has been a subject of much debate (Crile, 1968). The frequency of metastasis in the regional lymph nodes has cast doubt upon the hypothesis that they are defensive bastions. On the other hand, it may be argued that the tumor grows in and replaces a lymph node only after the node's hypothetical defensive potential is exhausted. More will be said of this subject in the discussion of immunity. For the present, it should be noted that the existence of gross or histologic tumor in a re-

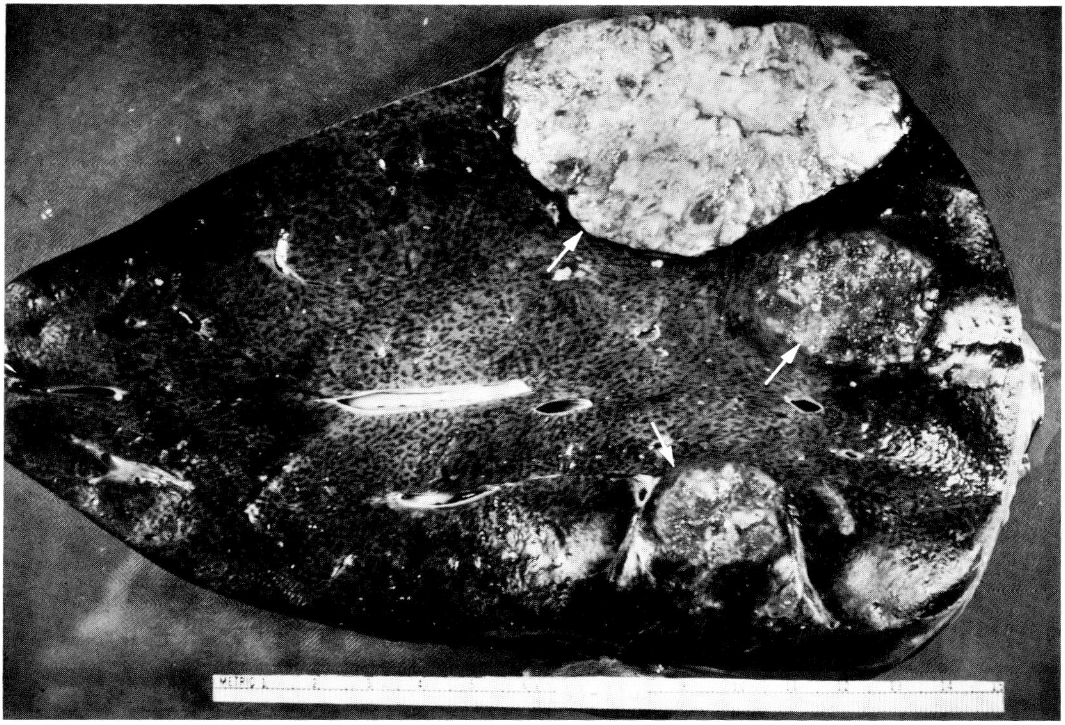

Figure 6-3. A cross section of liver from a patient with metastatic carcinoma from the colon. The vascular pattern in the liver is accentuated. The rounded masses (arrows) constitute nests of carcinoma cells arising from metastases distributed to the liver through the portal venous system.

gional lymph node is usually a grave prognostic sign indicating shorter patient survival. There are two reasons for this relationship: lymph node metastasis may indicate the more aggressive or malignant neoplasm; and it indicates a lesion that has already started to spread and may be widely disseminated.

C. Biology of the Neoplastic Cell

1. Chromosomal alterations

Since the neoplastic cell has a heritable defect, a study of the karyotypes of various tumors might reveal a distinctive lesion which directly results from or is

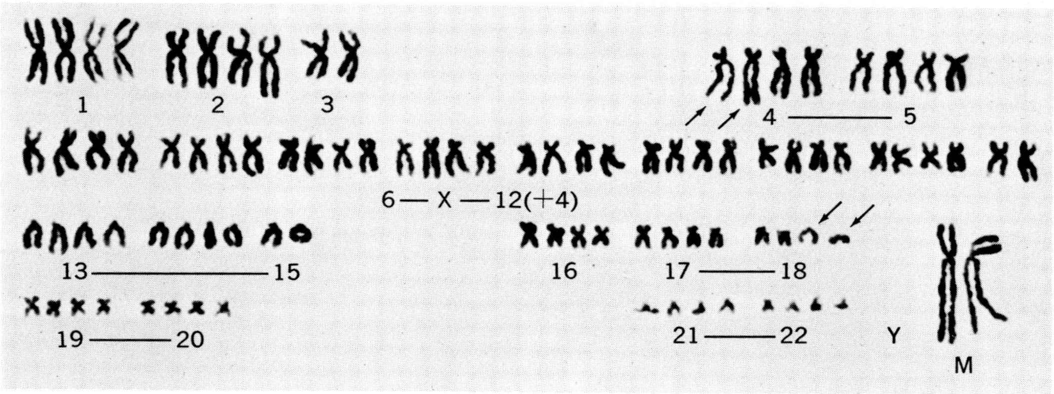

Figure 6-4. Karyotype from a lymph node cell in a patient with lymphoma. The cell is tetraploid with a total of 92 chromosomes. One extra abnormal chromosome is present as a pair (M). In addition, there are four additional chromosomes in group 6-7, loss of two no. 3 chromosomes, two group 13-15 chromosomes and two y chromosomes, and abnormalities of chromosomes in the 4-5 group and 17-18 group (arrows). Cells from some cancers show much more bizarre karyotypes than these. (Courtesy of Kajii, Neu, and Gardner, 1968).

the cause of the basic defect. With one remarkable exception, this does not appear to be the case.

It is true that virtually all malignant (and many benign) neoplasms show karyotypic abnormalities (Fig. 6-4). These cover a wide spectrum, including deletions, translocations, and more complex rearrangements in both aneuploid and euploid cells. No particular abnormality, with the one exception, seems to be associated with a particular type of neoplasm. Most neoplasms are aneuploid. Often more than one modal chromosome number is exhibited in a single lesion, although usually one mode predominates. A variety of abnormal chromosomes are frequently present. Occasional neoplasms, however, even some malignant ones, have perfectly normal chromosome complements, both by number and by quality, as far as present techniques reveal (Nowell, 1965).

The only exception we know of at present in which a specific chromosomal anomaly characterizes a particular type of neoplasm was discovered by Nowell and Hungerford. They found that in cases of chronic granulocytic leukemia, the neoplastic cells characteristically possess a small abnormal chromosome, the Philadelphia chromosome (Ph^1), apparently derived from a chromosome 21 through loss of approximately half of the longer arm (Fig. 6-5). This abnormality is limited to the leukemic cells and persists throughout the course of the disease, although additional karyotypic changes may be seen in the terminal phase. It has not been observed in other forms of leukemia nor in non-leukemic individuals. The significance of this chromosomal anomaly in chronic granulocytic leukemia remains unknown (Nowell, 1965).

In summary, although most neoplasms show chromosomal anomalies of one type or another, the usual lack of specific anomalies suggests that those that do exist may be a secondary result of mitotic events occurring during neoplastic growth. Thus, they probably have little etiologic significance but great importance in the process of neoplastic progression.

2. Neoplastic progression

It seems probable that no malignant neoplasm develops from the normal precursor tissue without intervening benign steps. The number of intervening steps is not definitely known and may be variable. Certainly, the length of time required to change patterns of differentiation and growth from normal to frankly malignant is highly variable. In some cases a benign neoplasm may develop which may never progress into a malignancy within the lifetime of the host animal. In other cases, transitory changes may occur in the progenitor cells which cannot be

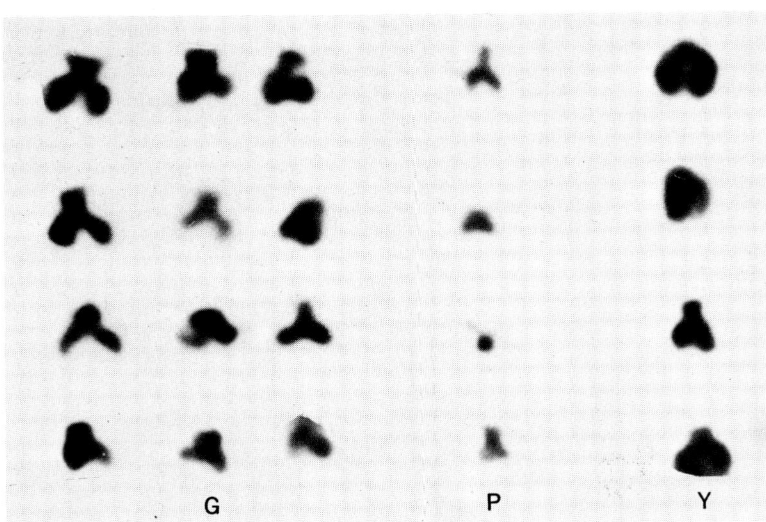

Figure 6-5. The Philadelphia chromosome. Normal chromosomes from group G and Y are compared with Philadelphia chromosomes from various patients with chronic granulocytic leukemia. (Courtesy of Richard L. Neu)

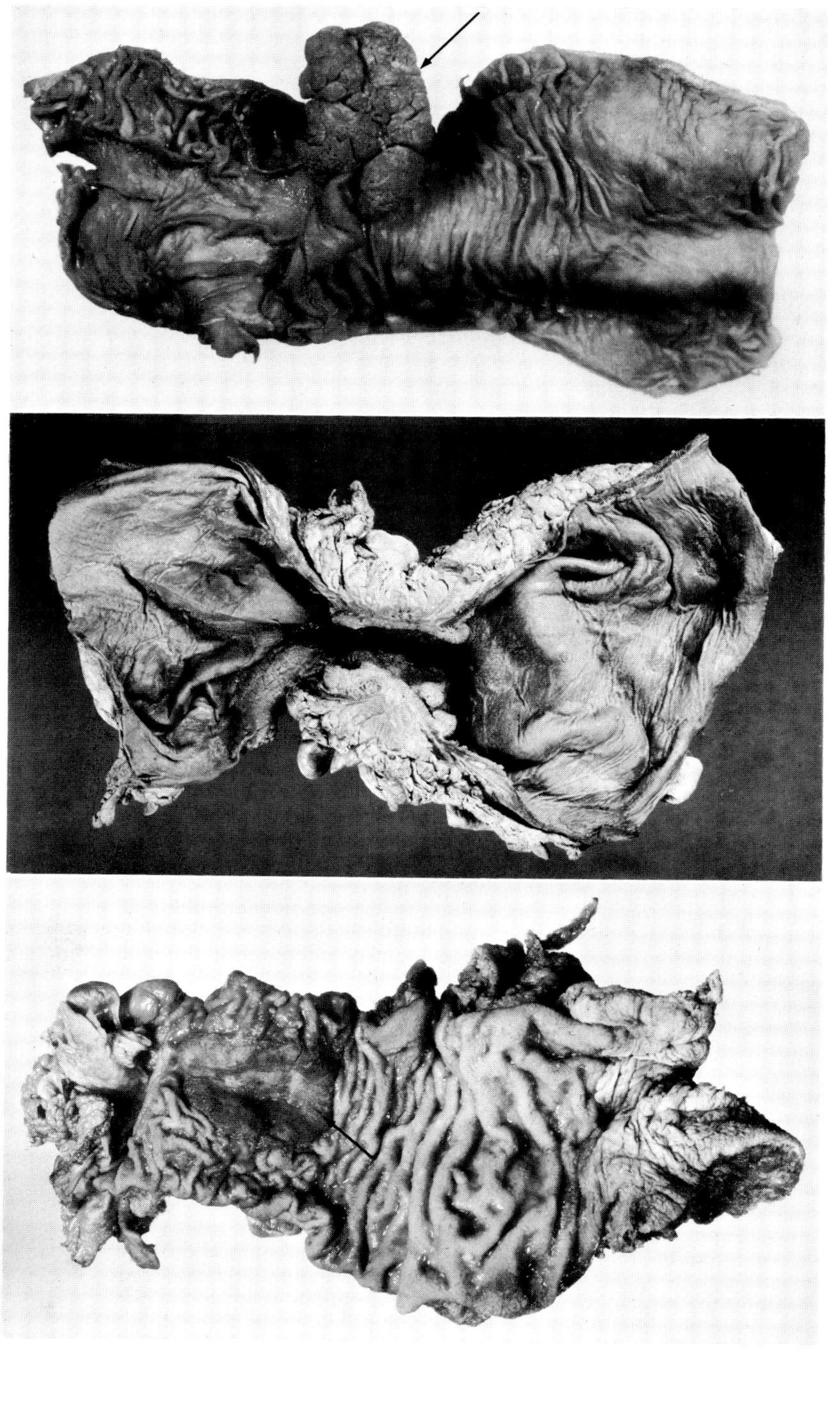

a

b

c

detected with our present tools until frank malignancy has appeared. It is probably safe to conclude that benign but aberrant phases precede the development of frank malignancy in most and perhaps all cases (Fig. 6-6a).

The change in the biologic attributes of the cells of a neoplasm over a period of time is termed *neoplastic progression.* Of course, most neoplasms are growing and spreading, but neither of these changes is an intrinsic part of progression—only the cellular changes per se are encompassed by the term (Foulds, 1954).

Just as the neoplasm begins as a result of heritable alterations in the involved cells, so too all of the varying attributes, morphological, biochemical, and behavioral, that in aggregate distinguish malignant from benign cells, are probably the result of progressive heritable alterations (Klein and Klein, 1957; Law, 1952; Patterson, *et al.,* 1969). There is a tendency for these varied attributes to behave in the manner of "randomly assorting" genetic characters. It is probable that in no two malignant neoplasms are the varied attributes assembled in identical proportions (Fig. 6-6b,c). Not only do neoplasms vary greatly from one to another, but even within a single lesion the variation from area to area may be great (Henderson and Rous, 1962). Therefore, when a neoplasm is graded histologically, the assessment must be made upon the basis of the most anaplastic microscopic field that can be found, for fields of this sort determine the malignant potential of the tumor.

The remarkable variation from area to area often seen in a single neoplasm may be a clonal phenomenon, i.e. each variant area may represent the progeny of a single deviant cell resulting from a relatively rare change analogous to, if not identical with, somatic mutation. It is possible, although it has been rigorously established in very few experimental systems, that all neoplastic progression may occur because of the random, chance appearance of clones of deviant cells and their subsequent amplification through the processes of natural selection (Klein and Klein, 1957).

If neoplastic progression occurs by the selection of randomly appearing, ever

Figure 6-6. a. An adenoma measuring approximately 2 cm in diameter (arrow) is attached to the mucosa of the large bowel by a stalk. Histologically, a section of this polypoid adenoma would be expected to bear resemblance to Figure 6-1a.

b. and **c.** Photographs of two carcinomas of the colon demonstrating varying growth patterns. In Figure 6-6b the tumor has taken on a "napkin ring" appearance. The tumor has completely encircled the bowel and caused stenosis with partial reduction of the lumen. In Figure 6-6c the tumor is an ulcerating tumor and has formed a small crater (arrows). Either of these tumors could give rise to metastatic lesions similar to those seen in Figure 6-3.

more deviant cells, is reverse progression (or perhaps it should be called retrogression) possible by a similar mechanism? It seems reasonable to suppose that a neoplastic cell population capable of giving rise to more malignant variants might also occasionally produce more normal variants. Variants of the latter type could not be observed unless the environment was such that they were not at their usual selective disadvantage. At present, this is little more than a speculation. However, some few neoplasms such as the Crown Gall of plants and the neuroblastoma of childhood seem able to resolve by becoming more normal or more differentiated. Perhaps this can be considered a form of reverse progression.

3. Biochemical features of progression

It is virtually axiomatic that the heritable alteration that produces a neoplastic cell has a biochemical basis. This biochemical basis has not yet been discovered although a number of hypotheses have been put forth.

The neoplastic cell possesses a number of characteristic biochemical features. Of most importance is *biochemical convergence,* extensively documented by Greenstein (Knox, 1967). The cells of each normal tissue type have a characteristic pattern of enzyme activity. Certain enzymes that are very active in kidney tissue have a low titer in liver and vice versa. In the neoplastic cell, these patterns tend to become less characteristic of the normal tissues of origin. A very malignant kidney cell neoplasm may be, in pattern of enzyme activity, more like a very malignant hepatocellular carcinoma than it is like normal kidney. There is a tendency for the varied normal patterns of enzyme activity to converge toward a common pattern in the more malignant lesions. This is simply the biochemical counterpart of the morphologic changes known as *anaplasia* which may prevent recognition of the site of origin of a neoplasm by its histologic features. The characteristic special features of a tissue give both morphologic and biochemical individuality. In the undifferentiated neoplasms these characteristics are much diminished.

Energy metabolism in relation to biochemical convergence has been investigated extensively since the observations of Warburg and his associates in the 1920's (Knox, 1967). Warburg established that the malignant cell has the capacity to produce large quantities of lactic acid from glucose and that this capacity is not markedly reduced in the presence of oxygen, i.e. the malignant cell exhibits an abnormally weak Pasteur effect. This high aerobic and anaerobic glycolysis was thought to be a characteristic of malignancies, but a number of exceptions, especially in well-differentiated neoplasms, has been described. A high anaerobic metabolism (usual range of 15-40 μl of lactic acid equivalent per milligram dry tissue per hour) is observed in most malignancies. With the exception of embryonic, placental, retinal, and cerebral cortical tissues, most normal tissues exhibit an anaerobic, glycolytic metabolism of only 10-20 per cent of that of most malignant neoplasms. In the presence of oxygen, glycolysis is reduced in malignant tissue to approximately 50 per cent of that observed anaerobically, while in most normal tissues glycolysis is nearly abolished in the presence of oxygen.

Warburg and his followers have argued that the degree of malignancy may be correlated with an increase in fermentation and a decrease in respiration, and that a defect in respiration is the root cause of the increased fermentation. Other investigators believe it would be accurate to state that the anaerobic glycolysis of malignancies is so high that a normal respiration and a normal Pasteur effect are incapable of reducing glycolysis to normal low levels. Despite much work by many investigators, the energy metabolism of neoplasia is still an area of considerable controversy primarily over two points: the role, if any, of defects in the respiratory apparatus in producing the usually high glycolytic activity of poorly differentiated neoplasms, and the basic significance of these metabolic abnormalities in the etiology of neoplasia.

Recently, a third biochemical characteristic of neoplasms has been described by Potter (1968). Using a series of rat hepatomas or hepatocellular carcinomas, he found that each neoplasm had a pattern of enzyme activity different from normal liver and characteristic of that individual lesion. The striking discovery was that the level of activity of any particular enzyme was much more invariable in the neoplasm, in the face of diurnal cycles or environmental stresses of various types, than in normal liver. The normal liver could adapt its enzyme levels to suit conditions; the neoplasms had less flexibility. All of the different stable levels of various enzymes in the various neoplasms were encompassed by the range of levels that could be produced in normal liver—but the levels in normal liver were much more easily varied. Pitot (1968) has advanced data to suggest that the varied levels of enzyme activity may be due not to variations in production of specific messenger RNA's, but to alterations in their stabilities or in the efficiency of translation of the particular message into protein. It seems that a crucial step in enzyme synthesis, probably that of translation, tends in the neoplasm to lose its normal regulatory flexibility.

In the previous sections it has been noted that neoplasms, once formed, tend to lose their specialized, differentiated characteristics. In terms of enzyme levels, however, the cells of the neoplasm seem to be more rigid, less adaptable, and thus perhaps in a sense more specialized than are the normal cells of origin. Perhaps they should really be considered superdifferentiated.

4. Inappropriate cell products

Malignant neoplasms, as we have seen, exhibit a loss or diminution of specialized products or functions. Thus a highly malignant carcinoma of the epidermis may make little or no keratin, or a rhabdomyosarcoma may make little myosin. However, in recent years, it has become apparent that many neoplasms may acquire to some extent the capacity to make products typical of a completely different organ or tissue. For example, some bronchogenic carcinomas make insulin. Inappropriate hormone production has been described in a variety of other neoplasms (Lebovitz, 1965). The organ-specific cellular antigens identified by heteroantibody may also be inappropriate (Olenov and Fel, 1968). Tumor cells are characteristically deficient in these normal antigens, but often there is also an apparent replacement with other antigens. A kidney carcinoma, for example, may be found to possess antigens characteristic of liver. In addition to acquiring inappropriate antigens characteristic of another organ, tumor cells acquire antigens that are not found in any other adult tissue. (These tumor-specific antigens will be discussed in some detail in the section on *Immunity*). Thus, in malignancy, differentiation is not only deficient but it may be abnormal as to type. It has been pointed out that each somatic cell, of whatever organ, supposedly possesses all of the genetic information contained in the egg cell itself. In malignancy, some of that information which is normally inactive is utilized in bizarre and unpredictable ways.

5. Dependency

Neoplasia may occur in organs or tissues that are undergoing physiologic hyperplasia. The early neoplasm, arising in such an area, is often composed of very benign cells that deviate only minimally from their normal counterparts. Like their normal counterparts but perhaps to a lesser degree, they may require a continued exogenous stimulus to continue the hyperplasia. It should be recalled that the definitions of neoplastic hyperplasia emphasized that the condition must be due, *at least in part,* to a heritable defect in the cells. In many early lesions that have undergone little progression, the heritable alteration is insufficient to maintain the hyperplastic state in the absence of a stimulus to ordinary physiologic hyperplasia. These lesions, although neoplastic, are thus *dependent* upon the exogenous stimulus. An excellent example is provided by some carcinomas of the breast (Boyland, 1961). Normal breast epithelium undergoes physiologic hyperplasia in rhythmic fashion during the estrus or menstrual cycle. Estrogens are particularly important as a hormonal stimulus. It is not surprising, therefore, that many breast carcinomas, especially relatively early in their natural histories, are dependent upon estrogen for their continued growth. They will undergo regression if this hormone is removed by ovariectomy, but with further progression the carcinomas lose this dependency. Similarly, ovarian neoplasms may be dependent upon gonadotrophins, thyroid neoplasms upon thyrotropin, etc. Although the term *dependency* is usually applied only to hormonal dependency, other types not so easily recognized undoubtedly exist in a variety of early neoplasms (Boyland, 1961).

A somewhat different form of dependency found in some neoplasms is of particular current interest because of its possible importance in therapy. This is dependence upon asparagine. Normal cells do not require exogenous asparagine for their growth and well-being. However, some neoplastic cells cannot grow without an exogenous supply. Such neoplasms may be treated by systemic administration of the enzyme asparaginase. This can effectively deprive the neoplastic cells of their required asparagine supply without harming most normal cells. It remains to be determined how many human neoplasms will prove to be dependent upon asparagine and for how long (Boyse *et al.*, 1967).

6. Growth in vitro

Neoplastic cells have certain behavioral characteristics *in vitro* that tend to distinguish them from their normal precursors. Most of these characteristics are the *in vitro* counterparts of behavioral features seen *in vivo*, but they are sufficiently distinctive to require special note. As is the case with *in vivo* characteristics, no single *in vitro* property is an absolute criterion either for neoplasia or for degree of malignancy.

One fairly general property of neoplastic cells is decrease of so-called contact inhibition of movement (Fig. 6-7). Many types of normal cells tend to be inhibited in their tendency to overlap other cells of the same type. They therefore tend to form monolayers over the bottom of a culture dish. Neoplastic cells are less inhibited by cell-to-cell contact and tend to crawl over one another to produce layers of randomly oriented cells. This property has been used to detect colonies of neoplastically transformed cells in cultures (Castor, 1968).

Another *in vitro* property which tends to distinguish the neoplastic cell from its normal counterpart is the ability to grow in very soft agar. Most normal cells, with the exception of hematopoietic cells, seem to require a firm substrate upon which to initiate growth. Many but not all neoplastic cells are able to initiate growth without a solid substrate (Stoker, 1968).

Perhaps the most important distinguishing characteristic is that neoplastic cells will proliferate *ad infinitum* under proper culture conditions. Normal cell

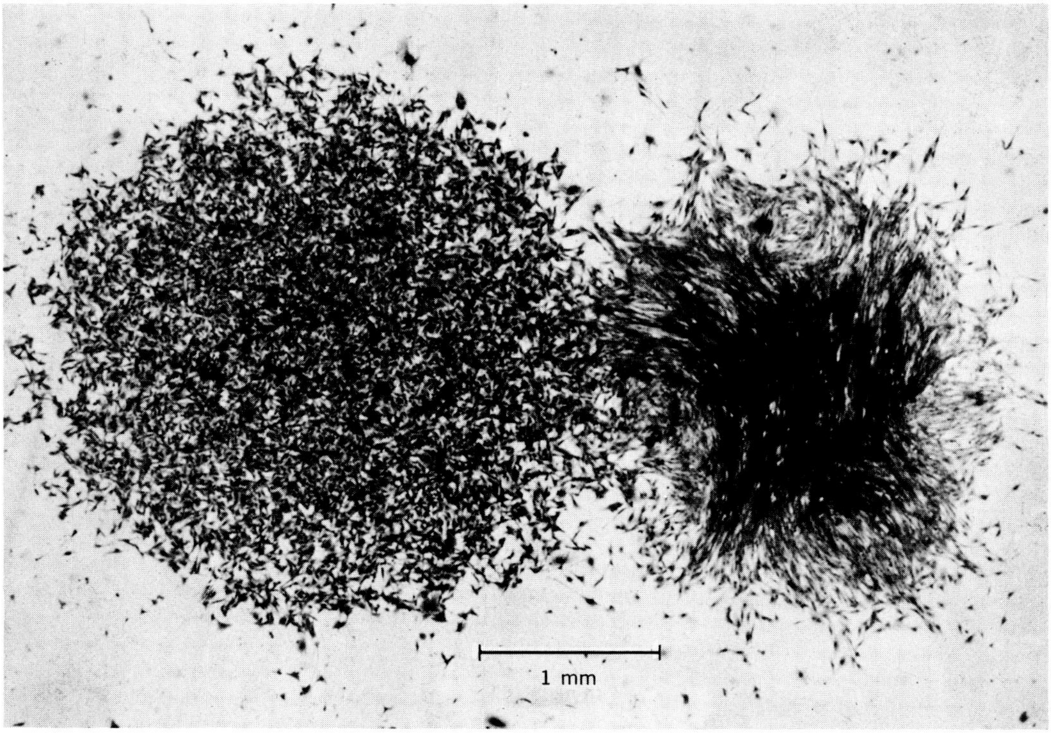

Figure 6-7. Hamster fibroblast cells in culture. The colony on the right has the normal configuration with cells lined up in parallel sheafs. On the left is a colony of malignant cells derived from the same explant after transformation by Rous sarcoma virus; the cells have a haphazard orientation and grow more widely. (Courtesy of MacPherson, 1965)

strains, in contrast, appear to have a finite lifespan characteristic of the cell type and species. This very important attribute does not seem to be a function of the culture conditions but rather an innate property of the cells themselves (Hayflick and Moorhead, 1961).

This finite lifespan of races of normal cells can also be demonstrated *in vivo.* Hematopoietic tissues can be serially transplanted in mice if the recipient mice have been depleted of blood-forming cells by lethal doses of X-irradiation. The transplanted bone-marrow cells will proliferate and replenish the marrow and spleen of the recipient. Serial transplantation can in this way be accomplished four to six times, but the cells will not multiply further. In contrast, leukemic cells exhibit no such exhaustion.

Likewise, a small fragment of mouse mammary ductal epithelium can be transplanted in suitably prepared recipient mice and proliferate into a normal-appearing ductal tree. This can be done serially but apparently only for a limited time before the cells lose their growth potential. Mammary carcinoma, on the other hand, can be transplanted indefinitely.

Thus, both *in vitro* and *in vivo* neoplastic cell lines seem to be immortal while normal somatic cell strains have a limited potential, perhaps related to the normal life-span of the animal.

D. Host Reactions

1. The stroma

The growth of most neoplasms is dependent upon an adequate, supporting connective-tissue stroma and blood supply (Fig. 6-8). These are normal tissues of the host that are induced to proliferate by the neoplasm. Most neoplasms cannot grow faster than the supporting vascular system. Many malignancies undergo extensive necrosis because they outgrow their blood supply or because the mechanical pressure of the tumor interferes with blood flow. The factors involved in the elicitation of a stroma and blood supply by the neoplasm are not known but are undoubtedly similar to those operative in normal tissues. Among experimental animal tumors there is great variation in the speed with which newly transplanted tumor fragments elicit a blood supply (Day, 1964).

The vascular system in malignancies is often abnormal. Rather than by a typical capillary bed, the tumor is sometimes supplied by a system of large thin-walled vascular sinuses. Blood flow is typically sluggish and gas exchange is inefficient. (Perhaps this is why neoplasms tend to develop a high anaerobic glycolysis.) The pH of the intercellular milieu is abnormally low. The vascular sinuses are fragile, and anoxia due to a temporary fall in blood pressure can produce extensive intratumoral hemorrhage.

Although most malignancies are supplied with a blood vascular network, induced stroma frequently lacks nerves and lymphatics. However, there appears to be a variation from tumor to tumor, some tumors being supplied with nerves or lymphatics or both. Also, the fact that the so-called nerve growth factor was first isolated from mouse sarcoma indicates that at least some tumors may stimulate nerve growth.

Certain malignancies, particularly scirrhous carcinomas of the human breast, stimulate an extensive desmoplastic reaction. Indeed, the fibrous connective tissue

a

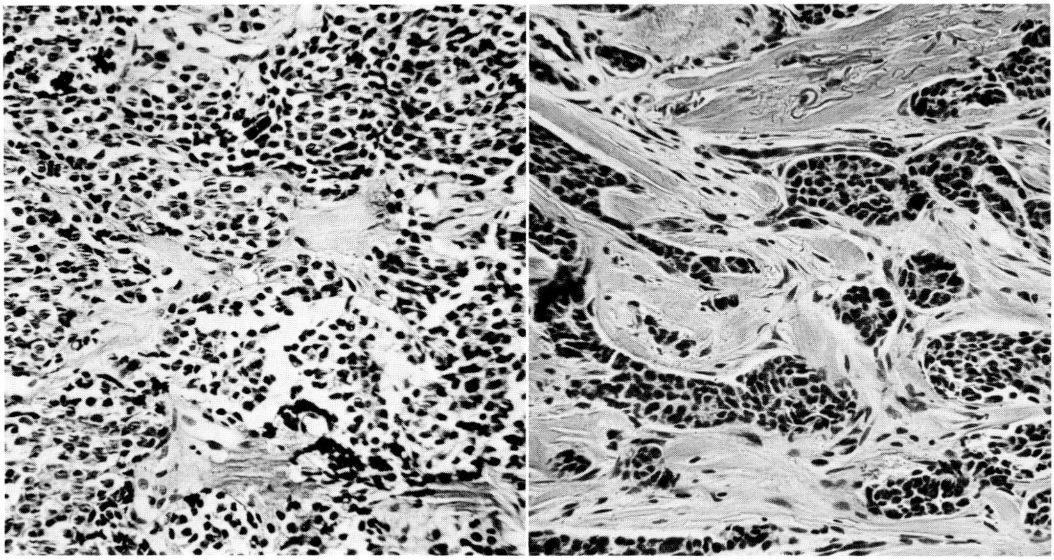

Figure 6-8. **a.** Photomicrographs of metastatic carcinoma of the prostate. The cells with dense small nuclei, mainly scattered in nests, are the carcinoma cells. Intermingled with these are delicate bands of fibrous stroma, which tend to separate the individual nests of tumor cells. Similar stroma is seen in Figure 6-1. In this stroma runs the vascular network which feeds and drains the tumor.

b. In this example of scirrhous adenocarcinoma of the breast, the stroma is very dense with large quantities of collagen. The cancerous epithelium is reduced to relatively small nests scattered in the stroma.

may constitute a much larger part of the gross tumor than do the neoplastic cells (Fig. 6-8b). Again, the chemical or physiologic basis of this reaction is not known.

Perhaps related to the qualitative abnormalities of the blood vascular supply is a characteristic abnormality in the inflammatory process. It has been observed in a number of experimental animal tumors that stimuli, such as foreign bodies placed within the neoplasms, fail to produce inflammation (Mahoney and Leighton, 1962). This interesting abnormality has not been further investigated and its basis is completely unknown. It may be a very important factor in the tendency of some tumors to become infected with bacterial agents and to harbor these agents chronically.

2. Physiologic effects

The most important physiologic effect of malignant neoplasia on the host animal is the production of cachexia. In the human being, weight loss is often one of the earliest symptoms of malignant disease. While it is found that the energy requirements of a tumor-bearing animal are greater than normal and that at the same time its dietary intake is usually reduced, these facts do not seem to account completely for the cachexia. A tumor appears to be a "nitrogen trap." A high nitrogen consumption in the diet appears beneficial in counteracting the effects of the neoplasm, which can be considered as a large parasite diverting amino acids from the metabolic pool for its own use.

Many malignancies have other widespread effects on the host animal apart from those of purely mechanical nature. One quite general effect in experimental animals is depression of liver catalase activity. This is not usually seen in human cancer, probably because the human neoplasms seldom reach the proportionate sizes seen in rodents. Anemia is a frequent feature of neoplastic disease even in the absence of bone-marrow replacement by the tumor. Not much is known about the basis of these effects although some workers have described possible toxic agents released by the tumor and have given these the name *toxohormone* (Nakahara, 1960).

3. Immunity

Many neoplastic cells are so sufficiently different in their surface characteristics from any normal cell that they are regarded as foreign by the host's immunologic mechanism. Thus, the level of host immunity is of vital importance in the biology of neoplasia. It is only recently that a mass of experimental data has overthrown the widely held view that immunity against neoplasia is theoretically impossible—the view that the neoplastic cell, as part of the "self," could not be the target of an immune reaction. Evidence now available suggests that most incipient neoplasms may be suppressed by an immune reaction before they reach macroscopic size. Clinical neoplasia, as seen by the physician, may well represent the remaining small minority of lesions that for one reason or another escape this defense (Klein, 1968a, 1968b).

The evidence for the importance of immunity is mainly of two types: (1) the demonstration that animals can be immunized using tumor tissue as antigen so that the growth of tumor transplants is markedly inhibited or prevented; and (2) the correlation between altered immunologic reactivity and the incidence of neoplasia under the altered conditions.

Experiments to demonstrate the antigenicity of tumor tissue and the anti-tumor effects of induced immunity are usually performed in inbred mice. Since all of the mice of a particular inbred strain are virtually identical genetically, it is possible to transplant normal or neoplastic tissues from one animal to another without encountering any immunity of the homograft type, i.e. immunity aroused by antigenic differences among the animals. Consequently, when an animal of such an inbred strain is inoculated with a suspension of killed tumor cells obtained from another animal of that same strain, the immunity to a subsequent inoculation of living tumor cells must be directed against tumor-specific antigens, i.e. antigens peculiar to the tumor and not shared with the normal tissues of the animal in which the tumor originated. This type of experiment is most conveniently carried out by transplanting tumor tissue from one mouse to another within the inbred strain. However, by means of immunization, immunity can be increased in the very animal in which the tumor first appeared, thus obviating even the slightest possibility that the immunity might not be directed against tumor-specific antigens. The growth of a neoplasm in its primary host may not always stimulate the maximum possible immunity in that animal (Klein, 1968a, 1968b).

The tumor-specific antigens that induce immunity to tumor growth are apparently located on the cell surface. They seem very similar to the homograft antigens that distinguish different, non-inbred animals of the same species. Thus far, their exact chemical nature is unknown, since efforts to extract them from the cell result in diminished antigenicity.

Tumor antigens frequently are characteristic of a specific tumor, and cross-reactivity cannot be demonstrated with antibodies to similar tumors in other animals, even when the two tumors are produced by the same stimulus in the same species. This is particularly true of tumors produced by chemical or physical agents. By contrast, many neoplasms produced by given virus will cross-react with antibodies to other tumors produced by the same virus. This makes it theoretically possible to immunize against tumors caused by a particular virus (Klein, 1968a, 1968b; Prehn, 1968).

Antigenic strength on the tumor cell surface varies greatly. Thus, some experimentally induced tumors immunize against themselves very well, others only slightly, if at all. In general, it seems that those neoplasms induced rapidly after an oncogenic stimulus, whether chemical, physical, or viral, tend to be highly antigenic in contrast to those with long latent periods. However, some etiologic agents tend to produce more or less antigenic neoplasms independent of variations in latent period. Within a single neoplasm there may be variation in antigenic titer among the cells. Consequently, immunoselection during tumor growth may gradually produce a progressively less antigenic neoplasm. While immunoselection has been convincingly demonstrated among chemically induced neoplasms, some viral neoplasms may be relatively resistant to this process.

Unfortunately, those animal neoplasms that occur spontaneously in low incidence seem to have little or no antigenicity. Perhaps it is owing to this fact that they escaped an immune reaction and were not suppressed in their incipiency. Neoplasms induced rapidly by chemicals or viruses escape not only because of their rapid growth but because the chemical oncogens, and perhaps some viral oncogens as well, seriously depress immune reactivity. (This subject will be discussed again in the section on etiology.) Furthermore, some neoplasms may induce a state of partial specific immunologic tolerance to the tumor cell antigens.

The immunity that is aroused by the tumor-specific antigens is mediated by lymphocytes and is thus analogous to delayed hypersensitivity. Except in the case of lymphomas, there is little evidence that circulating antibody participates in the suppression of tumor cells. In fact, there is much evidence that high levels of antibody may often make a tumor grow better. Somehow, the humoral antibody protects the tumor cells from the cell-associated type of immune reaction, a process called *tumor enhancement*. Some tumors are much more enhanceable than others. For this reason, if for no other, attempts at immunotherapy of tumors in man must be approached with the greatest circumspection.

Although all of the foregoing evidence concerning the antigenicity of neoplastic cells comes from animal studies, there is some evidence to suggest that human neoplasms have similar properties. Probably most suggestive is the histologic evidence. Many human neoplasms show a heavy lymphoid infiltration in and around the lesion. This is apt, especially in skin neoplasia, to be most prominent at about the time in tumor progression when invasion of surrounding tissues is commencing. Later lesions usually show a less prominent lymphoid reaction. This lymphoid reaction is very suggestive of the type of reaction seen in experimental neoplasms that have aroused an immune reaction. In human breast carcinoma, there is convincing evidence that a heavy lymphocytic reaction is associated with a relatively favorable prognosis. Evidence of a so-called sinus histiocytosis in the regional lymph nodes also suggests a good prognosis. Sinus histiocytosis probably reflects prolonged reaction to an antigenic stimulus.

Direct experimental evidence of tumor antigenicity in man is meager, though there have been a number of suggestive reports. The ethical difficulties in experimental manipulation severely limit progress in this area. Recently, however, this has been circumvented by a variety of *in vitro* techniques. It has been possible by immunofluorescence techniques to demonstrate an apparently common tumor antigen among cases of human melanosarcoma (Morton *et al.*, 1968). Another technique involves growing both tumor and lymphoid cells from the same patient in tissue culture. By this means an immune reaction of the lymphocytes, directed against a number of different tumors, can be demonstrated, while homologous (i.e. foreign) lymphoid cells usually fail to react or show a slower response (Hellstrom *et al.,* 1968).

The second basic approach to the study of the importance of immunity, namely, the correlation between alterations in immune capacity and susceptibility to neoplasia, has been explored extensively in mice and to some extent in man. In mice, immune capability can be reduced by neonatal thymectomy. Adult thymectomy combined with radiation can also produce immunologic deficiency. Either procedure leads to increased susceptibility of tumorigenesis.

In addition to showing that a decreased immune capacity increases susceptibility to oncogenesis, it has also been possible to demonstrate the converse: to increase resistance by non-specific stimulation of immune mechanisms. Administration of a derivative of B.C.G. has been shown to stimulate a variety of immune responses in mice and to inhibit mouse mammary tumor formation and skin papilloma development.

In the human, it has been observed that a variety of clinical syndromes known to be asociated with diminished immunologic capacity have predisposed to neoplasia, usually some form of lymphoma. Most striking is the development of neoplasia in kidney transplant recipients who have been maintained for long periods on immunosuppressive drugs.

A final link between alteration in immunocompetence and the development of neoplasia is suggested by the fact that the increasing incidence of neoplasia with advancing age is paralleled by age-associated lymphoid atrophy and a decline in general immunocompetence.

E. Etiologic Mechanisms

1. Threshold concepts

Since the fundamental molecular defect in the cancer cell is not yet known, a discussion of etiology must be confined to mere descriptions of environmental and genetic factors and to speculations concerning the precise details of how they work. Research on etiology has suffered, not from a dearth of etiologic factors, but from a plethora. Commonly, very diverse factors have an additive effect in tumor production so that it is incorrect to speak of the cause of any cancer. *Cancer is a multifactorial disease* (Heston, 1945).

This multifactorial etiology has perhaps been most clearly elucidated in the study of breast cancer of the mouse. The general principle applies, however, in varying degree to all neoplasms.

Historically, breast cancer in the mouse was considered a genetic disease because, by selective breeding, it was possible to obtain inbred strains with varying incidences of the disease, from virtually 0-100 per cent. In the 1930's, however, a series of studies at the Jackson Memorial Laboratory at Bar Harbor, Maine, under the general direction of C. C. Little, established that an "extrachromosomal factor" was also involved. In these experiments, reciprocal crosses between low and high tumor strains were bred, and then the mammary tumor incidences in the resulting two series of F_1 hybrids were compared. It was found that F_1 mice derived from the cross between high-tumor-strain females and low-tumor-strain males had a much higher tumor incidence than F_1 mice derived from the reciprocal cross between low-tumor-strain females and high-tumor-strain males. Since the genotypes of the F_1 mice of both series were identical, some non-genetic or extrachromosomal factor associated with a high-tumor-strain mother must have been involved. Three possibilities, not mutually exclusive, were considered:

1) the factor could be transmitted in the ovum of the high-tumor-strain female.
2) it could be transmitted across the placenta to the young.
3) it was present in and transmitted by the milk.

A further series of experiments using foster nursing established that the extrachromosomal factor was in the milk. If mice nursed upon high-tumor-strain mothers, their mammary tumor incidence in later life was high; conversely, the incidence was low if *all* the nursing was on a low-tumor-strain mother. Subsequent studies showed that the factor was an RNA-containing virus. Despite the importance of this virus, however, the genotype of the nursing mouse remained of great importance.

In the male mouse the mammary gland is rudimentary. Despite a favorable genotype and the presence of the milk agent, mammary cancer in the male is very rare. However, it can be brought up to the same level as in the female by the chronic administration of estrogens or prolactin. Conversely, the female ovariectomized in early life usually fails to develop tumors. Thus, not only are genotype and milk agent important, but estrogen is also an etiologic agent.

No one of these factors is of predominant importance in mouse breast cancer. Tumors occur in the absence of the milk agent if the hormonal stimulation and genotype are very favorable. In the presence of the milk agent, the other factors need be much less optimal. A variety of factors acting in conjunction must reach a certain threshold if a tumor is to occur.

There is no evidence that human breast cancer involves a milk agent, althought this possibility cannot be completely ruled out. The importance of the mouse system lies rather in its demonstration of the threshold concept. In the discussion that follows, various specific etiologic agents will be described. Although the threshold principle may not be reiterated in each case, it should be remembered that no one of the agents discussed can be considered *the* cause of any one neoplasm.

2. Oncogenic viruses

It seems certain that very soon a human malignancy will, for the first time, be proven to have a viral etiology. There are two leading candidates–the Burkitt lymphoma and carcinoma of the uterine cervix. The Burkitt lymphoma is predominantly a childhood disease prevalent in Central Africa. Its geographical distribution has strongly suggested transmission, possibly by an insect vector. Alternatively, malarial infection may alter the susceptibility to an oncogenic virus. Recently, immunologic studies have suggested a tumor antigen common to most cases and capable of inducing an antibody response. Herpes-type viruses have been implicated as the possible viral etiologic agents of both Burkitt's lymphoma and the supposedly quite unrelated disease, infectious mononucleosis (Henle *et al.,* 1968). The latter disease is a contagious, self-limiting, febrile illness often seen among young adults.

Whether Burkitt lymphoma and infectious mononucleosis are ever conclusively shown to have a common viral etiology, the fact that a single viral species can produce such very disparate types of disease is well established. Thus, Duran-Reynals (1950) showed that the Rous chicken sarcoma virus could produce either a hemorrhagic and inflammatory disease in young chickens or sarcomas in older ones, depending entirely upon the age and immunologic capacities of the birds at the time of virus injection. His work suggested that this particular oncogenic virus would only produce tumors if there was a moderate degree of immunologic resistance to the virus. If resistance were very low, the hemorrhagic disease occurred; if it were high, no infection was established or the tumors were only transient (Duran-Reynals, 1950).

The other leading candidate for a viral etiology, carcinoma of the cervix, has long been thought to be correlated with coitus and particularly coitus with uncircumcised males. Thus, the incidence of the disease is low among nuns and Jewish women. Only recently, epidemiologic studies have shown that it is not coitus *per se* that correlated with the incidence, but the number of *different* coital partners. The greater the number of different coital partners, the greater the pos-

Table 6-1 Best-Known Oncogenic Viruses

DNA	RNA
1. Polyoma	1. Murine leukemia viruses
2. Shope papilloma	2. Avian leukosis viruses
3. Simian virus 40	3. Rous sarcoma virus
4. Shope fibroma	4. Mouse mammary tumor viruses
5. Human adenoviruses (tumors in hamsters)	
6. Lucké frog kidney carcinoma	

sibility of carcinoma of the cervix. This fact strongly suggests that this disease is venereal and caused by an agent probably transmitted by some uncircumcised males. Again, a Herpes virus (not the same type found in so-called fever blisters) has been isolated from a high percentage of cases. Only time and more research will establish whether or not this is actually a causative agent.

In any case, it is virtually certain that many human neoplasms must have a viral cause. The viral etiology of many animal cancers has now been demonstrated and it is inconceivable that man might be unique in this regard (Eckhart, 1968).

The known animal oncogenic viruses can be divided into two major categories, RNA viruses and DNA viruses. The names of some of these are listed in Table 6-1. Many more will undoubtedly be discovered. These viruses will not be discussed in detail but rather a few examples will be discussed sufficiently to illustrate general principles.

The Rous sarcoma virus, which has already been mentioned, is the most thoroughly studied of the RNA viruses. In 1967, Peyton Rous of the Rockefeller University received the Nobel Prize, in large part for his discovery of this virus in 1910. As this long lag suggests, the viral theory of cancer is more popular now than it was then. In fact, at that time there was much opposition to accepting a chicken tumor as a "true" cancer. The very fact that it was caused by a transmissible agent was considered proof of its dubious qualifications.

Like other RNA viruses, the Rous virus particle is completed by budding from the surface of an infected cell, the viral coat being formed in the cell wall. Evidence now suggests that some strains of the virus are ordinarily "defective" in that they are unable to form a protein coat and replicate without help from another closely related virus, a "helper" virus. The defective Rous virus can produce neoplastic "transformation" of infected cells, i.e. it can somehow produce a neoplastic alteration. However, it cannot replicate itself without help. The viral genome remains in the neoplastic but non-viral-releasing cells as is proven by the fact that infectious virus can be "rescued" by superinfection with the helper (Rubin, 1964).

In the case of the DNA viruses, viral replication and release from infected cells is associated with cell lysis. Neoplastically transformed cells do not release virus. Why certain cells undergo only this abortive type of infection is unknown. Apparently, in some way the conditions in transformed infected cells are "defective" for viral replication (Dulbecco, 1966).

When cells in tissue culture are exposed to DNA viruses, it is found that only a small fraction of the cells actually undergo visible transformation. Also, this small fraction will not grow to produce a neoplasm when inoculated into appropriate animals. Further changes must first take place (a form of progression?) before the cells are sufficiently transformed. In all probability, the virus does no more than trigger the start of the process. Although a variety of studies demonstrate that virally coded messenger RNA is continually made in the transformed cells, the function of this RNA is unknown. Very early in cell infection, whether the infection be of a replicative and destructive or of an abortive and transforming type, a new antigen (so-called T or tumor antigen) is detectable in the nucleus of the cell. This antigen is probably coded for by the viral genome and thus serves as a marker for the continued presence of the virus. It is only later and presumably only in transformed cells that the "transplantation" antigen is formed on the cell surface. This latter antigen arouses host resistance to the tumor cells. Whether or not the genetic information specifying this antigen is contained in the viral or the cellular genome is not yet definitely known. Recent work, however, suggests that the surface antigen is probably specified by a cellular gene. The form of the viral DNA inside the transformed cell is also not clear but it is probable that it is integrated into the cellular genome.

It has already been pointed out that a number of host variables can determine the type of response to a virus. For example, it has been found that a number of human adenoviruses are capable of producing neoplasms in newborn hamsters. There is no evidence that these viruses are oncogenic in their natural host, man, although this remains a possibility. It is entirely possible that any virus could be oncogenic given the right type of host cell and suitable conditions. Also, many supposedly non-oncogenic viruses can potentiate the action of chemical agents that are themselves only weakly oncogenic or that are applied in suboncogenic doses.

It might be thought that the problem of whether a particular animal tumor is of viral etiology could be simply solved by analysis of the surface transplantation antigens. However, this is not the case. Although the known virally induced tumors are typically characterized by cross-reacting surface antigens induced by that particular virus, tumors of non-viral etiology may acquire cross-reacting antigens by virtue of infection with a passenger virus—one that had nothing to do with the initial transformation. Furthermore, if a neoplasm is caused by a virus that is ubiquitous in the animal population so that all the animals are infected at an early age, they may be rendered immunologically tolerant to both viral antigens per se and to virally induced cellular antigens. Under these conditions the cross-reacting surface antigen produced by the action of the virus will not produce an immune reaction in the animals and may be undetectable.

Whether a particular neoplasm involves a viral etiologic agent cannot be determined merely by the isolation of a virus from the lesion or its visualization by the electron microscope. Viruses are apparently quite ubiquitous in nature and mere passenger viruses unrelated to a tumor's etiology are commonly present in tumor tissue. Conversely, failure to isolate or visualize a virus hardly argues at all against a viral etiology, since viruses may disappear temporarily or permanently in a number of experimental virus-induced tumors. Considering these difficulties and the lack of persistent virus production in neoplasms of known viral etiology, it is probably not surprising that, more than half a century after discovery of the first oncogenic virus, viral malignancy in man is yet to be definitely identified.

3. Chemical agents

In the nearly two hundred years since the classical observation of Percival Pott that chimney sweeps were "peculiarly liable" to cancer of the scrotum, hundreds of chemical oncogens of a variety of types have been identified. Almost all of these have been found within the last half century. Although it was evident that the oncogenic factor in chimney sweeps' cancer was to be found in soot, this factor could not be isolated and identified for nearly a century and a half for the simple reason that, despite numerous attempts, tumors in experimental animals could not be produced with soots and coal tars. It was not until 1915 when Yamagiwa and Ichikawa had the patience to continue painting rabbits' ears with coal tar every two or three days for over a year that cancers were induced. Once an assay was available, the crude material could be fractionated and the active chemicals identified. In 1930, Kennaway and his associates isolated and identified the first known chemical oncogen. This was dibenz(a,h)anthracene, a polycyclic aromatic hydrocarbon with the formula:

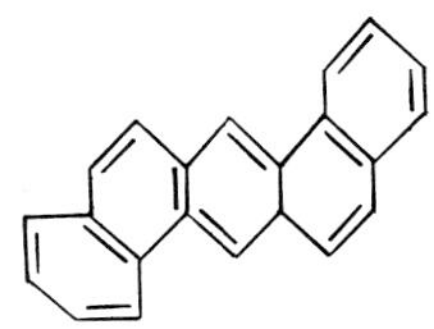

Numerous other somewhat similar agents were soon identified and made available for study. Some are remarkably powerful; microgram amounts are sufficient to produce skin cancers rapidly when applied topically to suitable animals. Chemically, these aromatic substances are fat-soluble. They often have a superficial resemblance to some of the steroids. For example, 3-methylcholanthrene, one of the most powerful, actually has some estrogenic activity. Whether or not these resemblances are of biologic significance is still not known. To this day, the aromatic polycyclic hydrocarbons are among the best studied but least understood of oncogenic agents.

These hydrocarbons are general oncogens, i.e. they can produce tumors locally in virtually any tissue to which they are applied or which they can reach. Adult liver is a notable exception, apparently because liver contains the necessary enzymes to convert the hydrocarbon to an inactive metabolite.

Some oncogens attack a much more restricted range of tissues and characteristically produce tumors at remote sites instead of the site of application. In general, if the chemical must be metabolized in a special way in order to serve as an oncogen, the range of susceptible target tissues may be reduced. A striking example concerns certain aromatic amines, especially 2-naphthylamine, which, when absorbed through the skin or inhaled by industrial workers in the dye industry, produce cancers primarily of the urinary bladder epithelium. Apparently, the aromatic amines are inactive as such and require conversion *in vivo* into a *proximate* oncogen. N-hydroxylation to the N-hydroxy derivative, which can be performed by bladder epithelium, has been shown to be a necessary metabolic step. Synthetically prepared N-hydroxy derivative is better able to produce tumors locally at a subcutaneous site of application than is the parent compound (Miller and Miller, 1969).

There is little point in discussing in detail the features of the vast variety of compounds that have some degree of oncogenic activity, although, as industrial hazards or contaminants of foodstuffs, many of them have considerable practical importance. It is almost certain that our environment, as it is progressively altered by technology, harbors more and more oncogens (Wogan, 1969).

Among the environmental oncogenic hazards, two have aroused sufficient interest in recent years to deserve special mention. In 1795, Soemmerring first noted the association between chronic pipe smoking and cancer of the lip, but only in the past two decades have the dangers of tobacco been widely recognized. The epidemiologic evidence now clearly implicates tobacco smoking, especially of cigarettes, in the causation of the growing pandemic of bronchogenic, squamous lung cancer. Tobacco probably also plays a role in the causation of cancer of the oral cavity and larynx, and possibly of the esophagus, kidney, and urinary bladder. The exact chemical oncogens in cigarettes and their interplay with other factors have not yet been elucidated.

Two widely separated epizootics in 1961 drew attention to another environmental oncogenic hazard. Hepatotoxicity due to ingestion of peanut meal killed thousands of turkey poults, ducklings, and chicks in England. Simultaneously, in the Pacific Northwest, trout hatcheries were plagued by an epidemic of hepatomas among the fish, which was also traced to the feed. It was soon determined that both conditions were due to contamination of the feed by the common fungus *Aspergillus flavus*. Four related compounds, all aflatoxins, were isolated from the contaminated feed. These, on a molar basis, are by far the most active known hepatocarcinogens, even more active than the aminoazo dyes that are the standard laboratory hepatocarcinogens. Recently, there has been a suggestion that the prevalence of hepatocarcinoma in man in Uganda and of stomach carcinoma in the Orient may be associated with high aflatoxin levels in the native diets.

When an aromatic hydrocarbon oncogen such as 3-methylcholanthrene is applied to the skin of a mouse in a vehicle such as acetone or olive oil, it accumulates in the hair follicles and sebaceous glands and has a toxic and destructive action on these epidermal appendages. Even a year or more later, however, long after its dissipation, a second application of the compound will still produce an additive oncogenic effect. Successive doses are at least somewhat additive no matter how widely spaced, but there does appear to be a threshold dosage below which no toxicity is evident and no cumulative oncogenic effect is seen. It is apparent that each effective dosage of the oncogen produces some long-lasting effect in the treated skin. The skin may look grossly and histologically normal between applications, but with each successive exposure to the hydrocarbon the probability of cancer formation increases.

When a chemical of this sort is first painted on an area of skin, many of the cells are killed. Very rapidly thereafter, a transitory, compensatory hyperplasia occurs. There is virtually no evidence in favor of a more direct mechanism of the hyperplasia production. With each successive application the epithelial cells show a greater and greater resistance to the toxic effect of the chemical, but the hyperplasia becomes more prolonged and abnormal. Eventually, carcinoma makes its appearance, usually in a quite localized focal area (Iversen and Evensen, 1962).

Against this picture of a gradual and progressive alteration is the evidence supporting the so-called two-stage theory (Boutwell, 1964). If mouse skin is treated with a suitable suboncogenic dosage of hydrocarbon, papillomas can be subsequently elicited by painting the same area with croton oil, a very weakly oncogenic but powerfully irritating substance. If the procedure is reversed, that is, if using the same dosages, the croton oil precedes the hydrocarbon, the papillomas are not produced. Berenblum (1970) suggests that these facts prove that the hydrocarbon and the croton oil act in qualitatively different ways. If this were not so, he argues, it would make no difference which one were applied first. He suggests that the hydrocarbon initiates and the croton oil promotes oncogenesis. According to this formulation, a complete oncogen like 3-methylcholanthrene can achieve both initiation and promotion, but in low dosage the initiating effect predominates. Croton oil, on the other hand, is predominantly a promoter, while ethylcarbamate (urethane), when applied to the skin, is a nearly pure initiator.

Initiation is apparently cumulative regardless of the intervals between initiating treatments; promotion is not. In the mouse, promoters must be applied at successive intervals of less than a week to be cumulative.

Berenblum (1970) postulates that the function of an initiator is to convert normal cells into latent tumor cells (mutation?). These then persist in the epithelium until exposed to the promoter. It is now quite clear that any procedure that causes transient hyperplasia, such as wound healing, can serve as a promoter. One final point needs to be made about the two-stage system in the skin: the papillomas produced are multiple, benign focal lesions that almost always regress. Very few progress to carcinomas. The regression is caused, at least in part, by an immune response mediated by lymphocytes. If more initiator and less promoter is applied, the number of papillomas decreases but the percentage that progresses to carcinoma increases. No dilution of dosage or alteration of schedule can enable one, using a complete carcinogen alone, to simulate the result achieved with the sequence of an initiator followed by virtually pure promoter.

How applicable the two-stage theory is outside the skin system is not known. The facts involved are very important, no matter how disputed their interpretation or possibly limited their applicability, because they must necessarily have a bearing upon theories of carcinogenesis.

Despite the plethora of oncogenic agents, it may now be a worthwhile exercise to search for common chemical and biological properties that might be clues to the mechanisms of neoplastic transformation by chemical oncogens. First, we can list the common biologic features:

1. All the oncogens that have been tested are apparently cytotoxic to the target tissue when used in effective dosage, and apparently for that reason, all produce hyperplasia.
2. Most of the "complete" hydrocarbon oncogens tested are more toxic to most normal cells than to most tumor cells (Vasiliev and Guelstein, 1963). This is not true of urethane, the seemingly pure initiator, or of certain alkylating agents. The exceptions are sufficiently numerous to cast doubt upon differential toxicity as an important general mechanism in chemical oncogenesis (Diamond, 1969).
3. Hydrocarbon oncogens and the azo dye and fluorenylamine hepatocarcinogens combine with a protein in the target tissue to produce physically similar conjugation products (i.e. the charge category is similar)—products that are diminished or absent in the resulting tumors. This may prove a general phenomenon of great importance.
4. Many, but not all, chemical oncogens are mutagens. It could perhaps be argued that the exceptions are due to lack of a proper test system. Not even known mutagens are mutagenic under all conditions and in all biologic systems. Perhaps all proximal oncogens will be shown to be mutagens. However, at present, this correlation is not very good.
5. All oncogens thus far examined, when used in oncogenic dosage, interfere with normal immunologic reactions (Prehn, 1963). In this connection it should be remembered that most neoplasms are probably at least slightly antigenic.

Looking back over this list it seems that #1 and #5 are the only two properties which have thus far failed to show exceptions; #3 has probably not been widely enough investigated to permit confident generalization. In #1, the production of compensatory hyperplasia after toxicity, it is probably the hyperplasia per se that is important since hyperplasia, as we shall see, also precedes oncogenesis by hormones. When hyperplasia occurs after hormone treatment, it is probably not a matter of compensation after toxicity. The importance of #5, interference with immune mechanisms, is further suggested by the fact that neoplasms produced by the chemical agents tend to be more antigenic than those produced by other modalities that may not seriously affect the normal immune reactivity. Thus, this property of the chemical oncogens may be an important facet of their activity.

Recently some progress toward elucidation of a common chemical mode of activity among the plethora of oncogenic compounds has been made. Many oncogenic amides and amines have been found to undergo N-hydroxylation to a "proximal" oncogen, which is then converted to a highly unstable, reactive, elec-

Figure 6-9.

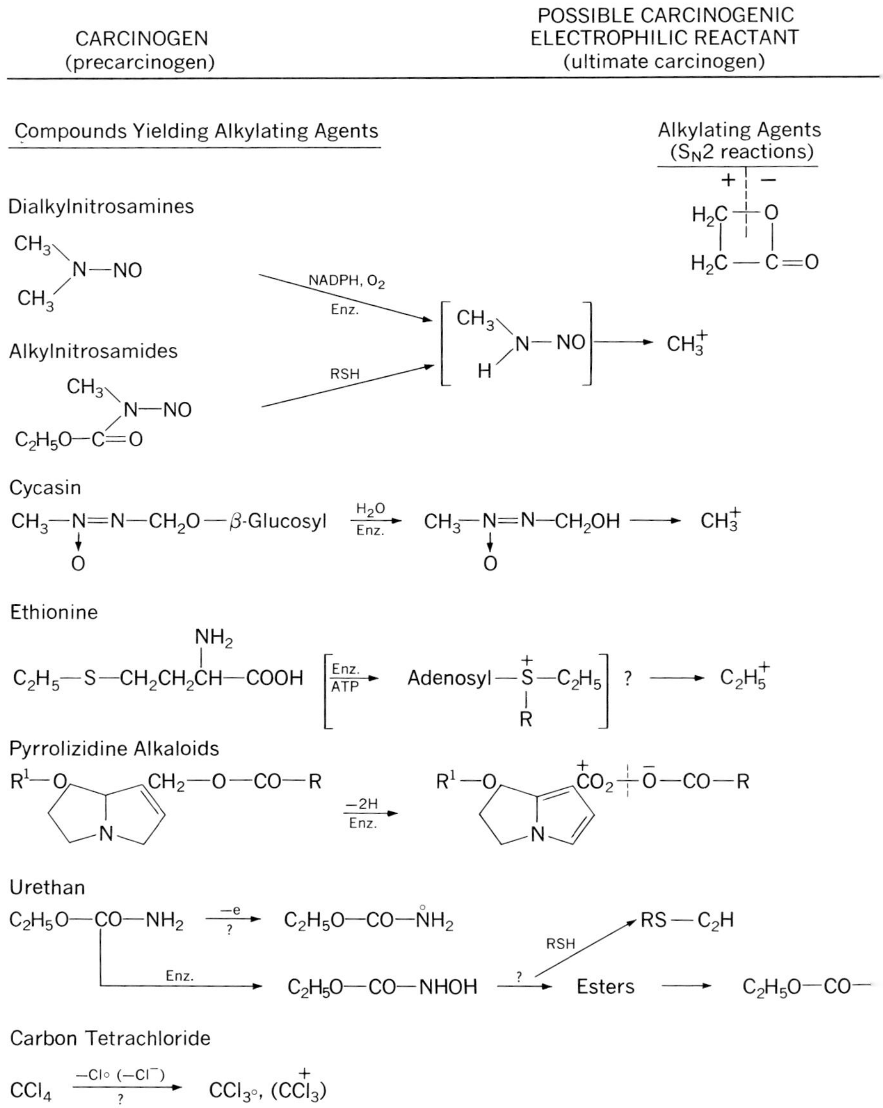
CARCINOGEN
(precarcinogen)
POSSIBLE CARCINOGENIC
ELECTROPHILIC REACTANT
(ultimate carcinogen)
Compounds Yielding Alkylating Agents
Alkylating Agents
(SN2 reactions)
Dialkylnitrosamines
NADPH, O2
Enz.
Alkylnitrosamides
RSH
Cycasin
CH3—N=N—CH2O—β-Glucosyl
H2O
Enz.
CH3—N=N—CH2OH
Ethionine
C2H5—S—CH2CH2CH—COOH
Enz.
ATP
Adenosyl—S—C2H5
Pyrrolizidine Alkaloids
−2H
Enz.
Urethan
C2H5O—CO—NH2
−e
?
C2H5O—CO—NH2
RSH
RS—C2H
Enz.
C2H5O—CO—NHOH
Esters
C2H5O—CO—
Carbon Tetrachloride
CCl4
—Cl∘ (—Cl−)
CCl3∘, (CCl3)

CARCINOGEN (precarcinogen)	POSSIBLE CARCINOGENIC ELECTROPHILIC REACTANT (ultimate carcinogen)

ompounds Yielding Arylating, Arylamidating, and Related Agents

omatic Amides and Amines

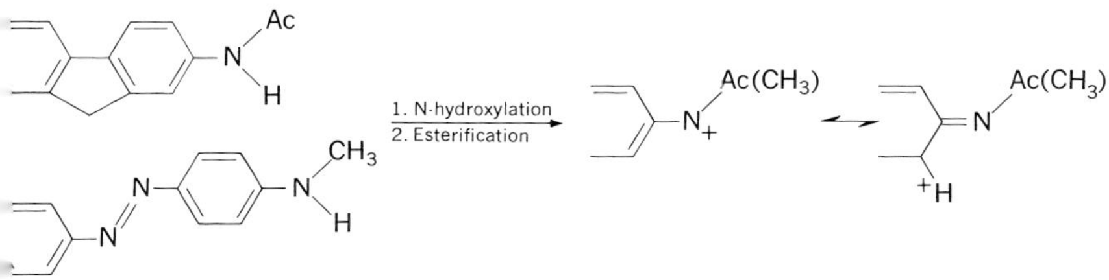

phenyl-N-nitroso Urea

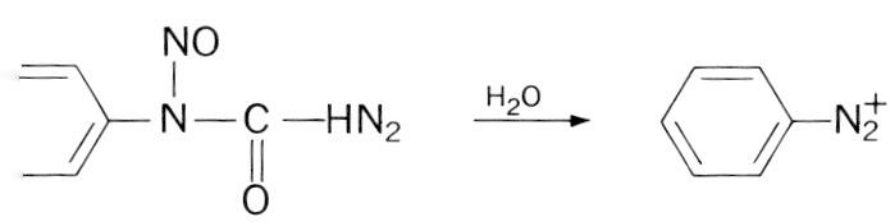

itroquinoline-l-oxide

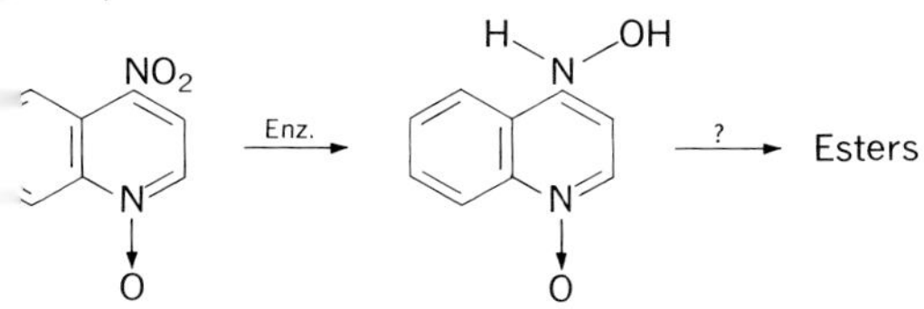

ycyclic Aromatic Hydrocarbons?

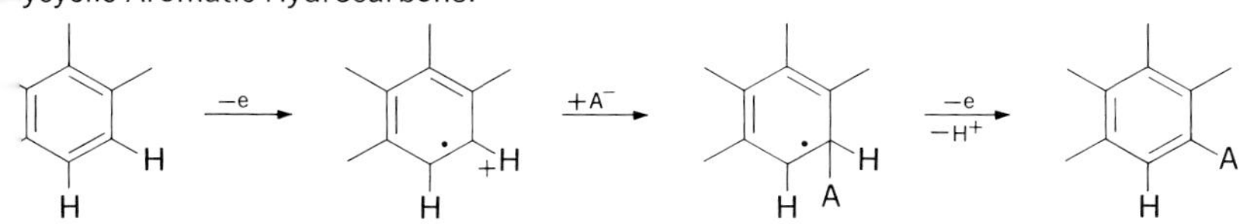

Radical cation

Carcinogenic Metals

Be^{++}, Cd^{++}, Co^{++}, Cr^{+++}, Pb^{++}, Ni^{++}

odified from Miller and Miller, 1969)

trophilic derivative. This derivative combines with nucleophilic groups in crucial cellular components, such as nucleic acids and proteins. Some suggested ultimate oncogenic electrophilic forms of various oncogens are given in Figure 6-9, modified from the Millers' work. Formulas in parentheses are conjectured (Miller and Miller, 1969).

The oncogenic polycyclic aromatic hydrocarbons form the only large group of chemical oncogens for which the nature of the probable reactive forms is still rather obscure. It seems probable, however, that the hydrocarbons also work via activation to electrophilic derivatives. It should be noted that the oncogenic hydrocarbons are relatively ineffective in primates. Thus, there may be profound species differences in the metabolism of these agents.

The knowledge of the ultimate reactive form of the various oncogens unfortunately does not delineate the target which could still be either protein, RNA, or DNA, or even all three. More will be said on this subject when various theories of oncogenesis are discussed in a subsequent section.

4. Hormonal agents

Although many hormones serve as important factors that contribute to the oncogenic activities of various other agents, it is clear that hormonal imbalance can produce neoplasia in the absence of any known viral or chemical agent. This is perhaps best exemplified by the hormonal production of ovarian neoplasms in rodents.

This system, which was developed by the Biskinds, involves a surgical manipulation to provide chronic excessive gonadotrophin for the ovarian tissues (Biskind and Biskind, 1949). The technique was to ovariectomize young adult mice or rats and then to make an ovarian graft to the spleen. Under these conditions, the grafted ovarian tissue in the spleen became hyperplastic and, after many months, neoplastic. The tumors that developed were initially often dependent upon excessive gonadotrophin but this dependence was usually rapidly lost by progression to more complete autonomy.

The mechanism of oncogenesis can be derived from the following facts:

1. The splenic transplant did not become tumorous if ovariectomy was incomplete.
2. Neoplasia was also prevented by implantation of ovarian tissue subcutaneously.
3. Hypophysectomy prevented the oncogenesis.
4. The pituitary also became hyperplastic and in some cases neoplastic.

5. Adhesions at the operative site between the spleen and body wall tended to prevent neoplastic transformation.

These and other facts support the theory that the neoplastic transformation in this system results from chronic stimulation of the transplanted ovarian tissue by excessive pituitary gonadotrophin. The feedback arc that normally regulates the production of pituitary gonadotrophin is broken by placing the only significant estrogen source in the hepatic portal system; the liver inactivates virtually all estrogen reaching it. Thus, in the experiment, estrogen from the intrasplenic transplant could not reach the pituitary. Without this estrogenic inhibition the pituitary produced excessive gonadotrophin, and the ovarian tissue was stimulated to hyperplasia.

This principle of hormonal oncogenesis is general. By chronic imbalance of the appropriate hormones, tumors have been produced in virtually all of the hormonally dependent organs. In all these organs, hormonally induced chronic hyperplasia may develop into neoplasia (Gardner, 1953).

5. Immunity as an oncogen

Immunity has thus far been considered only as an antineoplastic factor. This viewpoint is probably generally correct, but it is possible to produce lymphocytic neoplasms in mice by bringing about a chronic graft vs. host reaction. This can be done by inoculating F_1 mice with parental strain homozygous spleen cells. The transplanted immunologic mechanism of the parental strain is capable of reacting against F_1 tissue but for genetic reasons, the F_1 cannot react against the transplant. Thus, the host is subject to prolonged immunologic assault. Under these conditions the host lymphocytes may develop a lymphoma. This reaction is poorly understood, but it has been shown that immune attack can produce chromosomal abnormalities in target cells without necessarily being lethal (Fialkow, 1967).

6. Physical agents

The oncogenic effect of *ionizing radiant energy,* particularly X-rays, was discovered by tragic experience shortly after the discovery of X-rays themselves. Among early radiologists there arose numerous cases of chronic ulceration followed by squamous-cell carcinomas of the hands or fingers, making the new agent's potentialities only too evident. X-irradiation was probably the first environmental oncogen to be clearly identified.

Many cases of neoplasia have been induced by the physician. Infants who received radiation to the neck for a rather nebulous condition, enlarged thymus, suffered in later life from an unusually high incidence of thyroid carcinoma. Patients with Marie-Strumpels syndrome, a severe rheumatoid arthritis of the spine, were in the past often treated with large doses of radiation with a resultant increased incidence of lymphoma. Even today, there is mounting evidence that the small doses of radiation given in the course of diagnostic examination of the pelvis in complicated obstetrical cases can produce an increased incidence of leukemia later in the life of the children thus radiated *in utero* (Brues, 1954).

Radiant energy has been an industrial hazard as witnessed by the osteogenic sarcomas that were produced following radium ingestion by watch-dial painters. It has also become a hazard of modern warfare, causing the increased rate of leukemia in the survivors of Hiroshima and Nagasaki. Curiously, no other type of neoplasm has yet appeared in definite excess among these atomic bomb victims.

In experimental systems irradiation can increase the incidence of neoplasms due primarily to other agents, but does not appear to be a very potent oncogen in its own right. The marrow and lymphoid systems seem most sensitive to its toxic effects and it is in these tissues that neoplasia is most easily produced. In the mouse, X-irradiation can produce leukemias that are of virus etiology but which would not have appeared had it not been for the action of the radiation. Perhaps the virus is activated by the radiation.

In many experimental systems it appears that the action of the X-rays is indirect, i.e. the tissues that eventually become neoplastic need not have been directly radiated. This is particularly well demonstrated in mouse thymic lymphomas. Most mouse leukemia has its origins in the thymus gland and this is true of radiation-induced leukemia also. Using inbred mice, with various genetic markers, it is possible to show that transplantation of a radiated thymus gland into a non-radiated thymic reticulum, induces neoplasia in the non-radiated lymphoid cells of the recipient (Law and Potter, 1958).

The mechanisms by which ionizing radiation produces neoplasia are unknown. Of course, radiation is a known mutagen which can produce chromosomal aberrations; like chemical carcinogens, it depresses immune defenses, and it produces cell destruction and compensatory hyperplasia, especially in the marrow and lymphoid systems. Nevertheless, the intimate molecular events that produce neoplasia are just as obscure as in the case of chemical oncogenesis.

It is not really paradoxical that X-radiation is also a very important therapeutic modality for various kinds of cancer. It can destroy cells, especially rapidly dividing cells. In the cancer patient this property is far more important than the possible risk of inducing a new neoplasm in normal cells that survive the treament.

Radiant energy of yet another type is an important oncogen in man. It is quite clear that the vast majority of cases of skin cancer are the result of exposure to ultraviolet radiation. The oncogenic wave-lengths are the same as those producing skin destruction and sunburn, approximately 2900-3200 A. It is clear that skin pigmentation is markedly protective, and for this reason the incidence of skin cancer is low in the more heavily pigmented races. The visible effects of aging in the skin are largely the result, not of senescence per se, but of exposure to ultraviolet light. In view of these facts and the ready availability of vitamin D from other sources, the "health" fad of suntanning has no rationale in the twentieth century. Ultraviolet light is toxic, accelerating both aging and oncogenesis in the skin. It should be avoided.

The effects of *mechanical trauma* on oncogenesis have already been dealt with to some extent in the consideration of the two-stage theory. There is no question but that mechanical trauma can contribute to the neoplastic process. However, although chronic hyperplasia may in some circumstances be a complete oncogen, there is no evidence that acute trauma can do more than accelerate a process already under way. Clinical instances in which neoplasia has followed acute trauma are almost certainly not due to a causal relationship, but rather to the fact that trauma may call the patient's attention to an incipient neoplasm.

There is one interesting form of physical oncogenesis in rodents and related animals that may have little counterpart in man. This can be called *smooth-surface sarcogenesis* and consists of the induction of sarcomas around bakelite or cellophane films. The mechanism of the oncogenic effect of smooth films or foils is not known but a few features have narrowed the possibilities. It is known that a rather acellular, fibrous capsule develops around a smooth film after the foreign-body reaction subsides. Neoplasia arises from cells inside this capsule on the surface of the film. These cells are very flattened and thin, and perhaps this physical fact contributes to transformation. It has been shown that the environment inside the fibrous capsule is unusually conducive to the growth of tumor implants. If a chronic granulomatous reaction is maintained about the film, as it is about a rough film, fibrous capsule formation is diminished and oncogenesis is reduced.

There is little evidence that films and foils produce similar effect in man. The subcutaneous tissues of the rodent seem unusually susceptible to oncogenesis.

Another possibly related form of oncogenesis should be mentioned here. It is virtually impossible, for unknown reasons, to keep rodent cells that are grown in tissue culture from becoming neoplastic and growing as tumor when returned to an *in vivo* environment (Sanford, 1965). Primate cells, in general, seem to be much more resistant to neoplastic transformation under these conditions. The smooth surface upon which the cultures are grown may contribute to the oncogenic process in the rodent cells, but this is sheer speculation.

7. Aging

Cancer, with few exceptions, is a disease intimately related to aging (Doll, 1964). In human populations the probability of developing carcinoma of the prostate rises exponentially to approach 100 per cent in the very aged. A somewhat similar relation is seen for gastric carcinoma, bronchogenic carcinoma, and carcinoma of the breast, though in these cases the curve is not quite so steep. In mammary cancer there is a distinct hump in the curve around the age of menopause.

There are, however, certain cancers that are peculiar to childhood. Most prominent among these are childhood leukemia, neuroblastoma, Wilm's tumor, and retinoblastoma.

The reasons for the fairly general relationship of naturally occurring cancer to aging are not known, but they may be related to the possibility that the neoplastic cell may evolve by an accumulated series of random sequential alterations. In addition, the effectiveness of immunity decreases in old age.

8. Diet

There is an important and striking relationship, especially in experimental animals, between nutrition and the incidence of neoplasia. It is a general phenomenon that chronic caloric restriction reduces the incidence and delays onset of neoplastic disease. In this there seems to be an association between the effects of caloric restriction on aging and the effects on neoplasia. Although caloric restriction (and lowered body weight) inhibits the cancer incidence, there is no evidence that starvation alters or slows the course of an already established neoplasm.

F. Speculative Theories of Oncogenesis

Most theories concerning the nature of the neoplastic cell fall into two different categories, though some are intermediate. The basic, unresolved question seems to be whether the neoplastic cell should be regarded as a form of somatic mutation or as a form of abnormal differentiation, more akin to the variation that permits cells of identical genotype to become liver cells or kidney cells. All of the various etiologic factors that have been investigated, including the oncogenic viruses, can be accommodated under either theory. There is no logical necessity for a unitary hypothesis. Perhaps some neoplasms are of one type and some of another, and some may combine both elements. The difference between these two theories may actually not be very great. The term *somatic mutation* is often broadened for the purpose of this hypothesis to include any random heritable alteration, whether due to a change in a nuclear gene or not. Mutation-like processes in extragenic inheritance mechanisms thus qualify as somatic mutations. Many such systems are known at least in lower forms, and, in relation to cancer, have been assembled under the title of the *plasma gene theory* (Darlington, 1948). A real possibility along this line has been raised by the demonstration of the heritability of a surgically induced cell-surface change in paramecia (Sonneborn, 1964). If a random mutation-like change in the mammalian cell surface can also be heritable without gene mutation, one heuristically appealing hypothesis of neoplastic transplantation is obviously available. If the hypothetical cell-surface changes are actually somewhat less random, however, they may serve as a mechanism of normal differentiation. In that event the two theories virtually merge.

It seems that one of the essential features distinguishing the two theories is really the question of the randomness of the change. Does the change originate in a single cell or in a few cells on a random basis or, conversely, as the result of simultaneous and predictable change in all or many cells in a certain area? This question cannot be answered since only a limited amount of direct evidence is available. The histologic evidence suggests that a neoplasm often arises from an area, not from a randomly occurring abnormal progenitor. Conversely, the weight of experimental evidence tends to support the hypothesis of sporadic single-cell origin or at least origin from relatively few cells in a restricted area. It denies the general hypothesis that neoplastic growth ordinarily occurs by the continuous recruitment of newly transformed cells from the surrounding normal population, although this process may occur in some instances.

The histologic evidence to support the field theory comes from the observation that in many lesions, especially in skin and breast, there may be no recognizable dividing line between carcinoma and surrounding normal epithelial tissue. Instead there is often a gradation from areas of overt malignancy with the usual cytologic alterations through areas of less marked abnormality to areas of completely normal morphology. The appearance suggests the gradual conversion of cells from normal to malignant as the lesion expands. On the other hand, it is quite clear from transplantation experiments using cytologic, genetic, or antigenic markers, that most experimental animal tumors do not convert host cells to neoplastic cells. They behave as though derived from a single, abnormal ancestor. It will also be remembered that the usual explanation of the two-stage experiments is the production in the epithelium of randomly scattered, latent tumor cells.

Laboratory data have suggested a possible way to reconcile the histologic and experimental findings. It has been found that many carcinomas have the capacity to induce physiologic hyperplasia in a nearby normal epithelium (Argyris and Argyris, 1962). It has also been found that some epithelial neoplasms of the mouse breast regularly seem to contain a proportion of normal epithelial cells in some sort of symbiotic equilibrium with the neoplastic cells (Prehn, 1967). This normal component has apparently undergone an induced hyperplasia so that the cells are not distinguishable morphologically from neoplastic ones, but they have no heritable alteration. When separated from the neoplastic cells they revert to a normal morphology. Thus it is possible that neoplasia is essentially a clonal phenomenon which may, however, sometimes simulate a diffuse arisal in an oncogenic field by inducing morphologic alterations in the surrounding normal cells.

Perhaps a more important aspect of the original question is whether the varied changes seen in neoplastic cells represent altered patterns of normal gene expression or are the result of the acquisition of new genetic information, either by mutation or viral infection, not previously present in the ancestral cell line. Again, this is a question that cannot yet be answered with any certainty, and again, the theories are not mutually exclusive. Present evidence seems to favor the theory of altered patterns of normal gene expression rather than that of new genetic information.

Of course, it is becoming increasingly evident that many neoplasms have a viral etiology and that viral nucleic acid may be incorporated into the cellular genome. This is certainly new genetic information. However, it is not yet established that continued presence and activity of the viral genes are necessary conditions of the neoplastic state. Perhaps they are only some kind of trigger mechanism. Nonetheless, it must be admitted that the evidence for continued viral-gene activity in the neoplastic cells is at present the best argument in favor of the new genetic information hypothesis. Perhaps this will prove the better hypothesis for virally induced tumors.

Against the new genetic information theory, evidence has accumulated that neoplastic cells have no properties that are not found under other certain conditions in one or another line of normal cells. Neoplastic changes may be explained as stabilizations of abnormal patterns of expression in the normal genome. The recently acquired enzymatic evidence for this was discussed in the section on the biochemistry of the neoplastic cell (Pitot and Cho, 1965). The morphologic and behavioral features seem to be of a similar nature. Normal cells have the information necessary to undergo hyperplasia, but the neoplastic cell apparently becomes, to a varied degree, stabilized in that pattern of gene expression. Chronic physiologic hyperplasia may at times be difficult to distinguish morphologically from neoplasia and may even exhibit cytologic changes. Even invasiveness and the ability to metastasize cannot be considered evidence of new genetic information since many non-neoplastic cells exhibit these qualities. Blood cells, for example, tend to be free-living and invasive. Bone-marrow cells can "metastasize" in experimental animals under suitable conditions. Endometriosis may represent metastasis of otherwise normal cells. Migration of normal cells is a frequent occurrence during embryogenesis, and probably no neoplasm exceeds in its growth rate that of the embryo. All these qualities in a neoplasm may be abnormal stabilizations of various patterns of expression of the perfectly normal cellular genome. The new antigens seen in neoplastic cells may all turn out, as some already have, to be normal gene products that are usually expressed only during ontogeny. As of this writing, there is no unequivocal evidence that any of the new antigens that play a role in the behavior of virally induced neoplastic cells are encoded by viral genes. All of them may represent specific alterations in the expression of the normal genome. Perhaps even the immortality of neoplastic cell lines could be looked upon as an abnormal stabilization of a normal life-giving pattern of gene expression.

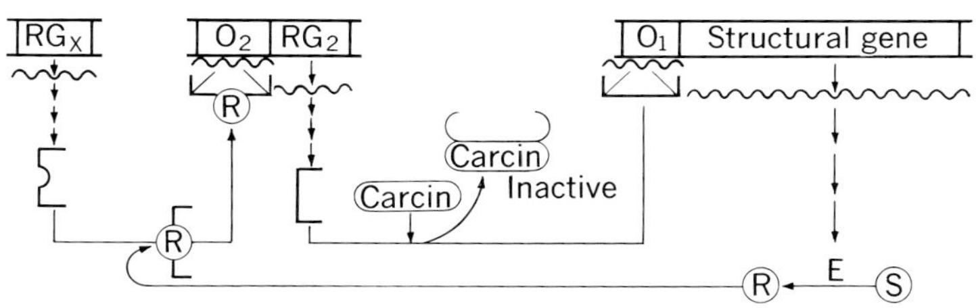

Modified product perpetuation circuit as a model for carcinogenesis. Carcin = carcinogen which combines with, and inactivates the product of, RG_2 which in turn allows synthesis of E, maintaining RG_2 in the inactive state.

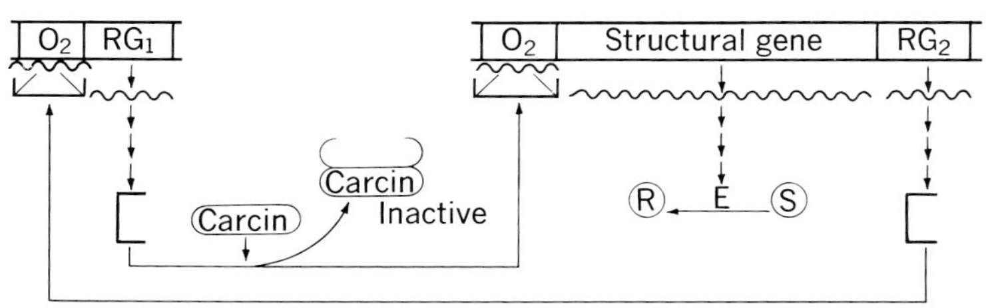

Product independent circuit.

Figure 6-10. Courtesy of Dr. H. C. Pitot.

If the basic alterations in the neoplastic cell need not involve changes in the genome, then theories concerning the mode of action of chemical agents need not involve reactions with DNA. An alternative way in which heritable alterations could be produced is through the reaction of the cell surface with lipoproteins. The basis for this hypothesis is the surgically induced heritable surface changes in paramecia already mentioned (Sonneborn, 1964). Another hypothesis, based upon the theories of gene regulation propounded by Jacob and Monod, has been put forward by Pitot and Heidelberger (Pitot and Cho, 1965). They suggest that the reaction of the oncogen with a repressor molecule could establish a self-perpetuating alteration in the regulation of an operator gene. Two such schemes are shown in Figure 6-10.

A third hypothesis of chemical oncogen action without the necessity of genic alteration can be called the *selectional hypothesis* (Prehn, 1964). It postulates that a variety of oncogen actions might alter the cellular environment so that spontaneously appearing neoplastic cells which would ordinarily lie latent or perish could proliferate to form a gross neoplasm. Among such actions might be interference with immune reactivity, greater toxicity to normal than to neoplastic cells, and production of extensive hyperplasia. It seems virtually certain that in most systems selective mechanisms are a necessary part of tumor production by a chemical agent. In some systems, in which the rate of spontaneous cellular variation may be high, selection might be a sufficient mechanism as well. Of course, selection would operate whether the basic neoplastic change were mutation-like or more akin to differentiation.

In view of the fact that immunoselection should reduce the antigenicity of tumors, the persistence of some degree of antigenicity even in long-transplanted neoplasms suggests that antigenicity is somehow an essential and intrinsic part of the neoplastic process. As cell-surface receptors of various types are probably important modulators of differentiation and tissue growth, it is possible that surface antigens represent an alteration in these receptors so that they no longer function properly in cell regulation. If these new antigens are a recapitulation of embryonic cell surface features, they may simply be inappropriate as regulators in the adult, or they may be actively involved in the more embryonal type of regulation exhibited by tumors, i.e. anaplastic properties and lack of growth stabilization. One could anticipate that immunoselection would gradually reduce tumor antigenicity to a compromise level between the hypothetical benefits to the tumor of antigenic surface changes and the disadvantages of an immune reaction.

The mechanisms of change in cellular antigenic titer or effectiveness are not known. A lowered antigenicity does not necessarily imply fewer antigenic sites on the cell surface. It has recently been proposed that the sialomucinous coating on the cell surface may serve to mask antigenic sites and thus regulate antigenic titer.

Apparently, cell-fixed acquired immunity first arises in phylogeny in the early vertebrates—it is seemingly a vertebrate adaptation. With the exception of Crown Gall and related diseases in plants, neoplasia also seems to be largely a vertebrate phenomenon. This phylogenetic coincidence of two major biologic traits has suggested to some investigators a causal relationship between them. They have speculated that acquired cell-fixed immunity may have arisen specifically because of the need for some mechanism to inhibit neoplasia in vertebrate animals. Conversely, perhaps a genomic instability that made the immune mechanisms possible is itself the cause of the increased incidence of neoplasia among vertebrates. The latter hypothesis seems to be at variance with what has been said previously about abnormal stability in the expression of the neoplastic genome. This is not necessarily so. The individual neoplastic cell apparently shows abnormally great stability, failing to respond normally to environmental stresses, but the population may show great adaptive ability because of a high mitotic rate and an abnormally great variation from one cell to another. It is this adaptive ability of the neoplastic cell population as a whole that has thus far frustrated long-lasting chemotherapeutic or hormonal therapy.

The probability that neoplasia usually represents some abnormality in differentiation leads to the speculation that an etiologic factor might be found in a derangement of those tissue relationships that are important in ontogeny. It is known that the development of many epithelial organs, such as the lung, kidney, and pancreas, are dependent upon a proper interaction with surrounding mesenchyme (Harris, 1964). The dependence of the epithelial component upon the connective tissue component is not necessarily completely lost in the mature organ. Recently it has been suggested that a disruption of the dermal-epidermal junction by 3-methycholanthrene, as seen with the aid of the electron microscope, might be the primary lesion in skin oncogenesis (Tarin, 1968). Dawe (1966) has shown that polyoma virus will only induce tumors in embryonic mouse salivary glands if both epithelium and mesenchyme are present.

Consideration will now be given to one speculative theory. Not only is there a phylogenetic correlation between the development of the immune response and neoplasia, but a third major biologic trait also appears for the first time in vertebrates: the loss of regenerative ability. Again, the relation to neoplasia may be purely coincidental.

It is well known that many lower organisms possess remarkable regenerative capacities. The hydra, for example, can regenerate an entire organism from a small fragment and regeneration in flat worms has been a classical object of study in developmental biology. As one ascends the phylogenetic tree, this regenerative capacity gradually becomes more restricted. In the vertebrates, limb and tail regeneration is found in some newts but not in the adult frog. In general, larval forms possess more regenerative capacity than adults—another example of ontogeny recapitulating phylogeny. Adult mammals if one excepts the deer whose antlers regenerate, possess very little regenerative ability, and what they do have is of a very restricted nature. To a considerable extent skin can be replaced, and the liver possesses the capacity to regain its original size after partial hepatectomy. In both of these cases, however, the process seems to be the proliferation of surviving differentiated tissues, probably a very different process from the regeneration of an amputated newt limb. In the newt limb, dedifferentiation appears to take place in the stump, and the new limb is then formed by a process of redifferentiation, analogous to that which occurs in embryologic limb formation.

Regeneration of the newt limb is preceded by formation of a tumor-like mass of undifferentiated tissue, the blastema of regeneration. For a variety of reasons, it is possible that a neoplasm may be a pathological counterpart of the regeneration blastema in an animal that has lost normal regenerative ability. Such a theory has the advantage, among others, of supplying a *raison d'être* for the existence of carcinoembryonic antigens in the tumor cells. In this formulation, neoplasia is again regarded as aberrant differentiation rather than somatic mutation. It raises the theoretical possibility of cure through differentiation, a process already known to occur in certain neoplasms arising from totipotent or near totipotent tissues, for example, Crown Gall in plants, neuroblastoma in children, and ovarian teratoma in mice. Frequent temporary regressions and rarer spontaneous cures of even advanced cancers suggest that few, if any, neoplasms are completely independent of host homeostatic mechanisms. These mechanisms include not only immunity and various types of dependency, but perhaps also mechanisms by which the host may may be able to induce tumor differentiation.

References

Andervont, H. B. (1945), The milk influence in the genesis of mammary tumors, *in* Mammary Tumors in Mice, F. R. Moultan, Ed., Publ. #22, p. 123, Am. Assoc. Adv. Sci., Washington.

Argyris, T. S., and Argyris, B. F. (1962), Differential response of skin epithelium to growth-promoting effects of subcutaneously transplanted tumor, Cancer Research, *22*:73.

Berenblum, I. (1970), The study of tumours in animals, *in* General Pathology, H. W. Florey, Ed., W. B. Saunders, Co. Philadelphia.

Biskind, G. R., and Biskind, M. S. (1949), Experimental ovarian tumors in rats, Am. J. Clin. Path., *19*:501.

Boutwell, R. K. (1964), Some biological aspects of skin carcinogenesis, Prog. Exp. Tumor Res., *4*:207.

Boyland, E. (1961), Human hormone-dependent tumors, Prog. Exp. Tumor Res., *2*:146.

Boyse, E. A. *et al.* (1967), Suppression of murine leukemias by L-asparaginase. Incidence of sensitivity among leukemias of various types: comparative inhibitory activities of guniea pig serum *L-asparaginase* and *Escherichia coli L-asparaginase, J. Exp. Med., 125*:17.

Brues, A. M. (1954), Ionizing radiations and cancer, Adv. Cancer Res., *2*:177.

Bullough, W. S. *et al.* (1967), The vertebrate epidermal chalone, Nature, *214*:578.

Castor, L. N. (1968), Contact regulation of cell division in an epithelial-like cell line, J. Cell. Physiol., *72*:161.

Crile, G., Jr. (1968), The natural history of metastases in lymph nodes, Am. J. Surg., *116*:1.

Darlington, C. D. (1948), The plasmagene theory of the origin of cancer, Brit. J. Cancer, *2*:118.

Dawe, C. J., Morgan, W. D., and Slatick, M. S. (1966), Influence of epithelio-mesenchymal interactions on tumor induction by polyoma virus, Int. J. Canc., *1*:419-50.

Day, E. D. (1964), Vascular relationships of tumor and host, Prog. Exp. Tumor Res., *4*:58.

DeCosse, J. J., and Gelfant, S. (1968), Non-cycling tumor cells: mitogenic response to antilymphocyte serum, Science, *162*:698.

Diamond, L. (1969), The interaction of chemical carcinogens and cells *in vitro,* Prog. Exp. Tumor Res., *11*:364.

Doll, R. (1964), Epidemiological observations on susceptibility to cancer in man with special reference to age, Acta Un. Internal. Contra Cancrum, *20*:747.

Dulbecco, R. (1966), Mechanism of cell transformation by polyoma virus, Perspectives in Biol. and Med., Winter, Vol. 9, p. 298.

Duran-Reynals, F. (1950), Neoplastic infection and cancer, Amer. J. Med., *8*:490-511.

Eckhart, W. (1968), Transformation of animal cells by oncogenic DNA viruses, Physiol. Rev., *48*:513.

Fialkow, P. J. (1967), Hypothesis: immunologic oncogenesis, Blood, *30*:388.

Foulds, L. (1954), The experimental study of tumor progression: a review, Cancer Res., *14*:327.

Gardner, W. U. (1953), Hormonal aspects of experimental tumorigenesis, Adv. Cancer Res., *1*:173.

Harris, M. (1964), Cell Culture and Somatic Variation, Holt, Rinehart and Winston, New York.

Hayflick, L., and Moorhead, P. S. (1961), The serial cultivation of human diploid cell strains, Exp. Cell Res., *25*:585.

Hellstrom, I., Hellstrom, K. E., Pierce, G. E., and Yang, J. P. S. (1968), Cellular and humoral immunity to different types of human neoplasms, Nature, *220*:1352-54.

Henderson, J. S., and Rous, P. (1962), The plating of tumor components on the subcutaneous expanses of young mice. Findings with benign and malignant epidermal growths and with mammary carcinomas, J. Exp. Med., *115*:1211.

Henle, G., Henle, W., and Diehl, V. (1968), Relation of Burkitt's tumor-associated Herpes-type virus to infectious mononucleosis, Proc. Natl. Acad. Sci., U.S., *59*:94.

Heston, W. E. (1945), Genetics of mammary tumors in mice, *in* Mammary Tumors in Mice, F. R. Moultan, Ed., Pub. #22, p. 55, Am. Assoc. Adv. Sci., Washington.

Iverson, O. H., and Evensen, A. (1962), Experimental skin carcinogenesis in mice, Acta Path. Microbiol. Scand., Suppl. #156, Vol. 55.

Kajii, T., Neu, R. L., and Gardner, L. I. (1968), Chromosome abnormalities in lymph node cells from patient with familial lymphoma, Cancer, *22*:218.

Klein, G. (1968a), Tumor-specific transplantation antigens; G. H. A. Clowes Memorial Lecture, Cancer Res., *28*:625.

Klein, G. (1968b), Summary: Antigens of chemically induced tumors; and search for tumor-specific antigens in other human tumors, Cancer Res., *28*:1354.

Klein, G., and Klein, E. (1957), The evolution of independence from specific growth stimulation and inhibition in mammalian tumour-cell populations, Symp. Soc. Exp. Biol., *11*:305.

Knox, W. E. (1967), The enzymatic pattern of neoplastic tissue, Adv. Cancer Res., *10*:117.

Laird, A. K. (1965), Dynamics of tumor growth: Comparison of growth rates and extrapolation of growth curve to one cell, Brit. J. Cancer, *19*:278.

Law, L. W. (1952), Origin of the resistance of leukemia cells to folic acid antagonist, Nature, *169*:628.

Law, L. W., and Potter, M. (1958), Further evidence of indirect induction by x-radiation of lymphocytic neoplasms in mice, J. Natl. Cancer Inst., *20*:489.

Lebovitz, H. E. (1965), Endocrine-metabolic syndromes associated with neoplasms, *in* The Remote Effects of Cancer on the Nervous System, Brain and Norris, Eds., p. 105, Grune and Stratton, New York.

MacPherson, I. (1965), Reversion in hamster cells transformed by Rous sarcoma virus, Science *148*:1731.

Mahoney, M. J., Leighton, J. (1962), The inflammatory response to a foreign body within transplantable tumors, Cancer Res., *22*:334.

Miller, J. A., and Miller, E. C. (1969), The metabolic activation of carcinogenic aromatic amines and amides, Prog. Exp. Tumor Res., *11*:273.

Morton, D. L., Malmgren, R. A., Holmes, E. C., and Ketcham, A. S. (1968), Demonstration of antibodies against human malignant melanoma by immunofluorescence, Surgery, *64*:233-40.

Nakahara, W. (1960), A chemical basis for tumor-host relations, J. Natl. Cancer Inst., *24*:77.

Nowell, P. C. (1965), Chromosome changes in primary tumors, Prog. Exp. Tumor Res., *7*:83.

Olenov, J. M., and Fel, V. J. (1968), The antigenic structure of tumor cells as material for a study of tissue differentiation, J. Embryol. Exp. Morph., *19*:299.

Papanicolaou, G. N. (1958), Historical development of cytology as a tool in clinical medicine and in cancer research, Acta Unio Internatl. Contra Cancrum, *14*:249.

Patterson, M. K., Jr., Maxwell, M. D., and Conway, E. (1969), Studies on asparagine requirement of the Jensen sarcoma and the derivation of its nutritional variant, Cancer Res., *29*:296.

Pitot, H. C. (1968), Some aspects of the developmental biology of neoplasia, Cancer Res., *28*:1880.

Pitot, H. C., and Cho, Y. S. (1965), Control mechanisms in the normal and neoplastic cell, Prog. Exp. Tumor Res., *7*:158.

Potter, V. R. (1968), Summary of discussion on neoplasms, Cancer Res., *28*:1901.

Prehn, R. T. (1963), Function of depressed immunologic reactivity during carcinogenesis, J. Natl. Cancer Inst., *31*:791.

Prehn, R. T. (1964), A clonal selection theory of chemical carcinogenesis, J. Natl. Cancer Inst., *32*:1.

Prehn, R. T. (1967), The significance of tumor-distinctive histocompatibility antigens, *in* Cross-reacting Antigens and Neo-antigens, p. 105, Williams and Wilkins Co., Baltimore.

Prehn, R. T. (1968), Tumor-specific antigens of putatively non-viral tumors, Cancer Res., *28*:1326.

Rubin, H. (1964), A defective cancer virus, Sci. Am., *210*:46.

Sanford, K. K. (1965), Malignant transformation of cells *in vitro,* Int. Rev. Cyt., *18*:249.

Sonneborn, T. M. (1964), The differentiation of cells, Proc. Natl. Acad. Sci., U.S., *51*:915.

Southam, C. M., Babcock, V. I., and Bailey, R. B. (1967), Selective localization of human cancer transplants in newborn rats, Transplantation, *5*:1.

Stoker, M. *et al.* (1968), Anchorage and growth regulation in normal and virus-transformed cells, Int. J. Cancer, *3*:683.

Tarin, D. (1968), Further electron microscopic studies on the mechanism of carcinogenesis: the specificity of the changes in the carcinogen-treated mouse skin, Int. J. Cancer, *3*:734.

Vasiliev, J. M., and Guelstein, V. I. (1963), Sensitivity of normal and neoplastic cells to the damaging action of carcinogenic substances: a review, J. Natl. Cancer Inst., *31*:1123.

Wogan, G. N. (1969), Naturally occurring carcinogens in foods, Prog. Exp. Tumor Res., *11*:134.

Zeidman, I. (1965), Fate of circulating tumor cells. 3. Comparison of metastatic growth produced by tumor cell emboli in veins and lymphatics, Cancer Res., *25*:324.

7

HEREDITY, DIFFERENTIATION, AND DEVELOPMENT

Robert H. Shikes, M.D.

A. Introduction

The biologic similarities which are common to all members of the human species are numerous and often quite obvious. Numerous, too, are the dissimilarities which distinguish individuals within the species. Individual variation in physiognomy, coloration, and physique enables us to recognize a friend in a crowd. Of medical significance are those differences that confer a biologic advantage or disadvantage upon the host.

Many of these differences are already present by the time of birth, i.e. they are inborn. The existence of inborn human variation has been recognized for at least as long as recorded history, and its nature and significance have provided a basis for much folklore as well as for scientific speculation and inquiry. For example, anatomists have for centuries assiduously recorded the multitude of variations in location, configuration, and vascular supply of human organs and structures; clinicians have long recognized the propensities of certain individuals to develop particular diseases.

Recent technical and conceptual advances in biochemistry, genetics, and molecular biology have expanded our knowledge of inborn human variation enormously. While many of these variations seem to have little or no effect upon the host, many others are associated with obviously deleterious effects in the fetus and newborn, or later, in the child and adult. These "birth defects" include the inherited disorders of metabolism, chromosomal disorders, and a variety of congenital malformations. In the United States alone, birth defects have been estimated to cause 500,000 fetal and 62,000 live-born deaths each year. Some 15 million Americans have various forms of disability due to one or more inborn variants (Apgar and Stickle, 1968).

Much of inborn human variation reflects individual differences in genotype. The anatomic, biochemical, and other properties by which we recognize and measure such genetically determined variants represent the phenotype. Other individual differences are not genetically determined but represent the consequences of environmental influences acting at other levels of biologic activity before birth.

B. Genetically Determined Biologic Variation

That a particular trait is genetically determined may be inferred from either of two observations:

1. Its occurrence within a family follows a pattern consistent with Mendelian genetics, i.e. it is inherited.
2. It is associated with a demonstrable chromosomal abnormality. Some of these are inherited; most, however, are acquired at some time during development.

Many of the inherited biologic variations are expressed as autosomal or sex-linked, and as dominant, recessive, or co-dominant traits. The heterozygote may show all, some, or none of the characteristic phenotypic manifestations. Some show differences in their degree of penetrance and/or expression; many are pleiotropic, i.e. they give rise to a variety of phenotypic alterations. Some individuals contain cells of two or more different genotypes (mosaicism); in these instances the phenotype depends not only upon the nature of the genotypic alteration but also upon how many and which of the individual cells are affected.

1. Protein polymorphism

It has been estimated that as many as 50,000 to 100,000 different species of protein molecules are present in the human organism (Pauling, 1964). Herein lies a vast reservoir of genetically determined heterogeneity in the form of protein polymorphism (Price, 1967; Harris, 1969). Each protein consists of one or more polypeptide chains characterized by a specific and unique sequence of amino acids. This sequence, in turn, is determined by a correspondingly specific sequence of nucleotides within the genome. Any alteration in nucleotide sequence, such as additions, deletions, substitutions, is expected to result in a corresponding alteration in the polypeptide which it codes.

Theoretically, one can detect all of the variations which exist in human proteins by sampling a large, representative population and by determining the amino acid sequence of each individual protein. For many reasons, such a study is at present impossible. Actually, most examples of protein polymorphism were discovered because of alterations in chemical and biologic activities of those proteins, resulting from changes in their primary structure. Thus, the substitution of one amino acid for another at a specific site may alter the configuration or electrical charge of the molecule in such a way as to confer upon it a different and unique electrophoretic mobility, antigenic specificity, or enzymatic activity. Finally, such a variation may result in abnormal host metabolism and disease.

The use of physical-chemical, biochemical, immunologic, and clinical screening has demonstrated protein polymorphism to be a widespread phenomenon in man. The serum protein, transferrin, is a case in point (Bearn and Parker, 1965). About 99 per cent of Caucasians have a transferrin which is electrophoretically homogeneous; in the remaining 1 per cent, transferrin is electrophoretically distinct from the "normal." Family studies demonstrate that this variant is inherited as a Mendelian co-dominant. Another electrophoretically distinct variant is found in 8 per cent of Navajo Indians and in 17 per cent of the Lacardan Indians of Central America. Altogether, eighteen different genetically determined electrophoretic variants of transferrin have been described in the human population, each variant presumably representing a different alteration in the genetic information which codes for this protein.

The search for protein polymorphism in the human population continues to yield an ever-increasing number of examples. In one study, Harris (1966) demonstrated protein polymorphism in several arbitrarily chosen enzymes in an unselected English population. One of these, erythrocyte acid phosphatase, occurred in five electrophoretically distinct and genetically determined varieties. A recent review (Childs and Der Kaloustian, 1968) cites eighty-four variants of hemoglobin, thirteen of haptoglobin, and twenty-five of glucose-6-phosphate dehydrogenase, as well as variants of lipoproteins, immunoglobulins, serum albumin, fibrinogen, and many enzymes.

The biologic significance of protein polymorphism is often unclear. The different forms of transferrin, for example, are equally active in their ability to bind and carry iron; none of the variants appear to confer any biologic advantage or disadvantage upon the host. Similarly, the various forms of erythrocyte acid phosphatase, although they appear to differ somewhat in their enzymatic activity, do not seem to have any significant effect upon the host.

2. Inherited disorders of metabolism

At the other end of the spectrum are those genetically determined variant proteins which have observable effects upon the host in the form of disease: the inherited disorders of metabolism.

Many of our present concepts relating to human genetic heterogeneity and disease are derived from the study of these disorders and ultimately from the observations and insights of Sir Archibald Garrod (Childs, 1970). Sixty years ago, this London physician introduced the one gene-one enzyme (or protein) concept and suggested the genetic basis for chemical individuality. He proposed that certain familial diseases were due to blocks at specific sites in metabolism, and that the metabolic block was determined by the loss of a specific enzyme. Such a block would result in the accumulation of substrate and substrate precursors and in a deficiency of product and product derivatives. Since the time of Garrod, a large number of diseases have been found which fulfill his criteria for inborn disorders of metabolism. Many of these are caused by a specific enzyme deficiency. Depending on the enzyme involved, such a deficiency may result in the impaired synthesis, degradation, mobilization, activation, secretion, absorption, excretion, or storage of one or more substrates or products. In addition to its direct effects, such a deficiency might have a variety of indirect consequences. These indirect effects can be seen in several of the enzyme-deficiency disorders.

In other cases, the defect is manifested by the appearance of a protein which is altered because of a mutational event leading to a base change in the DNA and to an amino acid change in the resulting protein. This type of defect which is at the basis of protein polymorphism may, in some cases, result in more or less severe disease.

a. Sickle cell disease

Sickle cell anemia is the best characterized of these inherited disorders of metabolism. This disease is seen almost exclusively in Negroes; in the homozygous state, its major manifestation is severe anemia exacerbated by episodes of hemolysis. Erythrocytes from these patients assume a distinctive crescent or "sickled" appearance, particularly under conditions of relatively low oxygen tension. These erythrocytes contain hemoglobin S, a variant which is electrophoretically distinct from normal adult hemoglobin A. Amino acid sequencing has demonstrated a specific molecular lesion in hemoglobin S: the substitution of valine for glutamic acid at position #6 in the beta chain. Certain conformational and other physical-chemical alterations can be predicted to result from this particular amino acid substitution (Murayama, 1967), leading to stacking of hemoglobin molecules and distortion of the erythrocyte which causes the phenomenon of sickling (Fig. 2-32a). This process is facilitated by deoxygenation; hence it is in the small peripheral blood vessels that the sequelae of sickling occur—hemolysis, stagnation of blood flow and thrombosis. Anemia, hypoxia, tissue ischemia, and infarction follow and produce the constellation of clinical features characteristic of this disease.

Given this demonstrated amino acid substitution, one can infer the corresponding genomic lesion in terms of the genetic code. The codon for glutamic acid is UAG and that for valine is UUG. Thus, the substitution of a single base—uridine for adenine—can ultimately account for this disorder. Other single amino acid substitutions have been demonstrated in many other variant hemoglobins; most of these can be accounted for by a substitution of a single base. Some profoundly alter the properties of hemoglobin and cause disease; others appear to have little effect on either molecule or host (Ranney, 1970).

In addition to full-blown sickle cell anemia some patients carry the sickle cell trait. These subjects are usually heterozygous and they have only about 40 per cent hemoglobin S with partial sickling. Patients with this trait are resistant to malaria but susceptible to venous thrombosis under reduced oxygen tension. Among West Africans the trait is quite common and this offers a biologic advantage to subjects living in an area where malaria is widely diffused. This may indeed be an example of a potentially harmful genetic change which may have developed in part as a defense mechanism.

b. Niemann-Pick disease

This disease is an autosomal recessive trait, seen in either sex and only in the homozygous state. It is a disorder of lipid metabolism, characterized by the intracellular accumulation of a specific complex lipid, sphingomyelin, in most tissues of affected children (Brady, 1966). The normal turnover of this important component of cell membranes is partially determined by sphingomyelinase, a lysosomal enzyme which acts at the initial step in its breakdown. This enzyme has been shown to be deficient in patients with Niemann-Pick disease and, in its absence, substrate accumulates within lysosomes. Unable to digest sphingomyelin, large and abnormally structured lysosomal derivatives crowd out other cytoplasmic organelles within neurons, hepatocytes, blood-cell precursors in the bone marrow, and other cells (Fig. 7-1). Eventually, this results in a multitude of clinical findings, including neurologic signs, hepatomegaly, and anemia.

Niemann-Pick disease is a prototype of many important inherited disorders of metabolism called "storage diseases" which are characterized by the accumulation of metabolites (Hers and Van Hoof, 1970). Other of these diseases are characterized by the accumulation of various lipids, glycogen or mucopolysaccharides (Fig. 2-28c,d).

c. Phenylketonuria

This is a disorder of amino acid metabolism manifested early in life by mental retardation, large excesses of phenylalanine in the blood, and the excretion of

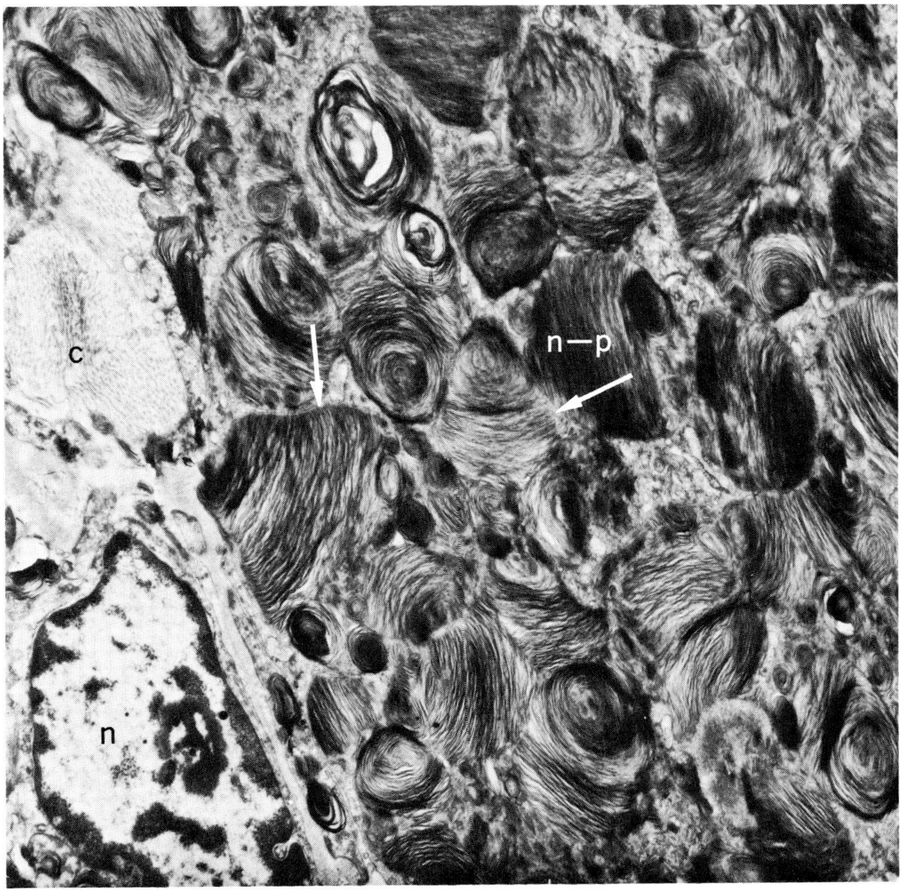

Figure 7-1. Electron microscopic appearance of the lipid deposition in hepatic cell of a child with Nieman-Pick disease. N—nucleus, C—collagen, N-P—characteristic lipid deposits with whorling configuration (sphingomyelin deposited within lysosomes).

large amounts of phenylpyruvic acid in the urine (Carpenter *et al.*, 1968). It is transmitted as an autosomal recessive trait. The deficient enzyme is phenylalanine hydroxylase, a liver enzyme which normally converts phenylalanine to tyrosine. When this major pathway of phenylalanine metabolism is blocked, the amino acid is channeled to an ordinarily minor alternate pathway, leading to phenylpyruvic acid and its derivatives. Phenylpyruvic acid can be detected in the urine by a single laboratory test which is now routinely done on most newborns; the early diagnosis of this disease is of particular importance since the prompt withdrawal of dietary phenylalanine prevents the development of this form of mental retardation. The reason for the development of mental retardation is not clear, but it appears that the metabolic alteration impairs normal postnatal myelinization.

d. Galactosemia

In this disease, a deficiency of galactose-1-phosphate uridyl transferase blocks the normal conversion of galactose to glucose (Hsia, 1967). Of particular importance is the failure to form UDP-galactose, an intermediate necessary for the incorporation of galactose into many large and important carbohydrate-containing molecules. The diversity of molecules so affected probably accounts for the pleiotropic effects of galactosemia, which include mental retardation, cataract formation, and cirrhosis. An autosomal recessive transmission is the trait in both this disease and the one immediately following.

e. Hereditary orotic aciduria

This is a disorder of pyrimidine metabolism characterized by the development, in infants, of megaloblastic anemia and developmental retardation (Smith *et al.*, 1966). In this disorder, two enzymes are deficient; these enzymes are responsible for sequential steps in the conversion of orotic acid to uridine monophosphate (UMP). UMP is an important precursor of RNA and of certain coenzymes. A good therapeutic response is achieved by dietary supplementation with uridine, thus by-passing the metabolic block.

f. Lesch-Nyhan syndrome

Lesch-Nyhan syndrome (Proceedings, 1968) is an X-linked recessive disorder and is observed only in males. The disease is manifest in childhood by mental and growth retardation, abnormal motor activity, and a peculiar behavioral pattern characterized by compulsive automutilation of fingers, toes and lips. The deficient enzyme is hypoxanthine-guanine phosphoribosyl transferase. In its absence, hypoxanthine cannot be utilized in nucleotide synthesis, and there is a marked increase in the production of its catabolite uric acid. The increase in uric acid accounts for the gout seen in some of these patients; the other clinical manifestations cannot be explained on the basis of the known metabolic defect.

g. Miscellaneous disorders

Other inherited disorders of metabolism have been more or less well defined in terms of their clinical manifestations, patterns of inheritance, and specific metabolic and molecular alterations. In addition to the examples cited above, specific enzyme deficiencies have been demonstrated in various disorders involving carbohydrate, amino acid, lipid, purine, porphyrin, and hormone metabolism. Wilson's disease, an inherited disorder of copper metabolism, is associated with a deficiency of the serum protein, ceruloplasmin. The inherited disorders of coagulation are due to deficiencies of specific coagulation factors. The active transport of specific molecules across biological membranes appears to depend upon certain ill-defined "receptors" and "carriers"; abnormalities of such factors have been suggested in certain diseases with defective absorption, secretion, or excretion. Examples include some of the hereditary intestinal malabsorption syndromes and the renal aminoacidurias (Scriver, 1969b), and one form of hereditary hemolytic anemia may be due to a deficiency of erythrocyte Na-K dependent ATPase (Oski *et al.,* 1969).

The basic metabolic defect involved in a number of the inherited disorders of metabolism is completely unknown. An outstanding example is pancreatic cystic fibrosis, a fairly common disease. It has been suggested that some of the inherited disorders of connective tissue may be due to deficiencies of enzymes or other factors responsible for the synthesis or cross-linking of collagen or elastin; genetically determined alterations in the primary structure of these proteins may also occur. Some of the inherited disorders of metabolism may actually represent a variety of different biochemical lesions which give rise to a common clinical picture. Diabetes mellitus and gout are two examples; each will probably prove to consist of a group of genetically, etiologically and pathogenetically distinct metabolic disorders. A small percentage of cases of gout is distinguished from the great majority by the genetically determined deficiency of a specific enzyme involved in purine metabolism (Kelley *et al.,* 1969).

Of major clinical significance are genetically determined individual differences in the response to drugs. Pharmacogenetics refers to the study of such variation in terms of response and the metabolism and excretion of various drugs and their bio-derivatives (LaDu, 1969). Use of the antimalarial primaquine causes hemolytic anemia in some persons; about ten per cent of Negro males are at risk because of an X-linked defect. This unique response is associated with certain variants of erythrocyte glucose-6-phosphate dehydrogenase. Inherited variations in drug metabolizing enzymes have been demonstrated or implicated in untoward responses to a variety of drugs, e.g. isoniazid (antitubercular agent), succinylcholine (muscle relaxant), diphenylhydantoin (anticonvulsant), and dicumarol (anticoagulant).

h. Genetics and the immune response

Antibody specificity is at least partially due to variations in the primary structure of immunoglobulins; one theory of immunogenesis holds that some of this specificity is inborn and genetically determined. Examples of genetically determined individual variation within immunoglobulins have been demonstrated (Franklin, 1967). However, it is not yet known whether such polymorphism is related to individual differences of response to antigenic stimulation, such as occurs in asthma and allergies. Inherited defects in antibody synthesis or cellular immunity account for some of the immune deficiency diseases (see Chapter 5). Genetically determined individual variations in cell-surface antigens have been extensively studied, particularly with regard to blood types and organ transplantation. Fetal-maternal immunologic incompatibility, most clearly demonstrated in erythroblastosis fetalis, may account for a significant portion of other forms of fetal wastage and disease (Brent, 1966).

i. Variations in the inherited disorders of metabolism

In addition to the "typical" examples, many of the inherited disorders of metabolism present a variety of clinically and/or biochemically "atypical" forms (LaDu, 1967). Each of the five enzyme-deficiency diseases we have discussed has shown one or more genetically determined variant form. Thus, cases of phenylketonuria have been described in which there has been little or no mental retardation, and various degrees of phenylalanine hydroxylase deficiency have been reported (Carpenter *et al.,* 1968). Such biochemical and clinical heterogeneity can be ascribed to the heterogeneity of genetically determined molecular alterations. Depending on the nature of the amino acid substitution and its location within the polypeptide chain, alterations in primary structure might have profound, minor, or no effects on the biologic activity of the protein and result in severe disease, mild disease, or none at all.

Such a situation may be operative in the Duarte variant of galactose-1-phosphate uridyl transferase (Mathai and Beutler, 1966). Individuals homozygous for this variant show 50 per cent of normal enzyme activity and none of the stigmata of galactosemia. The variant is electrophoretically distinct from the normal enzyme and was incidentally discovered in a survey of a phenotypically normal unselected population. Whether such variants do indeed reflect different amino acid substitutions awaits sequence analyses such as those which have been applied to hemoglobin.

j. Inherited disorders of control mechanisms

As was pointed out in Chapter 1, one becomes aware of injury when an enzymatic activity is affected. This may be due to alterations in the structure of the enzyme (reflecting a genetic lesion in a structural gene), but it may also be due to the amount of the enzyme, or to various necessary non-enzymatic components of a reaction. The control mechanisms which have been so expertly investigated and described in microbial organisms may have identical or at least analogous counterparts in animal cells (Dreyfus, 1969). Thus, loss of enzyme activity might be due to a lesion in an operator or promoter segment of the genome or in a gene which codes for a particular inducer or repressor. Genetically determined defects could act at the level of protein synthesis (translation), in the transport and packaging of proteins, or in the attachment of important carbohydrate or lipid moieties within cytoplasmic organelles. Still another possibility lies at the level of the biologic activity itself, with deficient activity due to the lack of a specific activator or co-factor.

A role for controlling factors in determining genetic heterogeneity is implied in several inherited disorders of metabolism. One of these, beta thalassemia, is characterized by severe anemia and growth retardation, terminating in death during childhood or adolescence (Weatherall, 1967). Erythrocyte precursor cells from these patients have a greatly reduced ability to synthesize normal adult hemoglobin, specifically the beta chain component. The small amount of beta chain which is synthesized is of normal amino acid sequence. Thus, unlike the other hemoglobinopathies, the genetically determined defect is a quantitative rather than a qualitative one. The implication is that the genetic lesion lies in some factor which controls the synthesis of beta chains (Clegg *et al.,* 1968), perhaps at the level of translation.

In the case of hereditary orotic aciduria, it will be recalled that two enzymes are deficient, and that these enzymes act at sequential steps in pyrimidine metabolism. This phenomenon seems similar to mutations of operator genes in microorganisms. More direct evidence for a genetic lesion of a controller factor lies in the observation that the deficient enzymes can be "turned on" when cells from these patients are maintained *in vitro* and grown under certain conditions (Pinsky and Krooth, 1967).

Acute intermittent porphyria, a disease transmitted as an autosomal dominant disorder, may illustrate still another type of genetic lesion of control mechanisms. In this condition, characterized by episodes of neurologic dysfunction, a marked excess (up to sixty-fold) of the enzyme delta aminolevulinic acid synthetase (ALA synthetase) is regularly found. The reaction catalyzed by this enzyme is normally a rate-limiting one in the synthesis of porphyrins from succinate; an excess of the enzyme thus leads to an excess of porphyrin intermediates, especially delta aminolevulinic acid and porphobilinogen. This phenomenon seems most likely to involve a constitutive mutation of the operator gene, resulting in lack of ability to repress the structural gene for ALA synthetase: synthesis of the enzyme thus is uncontrolled (Tschudy, 1969).

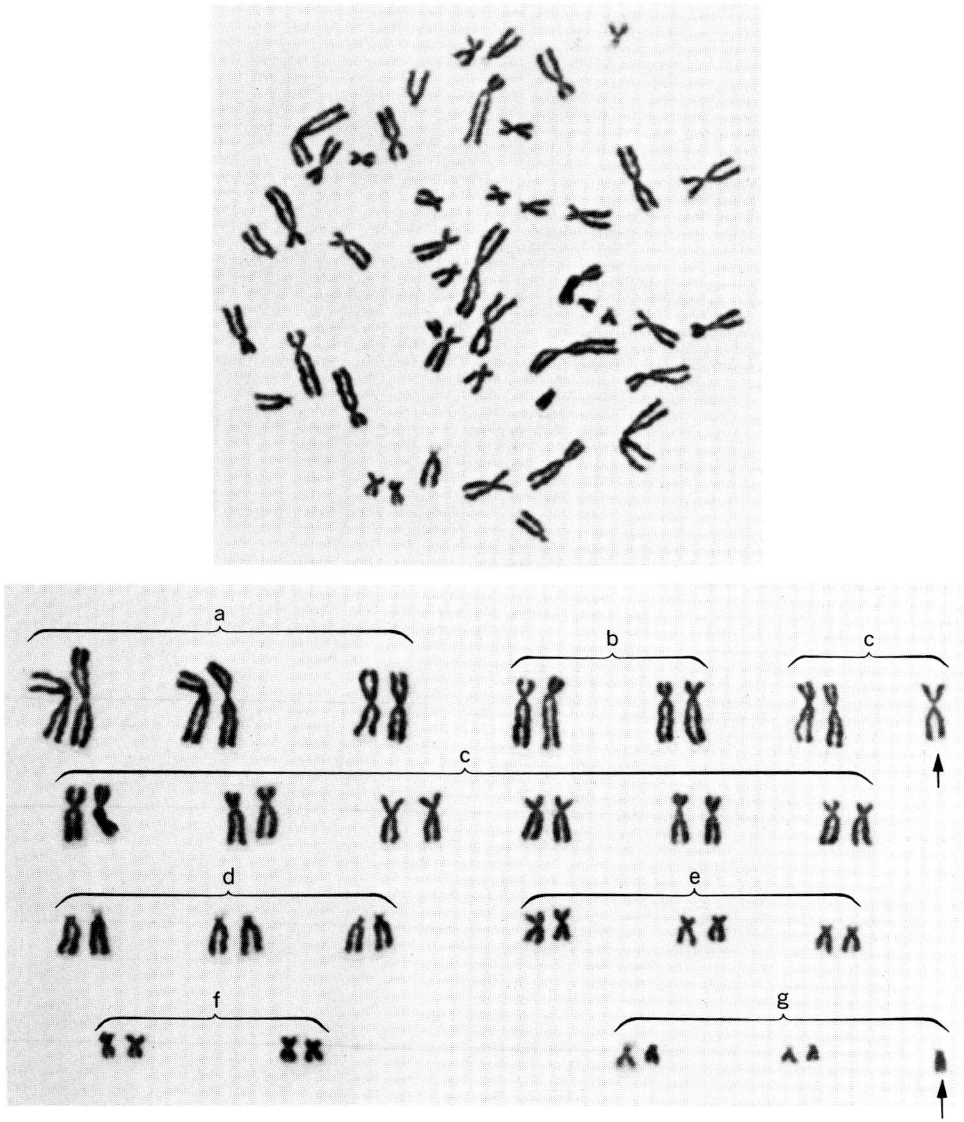

Normal Male

Figure 7-2. Normal male and female karyotypes. Karyotypic analysis involves the examination of a large number of such metaphase spreads obtained from cultured blood or amniotic cells or fibroblasts. One or more representative cells are photographed and the photographed chromosomes are arranged, in pairs, according to the accepted system of classification. Any deviations from normal number, size, and morphology are noted.

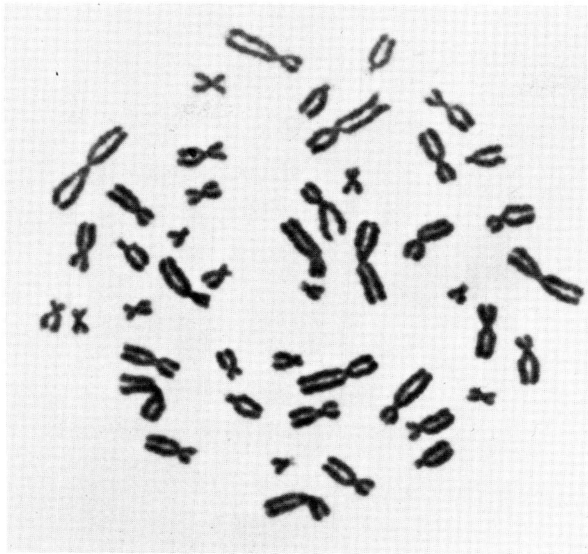

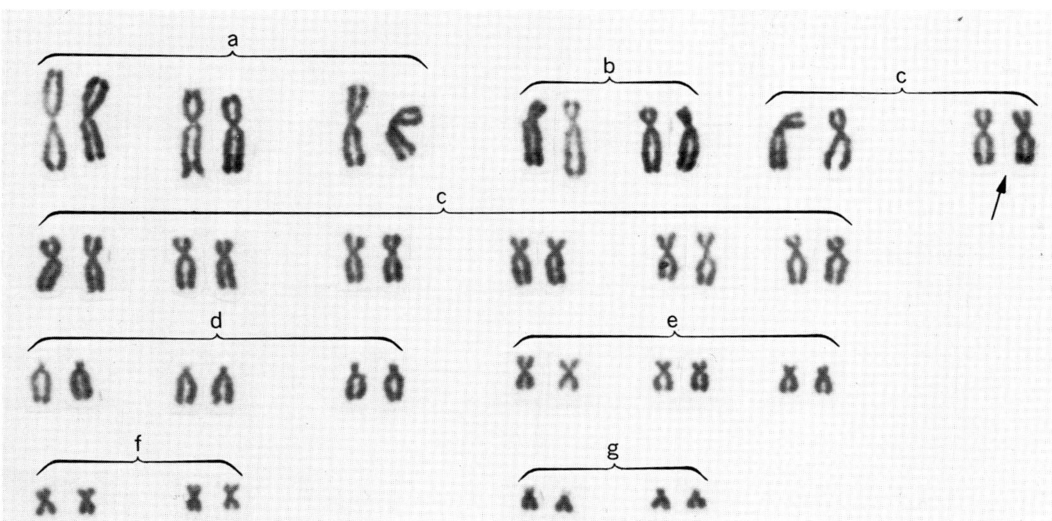

Normal Female

In the male karyotype the X chromosome is in group C (arrow) and the Y chromosome in group G (arrow). In the female karyotype the X chromosomes are in group C (arrow).

Courtesy of Dr. Arthur Robinson.

3. Chromosomal abnormalities

In recent years advances in cytogenetic techniques have allowed the partial characterization of the human somatic cell set of chromosomes. Large numbers of mitotic preparations derived from unselected populations have been examined by light microscopy, and from this has arisen a generally accepted description of the normal human karyotype, based upon chromosome number, size and morphology (Chicago Conference, 1966). Using these criteria, the human somatic cell complement of twenty-two pairs of autosomes and two sex chromosomes has been divided into seven groups designated A, B, C, D, E, F, and G. Group A includes the three large pairs of autosomes and Group G the two smallest pairs plus the Y chromosome in the male. Within some groups individual homologous pairs can be distinguished, and within group A, for example, each pair is designated as 1, 2 or 3. Within other groups, such as Group C, such a distinction is not possible (Fig. 7-2).

All human cells contain a single genetically active X chromosome. If one or more additional X chromosomes are present, they are genetically inactive. By light microscopy, such genetically inactive X chromosomes are represented by discrete foci of heterochromatin adjacent to the nuclear membrane (Barr bodies). The number of Barr bodies is one less than the total number of X chromosomes contained within a given cell. Analysis of human material for Barr bodies provides a rapid and easy method for determining an individual's complement of X chromosomes and for establishing sexual genotype (Fig. 7-3).

The application of karyotypic analysis has resulted in an extensive literature describing many human chromosomal variations involving both autosomes and sex chromosomes (Redding and Hirschhorn, 1968; Carr, 1969a; and Jacobs, 1969). Many of these variations appear to occur during gametogenesis or early development and others are transmitted through succeeding generations. Some are associated with no apparent phenotypic abnormalities, while others consistently give rise to significant disease, usually in the form of developmental aberrations of particular organs and other anatomic structures. Some chromosomal abnormalities are characterized by fairly specific constellations of congenital abnormalities in the form of syndromes. The chromosomal abnormalities seen in cancer cells were discussed in Chapter 6.

Chromosomal abnormalities account for a significant proportion of human disease. Karyotypic analyses of fetuses that have died spontaneously *in utero* have shown abnormalities in about 20 per cent (Carr, 1969c). In newborns with obvious congenital malformations the incidence of chromosomal abnormalities is 4 per cent (Stewart *et al.,* 1969) and in phenotypically normal newborns it is

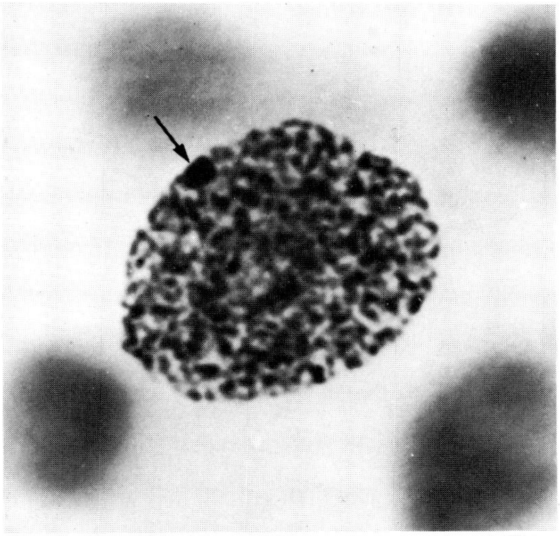

a

Figure 7-3. Barr bodies

	Number of Barr bodies	Number of X chromosomes
upper left	1	2
middle	2	3
lower right	3	4

Courtesy of Dr. Arthur Robinson.

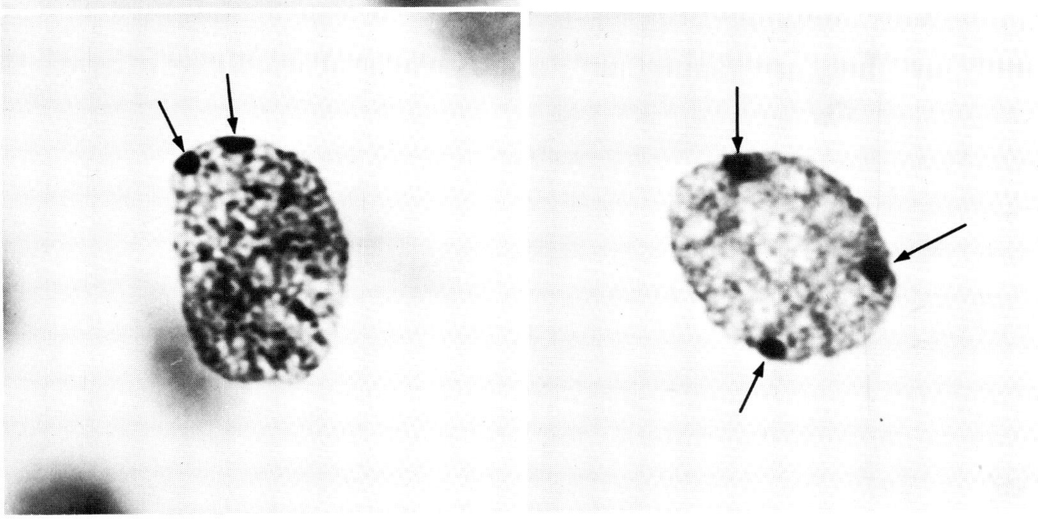

b c

about 0.5 per cent (Walzer *et al.,* 1969). Such abnormalities are said to account for 20,000 new cases of mental retardation each year in the United States (Carr, 1969b).

a. Additions

The most frequently observed human chromosomal variant is the presence of an extra chromosome (trisomy), and the first disease to be associated with a

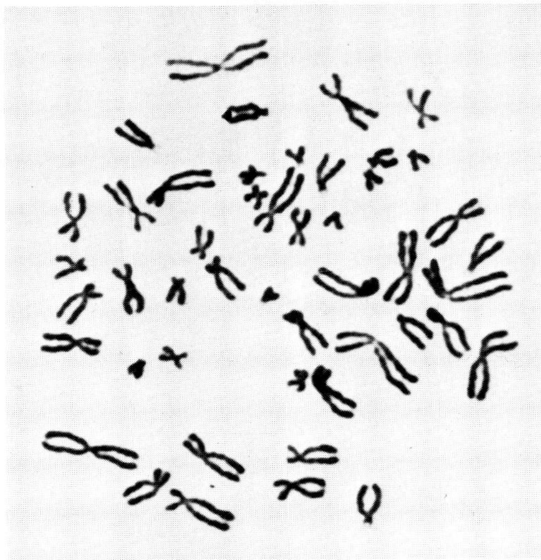

Down's Syndrome

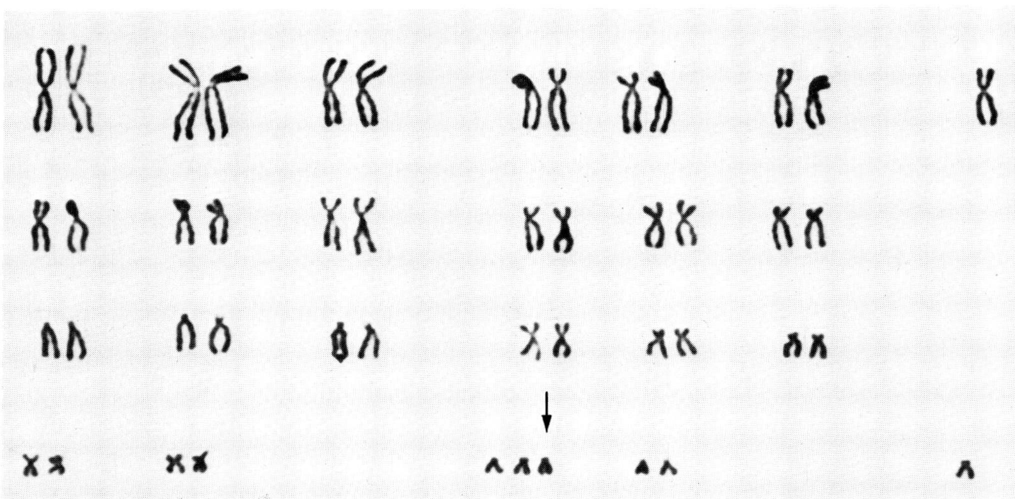

Figure 7-4. Down's syndrome. This patient's karyotype shows 47 chromosomes. There is an additional G group chromosome (arrow). Such a patient would be expected to show the phenotypic features of Down's syndrome.

Courtesy of Dr. Arthur Robinson.

chromosomal abnormality was Down's syndrome (Fig. 7-4). Nearly all patients with this syndrome have an extra G group chromosome (Trisomy G). The birth defects which comprise this clinical syndrome were described long before the chromosomal defect; it includes a characteristic so-called Mongoloid facies, mental retardation, congenital heart disease, and a variety of other less constant developmental anomalies.

Trisomies involving other autosomes are almost exclusively limited to severely malformed aborted fetuses. Trisomy D and trisomy E are occasionally seen in live births, but these infants usually have severe congenital malformations and die early in life.

Additions of sex chromosomes are seen more frequently than the autosomal trisomies. When a Y chromosome is present, the person is a gonadal male regardless of the number of X chromosomes; in the absence of a Y, phenotypic development follows the female pattern. In either situation, however, there is usually retarded sexual development and sterility, and there may be mental retardation and other phenotypic abnormalities as well. In patients with Klinefelter's syndrome (XXY), for example, the testes remain anatomically and functionally immature after the age of puberty, and the secondary sex characteristics of the adult male fail to develop. The XYY genotype has been associated with an increased incidence of tall stature and sociopathic behavior, and has received much publicity in the past year or two, particularly in connection with sexual crimes. A recent study indicates that this chromosomal abnormality occurs much more frequently than was thought, without clinical manifestations, and thus casts doubt on its sociopathic role.

b. Deletions

The deletion of an entire autosome is a rare phenomenon associated with severe malformations and intrauterine death. A few cases of monosomy G have been reported in infants. More frequently seen, though still rare, are partial autosomal deletions. Of these, the most common is deletion of the short arm of a B group chromosome, which results in the *cri-du-chat* syndrome. Infants with this disease are characterized by mental and growth retardation, microcephaly, abnormal facies, various other congenital malformations, and a typical plaintive cry which resembles the mewing of a cat. Other partial autosomal deletions have been associated with all sorts of phenotypic abnormalities.

The presence of a single X chromosome (XO, Turner's syndrome) is associated with phenotypic "femaleness," but with immature ovaries, infertility, and a variety of other findings including short stature, webbed neck, and mental retardation (Fig. 7-5). The YO genotype has not been observed.

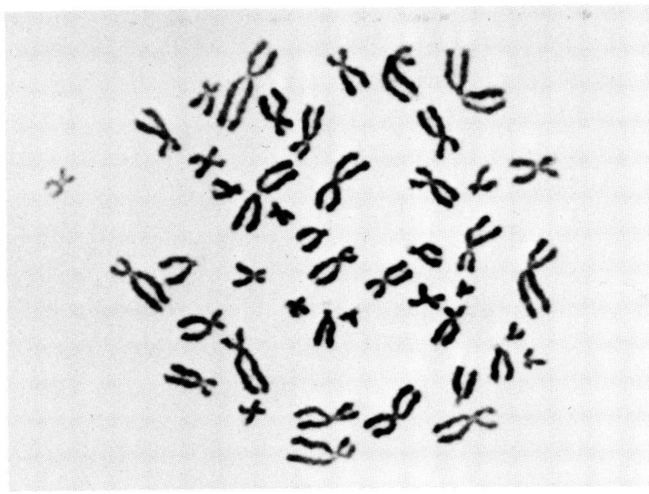

Turner's Syndrome

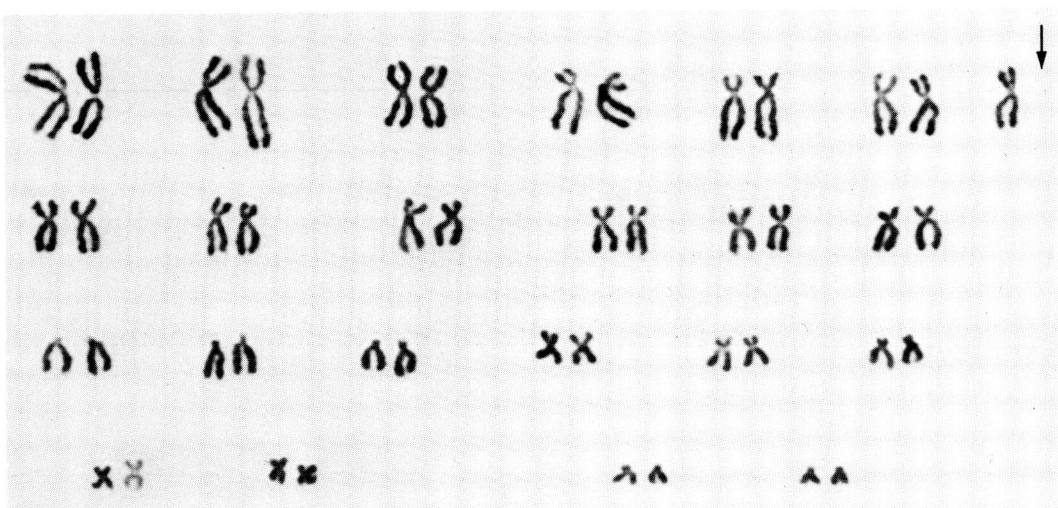

Figure 7-5. Turner's syndrome. This karyotype shows only 45 chromosomes and although such patients are phenotypic females, there is only one X chromosome (arrow). As expected, cells from such patients show no Barr bodies.
Courtesy of Dr. Arthur Robinson.

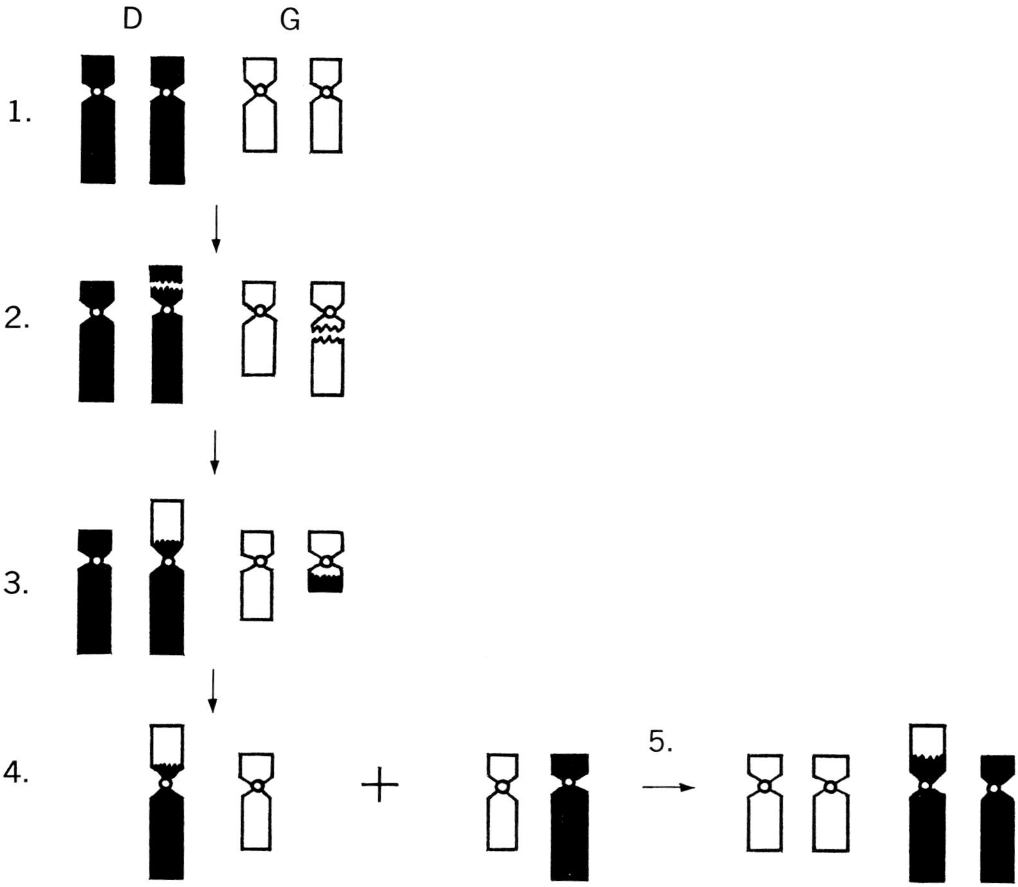

Figure 7-6. Translocation

1. Normal diploid cell containing 2 homologous pairs of D and G chromosomes.

2. Fragmentation of one member of each pair.

3. Balanced translocation. Fragments have been exchanged between D and G chromosomes.

4. Meiotic reduction division. Three patterns of segregation are possible. In this one, the gamete contains an intact G chromosome plus a D chromosome to which has been added a large segment of G chromosome.

5. Fertilization adds still another homologous G chromosome; the resultant zygote contains essentially three homologous G chromosomes—trisomy G.

This is one form of translocation; the treating and joining of chromosomes can result in a variety of other forms of genetic rearrangement and translocation.

c. Rearrangements

Many chromosomal abnormalities appear to result from chromosome or chromatid breaks and subsequent fusions which occur during meiosis and mitosis. Broken fragments may rejoin to form an intact chromosome, or one in which there is an internal rearrangement in the sequence of genetic material. A fragment may be irretrievably lost, or it may unite with another broken chromosome (translocation) (Fig. 7-6). Fragments may be exchanged between homologous or non-homologous chromosomes. Obviously, the variety of genomic rearrangements which can result is enormous. Many of the morphologic aberrations which have been described in autosomes and sex chromosomes are presumed to be due to the consequences of such chromosomal breakage and fusion.

When an exchange of fragments between non-homologous chromosomes is not accompanied by significant loss of genetic material, the resulting translocation is said to be balanced and the host is usually phenotypically normal. The host's offspring, however, are subject to genetically unbalanced situations. For example, one form of translocation has been frequently described which results in the formation of a hybrid chromosome consisting of a large segment of chromosome #15 to which a large fragment of a G group chromosome has been attached. This results in no significant loss of genetic material in the host, who is phenotypically normal. A certain percentage of the host's gametes, however, will contain both this hybrid chromosome and an intact G group chromosome homologous to the G group fragment contained in the hybrid. Fertilization results in a zygote which has a triple dose of this G group chromosome, effectively trisomy G. These patients show the phenotypic manifestations of Down's syndrome and account for about 5 per cent of the cases of this disorder.

d. Minor abnormalities

Included in this heterogeneous group are individuals who show variation in the size or shape of particular chromosomes, or abnormalities of secondary constrictions or satellites. They are termed *minor* because they are usually unassociated with any phenotypic abnormality; many are inherited in Mendelian form.

e. Pathogenesis of phenotypic abnormalities

Gene dosage and the site of genomic lesions are important in determining the phenotypic features of the chromosomal abnormalities.

Gene dosage. Birth defects due to chromosomal abnormalities are almost always due to the addition or deletion of a portion of the genome, regardless of whether the alteration is a trisomy or a monosomy, a partial deletion or an unbalanced translocation. Any deviation from the diploid state apparently results in genetic imbalance sufficient to preclude normal development. How such deviations give rise to the various congenital malformations is unknown.

Site of the genomic lesion. A chromosomal addition or deletion of sufficient size to be detected by light microscopy must affect a very large number of genes; hence, the phenotypic heterogeneity of these abnormalities. Such massive chromosomal lesions, when they occur in most autosomes, are incompatible with fetal survival. Many theoretically possible autosomal additions or deletions have not been found, even in fetuses; if they occur, they must cause death very early in development and may account for a large number of unrecognized, unsuccessful pregnancies.

The relatively mild effects associated with additions of the X chromosome are consistent with the Lyon hypothesis, i.e. no matter how many X chromosomes a cell might contain, only one is expressed. Nevertheless, at least a portion of the second X must be expressed at least some time during development; the genotype XO is phenotypically abnormal, and some effects, however mild, are seen with additions of X chromosomes.

f. Pathogenesis of chromosomal abnormalities

Two major mechanisms have been implicated in the pathogenesis of inborn chromosomal errors: non-disjunction and chromosomal breakage. Non-disjunction refers to the failure of the members of a particular pair of chromosomes (or chromatids) to segregate independently during meiosis or mitosis (Fig. 7-7). In meiotic non-disjunction, the resulting gametes contain either both members or neither member of a homologous pair and the resultant zygote is either trisomic or monosomic. The incidence of trisomy has been statistically correlated with advanced maternal age and presumably with aging of the ovum. In any human ovum, the process of meiosis is interrupted for a period of many years before fertilization, and this hiatus is even greater in ova of women conceiving late in reproductive life. The passage of time increases the risk of injury and may allow for the accumulation of injuries which, in turn, facilitate aberrant cell division in the form of non-disjunction.

Non-disjunction has been observed in mitotic cells as well and its occasional occurrence in zygotic mitosis cannot be ruled out. That it also occurs early in embryonic development is confirmed by numerous instances of individuals of various combinations of monosomic, disomic and/or trisomic cells. Individuals mosaic for Trisomy G have shown all, some, or none of the phenotypic features of Down's syndrome (Kohn *et al.*, 1970).

Chromosomal breakage is a widespread biologic phenomenon, and the re-

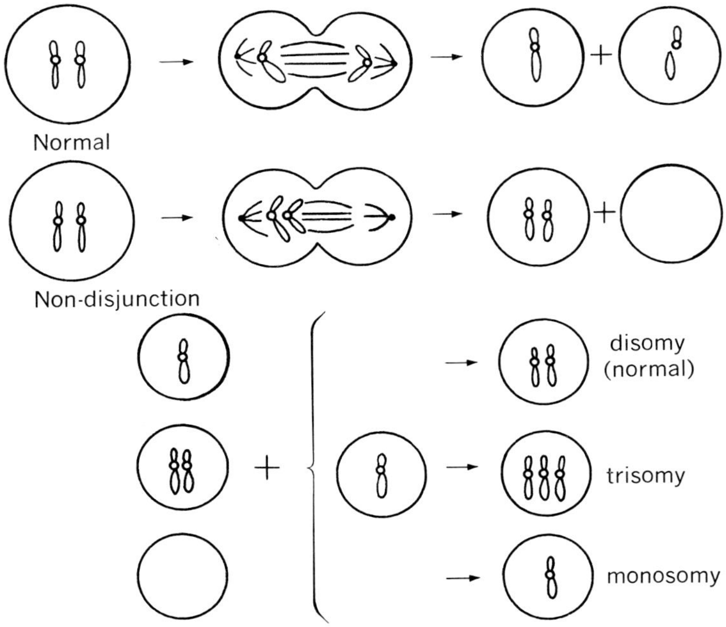

Figure 7-7. Non-disjunction during meiosis of developing gametes. This can also occur during mitosis.

combinations of genetic information which result are important in the evolutionary process. Although most breaks probably heal spontaneously and are without consequence, they can, as we have seen, result in chromosomal rearrangements with deleterious effects upon the host or his offspring. Mosaics may occur in this situation too, again apparently representing errors occurring during mitosis in the early embryo.

Cells derived from patients with two inherited diseases, Bloom's syndrome and Fanconi's anemia, show a remarkable propensity for the development of chromosomal breakage and all sorts of aberrant and rearranged chromosomes (German, 1969). Although these diseases are quite different in their clinical manifestations, they have another feature in common: both often lead to the development of leukemia or malignant neoplasms relatively early in life.

g. Etiology

Experimentally, various agents have been shown to cause chromosomal abnormalities in normal mammalian cells (Nowell, 1969); these agents include ionizing radiation, viruses, chemicals, and immunologic injury. Some of these agents are likely to have a role in the pathogenesis of inborn human chromosomal abnormalities, but evidence for such relationships is as yet indirect and far from conclusive.

Irradiation of the gonads of experimental animals has been shown to cause inborn chromosomal abnormalities in their offspring. An increased incidence of trisomy in the children of women who have had diagnostic abdominal irradiation before pregnancy suggests an analogous mechanism in humans (Uchida *et al.,* 1968). Suggestive, too, is a study which shows an increased occurrence of various chromosomal aberrations in cells derived from persons who had been exposed *in utero* to radiation from atomic explosives (Bloom *et al.,* 1968).

Many viruses have been shown to be potent inducers of chromosomal lesions experimentally and, as in the case of neoplasia, a viral etiology for human inborn chromosomal abnormalities has been suggested (Nichols, 1966). It is certainly possible that clinical or subclinical maternal infection could give rise to aberrant meiosis in the ovum or aberrant mitosis in the zygote or early embryo. Reports of seasonally related space-time clusters or "outbreaks" of inborn chromosomal abnormalities are consistent with such a hypothesis (Day, 1966). Epidemiologic data have been interpreted as demonstrating a relationship between "epidemics" of infectious hepatitis and the increased incidence of Down's syndrome in infants born nine months after such epidemics (Stroller, 1969).

Although a wide spectrum of biologic and non-biologic chemicals have been shown to cause a wide variety of chromosomal abnormalities in mammalian cells, there is as yet no direct evidence that any chemical is responsible for inborn human chromosomal aberrations. Altered maternal immune mechanisms have also been suggested as a factor in the etiology of chromosomal aberrations; it has been reported, for example, that mothers of Down's syndrome patients have an increased incidence of thyroid auto-antibodies (Fialkow, 1966).

The obvious difficulty in establishing an etiological role for these and other suggested agents of inborn chromosomal abnormalities reflects the difficulties inherent to the study of early normal and abnormal mammalian and human development. Unless such an etiologic relationship is overwhelmingly clear, interpretations of retrospective and even prospective studies are fraught with danger. Some of these difficulties may be circumvented by the study of early mammalian development *in vitro.* Mammalian ova, zygotes, and very early embryos have been successfully maintained in culture and, in one instance, a specific agent (the antibiotic, Streptonigrin) has been shown to enter the immature mouse ovum and cause chromosomal abnormalities during meiosis (Jagiello, 1967). The successful application of such techniques to human material (Edwards *et al.,* 1969) will undoubtedly be exploited along these lines.

4. Challenge of the future

The past two decades have witnessed a steady progression in our understanding of basic biological mechanisms in terms of cellular, subcellular, and molecular structure and function. The use of ever more refined methods of morphologic, genetic, biochemical, and physical-chemical analysis continues to define the nature and arrangement of genetic information, the mechanisms by which this information is replicated and expressed, and the system of controls which affect and effect these phenomena. Much of this knowledge is derived from the study of the microbial systems.

The application of the spectacular successes of microbial biology to human genetics presents an exciting prospect to the human biologist. The difficulties of such an endeavour are obvious, but, some of them may be circumvented by the use of cell culture (Priest, 1968; Mellman and Kohn, 1970). Lines of "fibroblast-like" cells derived from human biopsies can be maintained *in vitro.* These cells retain the chromosomal and biochemical properties of the host's fibroblasts, and they can be manipulated under controlled conditions in ways similar to bacterial cultures.

The study of microbial molecular biology has been facilitated by the inspired exploitation of naturally occurring and experimentally induced genetic markers or mutations. As we have seen, there are abundant examples of such genetic markers in the human population in the form of protein polymorphism, inborn disorders of metabolism, and chromosomal abnormalities. Many of these markers are carried over to cells in culture, where they can be used to elucidate normal, variant, and pathologic genetically determined biologic functions.

Thus far, the major effort in cell culture has been applied to the demonstration of specific metabolic or chromosomal aberrations. Cultured fibroblasts obtained from patients with Niemann-Pick disease are deficient in sphingomyelinase, and cells obtained from patients with Trisomy G contain an extra G group chromosome. Cells from patients with Lesch-Nyhan syndrome have been used to elucidate the specific enzymatic defect characteristic of that disease. Cells from patients with certain of the inherited disorders of metabolism stain metachromatically with toluidine blue. This characteristic is also seen to a lesser degree in cells derived from heterozygotes and is used in the identification of such phenotypically normal carriers. The prenatal diagnosis of inherited disorders of metabolism and chromosomal abnormalities is accomplished by the demonstration of these defects in cultured amniotic cells (Nadler, 1969).

The use of genetic markers will eventually achieve the goal of mapping the human genome, possibly through the use of selective cell hybridization or the experimental induction of specific chromosomal deletions and recombinations (Renwick, 1969).

The prevention and therapy of the diseases associated with genetically determined inborn variation are major goals of biomedical science. Prevention of the disease states themselves is limited, as yet, to genetic counseling of prospective parents and therapeutic abortion of demonstrably affected fetuses. In a few of the metabolic disorders, early diagnosis and treatment can prevent some of the significant clinical manifestations. Deletion of phenylalanine from the diet of infants with phenylketonuria significantly retards the development of mental retardation, and supplementation of the diet of patients with hereditary orotic aciduria corrects the anemia associated with this disease. Few of the metabolic disorders and none of the chromosomal abnormalities are at present amenable to therapy and most are progressive and invariably fatal.

A number of possible approaches to prevention and therapy warrant investigation (Lowe, 1969; Scriver, 1969a). The enzyme (and other protein) deficiencies, for example, may be treated by administration of the deficient enzyme, as in the treatment of diabetics with insulin. For a variety of reasons, this most obvious and direct approach has not been feasible. Many of the enzymes in question have been only partially purified, are not readily available, and are rapidly degraded *in vivo*. Some of these difficulties may be avoided by using new techniques of *in vitro* protein synthesis to produce polypeptides with the desired enzymatic activity and with increased biologic lifespans. Another possibility involves the administration of enzymes in a "protected" state. Catalase molecules, for example, have been enclosed within semipermeable microcapsules consisting of a synthetic polymer. The capsule protects the enzyme from degradation but allows the entry of small molecules such as the substrates of catalase. This technique has been successfully applied to the treatment of a genetically determined deficiency of catalase in mice (Chang and Poznansky, 1968); it has not been used in human acatalasemia.

In the enzyme deficiencies which are due to abnormalities of control mechanisms, one might hope to be able to bypass the defective controller and "turn on" the deficient enzyme activity. An example of this possibility has been previously discussed in the case of hereditary orotic aciduria, in which production of the deficient enzymes can be induced in cell culture.

Ultimately, one hopes to replace an absent or defective segment of the genome in a process analogous to bacterial transformation. Small segments of intact template will be inoculated into deficient cells in culture and the cultured cells returned to the host. The introduction of small segments of genetic material may be accomplished by using innocuous "carrier" viruses. Another possibility is the *in vitro* mating of enzymatically sufficient and deficient cells, and the selection of sufficient progeny for administration. The problems involved in such feats of genetic engineering are obviously quite formidable.

The chromosomal abnormalities are acquired during gametogenesis or during mitosis in the zygote or its immediate derivatives, and many of their manifestations are already present very early in development. Their eradication rests upon an increased understanding of such processes as chromosomal replication, breakage, repair, and segregation, and upon the identification and elimination of etiologic factors which cause disarrangements in these processes.

C. Non-Genetic Biologic Variations: Teratology

Thus far, inborn human variation has been discussed in terms of genetically determined alterations. A great deal of human variation, however, is the consequence of alterations at other levels of biologic activity. These account for a large percentage of birth defects. In these instances, the presence of genetic damage is tentatively excluded by the failure to demonstrate chromosomal abnormalities or inheritance of the variant trait. It must be emphasized, however, that the absence of such findings does not completely preclude the participation of genetic phenomena; genetic damage may play a role which is simply undetectable at present.

The emergence of the newborn is the culmination of an exquisitely timed series of integrated anatomic and biochemical events. Although this process occurs within a relatively well protected environment, even this environment is not free of hazards (Ferreira, 1969). Alterations of the environment may occur at any time between formation of the gamete and birth. Their effects are most obvious when they produce injury or death. Injuries occurring during fertilization, implantation, or early embryogenesis probably account for a large number of unsuccesful pregnancies. Since they occur so early in development, they are usually unrecognized and their true incidence is unknown. Lethal injuries occurring later in pregnancy are recognized as spontaneous abortions and as many as 25 per cent of all detectable pregnancies terminate in this way. Sublethal injury may occur in the fetus or newborn because of hypoxia, malnutrition, hormonal, vitamin, or electrolyte imbalance, and so on, and can result in a variety of more or less well defined anatomic and physiologic abnormalities.

Teratology refers to the study of congenital malformations: anatomic abnormalities which result from aberrant morphogenesis of specific tissues, organs, and organ systems. As we have seen, teratologic malformations are a frequent manifestation of inherited and acquired genetic lesions; frequently, however, environmental alterations and injury occurring during critical periods of development are responsible. Specific tissues and organs are particularly susceptible during periods of accelerated growth or when they are undergoing the alterations and rearrangements implicit to the formation of new anatomic structures. The heart and its attendant great vessels undergo profound changes during the fourth and fifth weeks of gestation; sublethal injury occurring at this time can result in a wide variety of congenital cardiac and vascular malformations.

In addition to timing, the nature of the environmental alteration is of obvious importance in determining the type and extent of fetal injury. Some agents may act only on specific targets, while others may be unselective in their ability to cause injury. A particular agent which is target-selective may produce no injury if it appears at a time when the target is not susceptible. Conversely, an unselective agent which is present over a long period of gestational time may give rise to a variety of congenital malformations involving multiple organs.

The catalogue of congenital malformations in man is enormous and includes almost every structure in the body. Some malformations are incompatible with prenatal life and others with postnatal survival. Some are compatible with life but cause severe disability, and still others are of no apparent consequence and may be incidental findings at autopsy in nonagenarians. Congenital malformations may occur singly or in random association, and sometimes they are found in characteristic patterns within individuals.

The true incidence of congenital malformations is unknown, and reports vary with the source of material (abortuses, newborns, adults), means of investigation (clinical, autopsy, death certificate), and location of the study (geography, hospital population, socio-economic groups). One meaningful statistic is that 2-3 per cent of all liveborn babies have malformations which are clinically recognizable at birth and are of some medical significance (Warkany and Kalter, 1961). Additional defects become manifest later in life, and by one year of age this figure has risen to 5 per cent. The incidence in abortuses and stillborns is much higher. The frequency with which congenital malformations occur in the general population is indicated by their discovery in nearly half of a large series of unselected autopsies; of these about 50 per cent were considered to be of clinical significance (Sotelo-Avila and Shanklin, 1967).

An extensive list of environmental alterations and specific agents or teratogens have been implicated in the etiology of non-genetically determined congenital malformations. Many have been shown to cause malformations in experimental animals, and some of these serve as experimental models for similar or identical malformations in humans. In addition, there are several examples of human malformation in which a clear-cut etiologic relationship has been established; of these, perhaps the best studied is rubella syndrome (Cooper, 1968)

1. Intrauterine infection

A relationship between maternal rubella and the occurrence of congenital malformations was first recognized in 1941 by Gregg, an Australian ophthalmologist; this relationship has been subsequently confirmed by extensive epidemiologic analyses, by serologic studies, and more recently, by isolation of the virus from the tissues of affected fetuses and newborns. The clinical syndrome includes cataracts, congenital heart disease, and a variety of other malformations. The fetus of a mother who is infected during the first trimester runs a high risk of being diseased. The consequences may range from spontaneous abortion of a severely malformed fetus to birth of an infant with little impairment. It has been estimated that the rubella epidemic which occurred in the United States in 1964 resulted in as many as 30,000 malformed babies.

When pregnant experimental animals are inoculated with rubella virus, the results are fetal infection and the production of malformations similar to those which occur in humans. This virus does not appear to be particularly cytopathic, either *in vivo* or in tissue culture; it does, however, appear to cause significant retardation of cell growth (Plotkin and Vaheri, 1967). Such growth retardation, occurring during critical periods of development, presumably accounts for at least part of the spectrum of congenital malformations. Rubella also gives rise to chronic infection and can exert its effects over long periods of time; it has been recovered from children years after the initial intrauterine infection.

The demonstration that maternal infection with rubella can be transmitted to the fetus and can cause congenital malformations has led to intensive searches for other examples (Elizan and Fabiyi, 1970; Sever and White, 1968). Herpes virus and cytomegalovirus, as well as toxoplasma have been shown to cause human congenital malformations; other infectious agents have been implicated as well. The potential role of maternal infection in causing fetal disease is becoming increasingly apparent. Perhaps 5 per cent of all pregnancies are complicated by one or more clinical infections in the mother (in addition to the common cold), and this figure is amplified to an unknown extent by inapparent subclinical or chronic infection. Furthermore, organisms which are ordinarily non-pathogenic for adults can have a significant effect upon the fetus. Recent serologic studies suggest that fetal infection is a far more common phenomenon than has been suspected.

2. Chemical and environmental teratogens

A broad spectrum of exogenous chemicals has been shown to cause congenital malformations in animals and occasionally in man (Smithells, 1966). Thousands of cases of severe malformation have been ascribed to the administration of the sedative thalidomide to pregnant women in Europe. Anomalies of the limbs were particularly prominent in these cases, and the occurrence of these anomalies has been correlated with administration of the drug during a particular two week period in gestation (Nowack, 1965). During this period, limb morphogenesis is particularly active and apparently susceptible to injury.

Other experimental teratogenic agents include various antibiotics and antimetabolites, anti-thyroid drugs, and corticosteroids; for some of these, a role in human malformation has been demonstrated. Even the ubiquitous acetylsalicylic acid (aspirin) can, under certain conditions, produce malformations in mice and rats, but teratogenic effects in humans have not been demonstrated. Possible teratogenic effects of LSD and other psychoactive drugs are being intensively investigated.

Other exogenous agents may play a significant role in the etiology of fetal diseases and malformation; these include food additives and preservatives, cigarette smoke, herbicides and pesticides, industrial waste products, and other environmental pollutants. In the Minimata Bay area of Japan, a correlation has been demonstrated between a congenital neurologic disorder and the ingestion, by pregnant women, of seafood from the bay. This seafood was heavily contaminated by neurotoxic industrial waste products, methyl mercury compounds (Matsumoto *et al.,* 1965). Another exogenous agent, radiation, is usually discussed in terms of chromosomal damage; yet its injurious effects are extragenomic as well. It may prove to be a significant cause of non-genetic fetal disease (Brill and Forgotson, 1964).

3. Maternal factors

The fetus depends upon an intact maternal metabolism, and changes in maternal health can have profound effects upon the developing fetus. Toxemia of pregnancy, maternal diabetes, malnutrition, and cardiac and renal disease increase the likelihood of fetal death, prematurity, growth retardation and malformation. The fetal-placental-maternal hormonal relationship is a delicate and highly integrated one in which a single alteration can be expected to affect the fetus in a variety of ways (Solomon and Friesen, 1968). Any factor, exogenous, maternal, or placental, which reduces oxygen or nutrient supply or the elimination of wastes, or upsets delicate metabolic balances will also affect the fetus (Gruenwald, 1968). Morphologic alterations in the placenta are known to take part in the pathogenesis of fetal disease. It has become increasingly apparent that this organ plays an active role in fetal homeostasis, such as in the active transport of specific molecules and the synthesis of hormones and other important compounds. Disorders of specific placental functions will become apparent as mechanisms of normal function are elucidated.

Fetus and trophoblast have an immunologic status similar to that of a homograft since they contain paternally determined antigens, some of which are foreign to the mother (Lanman, 1965). Although the fetal homograft is protected by the anatomic separation of the fetal-maternal circulations, this separation is not absolute, and cells have been shown to cross this barrier in either direction. While immunologic rejection of the fetus has not been observed, it must be considered as a possibility in the etiology of fetal wastage and malformation.

4. Conclusion

Genetic and non-genetic influences may so damage human development that the biologic variation produced is responsible for much disease, disability, and death. On the other hand, very minor variations can be identified which seem to have no effect on the ability of the host to function in his milieu.

Somewhere between these two extremes may lie a spectrum of inborn human variation whose existence is unproven, whose nature is unknown, and whose effects upon the host are undetermined. It may be genetically and/or non-genetically determined. Its effects may be indirect, subtle, or delayed. Its expression may depend upon a unique concert of other inborn as well as postnatal environmental factors, without which the variant may never have an opportunity for expression. Such a hidden interplay between genetic and environmental factors is illustrated by experiments in which the administration of cortisol to pregnant mice results in cleft-palate in the offspring. This effect, however, is seen only in certain inbred strains of mice and not in others (Smithberg, 1967).

Individual propensities for the development of certain diseases later in life may be a function of inborn variation; such variation might provide the correct setting for the action of various extrinsic agents in the etiology of such diseases as cancer, atherosclerosis, emphysema, hypertension, and mental illness. Environmentally conditioned inborn variation may, in addition, play a role in determining individual uniqueness with regard to various biologic, psychologic, and social functions—aging, intelligence, specific aptitudes, talents, and so on. Provocative hints of such remote relationships are beginning to appear (Brozek, 1966). The documentation of additional examples of inborn variation and of their significance in postnatal as well as prenatal life will undoubtedly be forthcoming.

References

Apgar, V., and Stickle, G. (1968), Birth defects: their significance as a public health problem, J. Am. Med. Assoc., *204*:371.

Bearn, A. G., and Parker, W. C. (1965), Genetics and evolution in three human serum proteins, *in* New Directions in Human Genetics. Birth Defects Original Article Series, *1*:57.

Bloom, A. D. *et al.* (1968), Cytogenetics of the *in utero* exposed of Hiroshima and Nagasaki, Lancet, *II*:10.

Brady, R. O. (1966), The sphingolipidoses, New Eng. J. Med., *275*:312.

Brent, R. L. (1966), Immunologic aspects of developmental biology, Adv. Teratol., *1*:82.

Brill, A. B., and Forgotson, E. H. (1964), Radiation and congenital malformations, Amer. J. Ob. Gyn., *90*:1149.

Brozek, J. (1966), The biology of human variation, Ann. N.Y. Acad. Sci., *134*:497.

Carpenter, G. G., Auerbach, V. H., and DiGeorge, A. M. (1968), Phenylalaninemia, Ped. Clin. N. Amer. *15*:313.

Carr, D. H. (1969a), Chromosomal abnormalities in clinical medicine, Prog. Med. Gen., *6*:1.

Carr, D. H. (1969b), Chromosomal errors and development, Amer. J. Ob. Gyn., *104*:327.

Carr, D. H. (1969c), Lethal chromosome errors, *in* Comparative Mammalian Cytogenetics, K. Benirschke, Ed., Springer, New York.

Chang, T. M. S., and Poznansky, M. J. (1968), Semipermeable microcapsules containing catalase for enzyme replacement in acatalasemic mice, Nature, *218*:243.

Chicago Conference (1966), Standardization in Human Cytogenetics, Birth Defects: Original article series, Vol. II, No. 2.

Childs, B., and Der Kaloustian, V. M. (1968), Genetic heterogeneity, New Eng. J. Med., *279*:1205, 1267.

Childs, B. (1970), Sir Archibald Garrod's conception of chemical individuality: a modern appreciation, New Eng. J. Med., *282*:71.

Clegg, J. B. *et al.* (1968), Hemoglobin synthesis in betathalassemia, Nature, *220*:664.

Cooper, L. Z. (1968), Rubella: a preventable cause of birth defects, Birth Defects: Original article series, Vol. IV, No. 7, p. 23.

Day, R. W. (1966), The epidemiology of chromosome aberrations, Am. J. Hum. Gen., *18*:70.

Dreyfus, J. C. (1969), The application of bacterial genetics to the study of human genetic abnormalities, Prog. Med. Gen., *6*:169.

Edwards, R. G., Bavister, B. D., and Steptoe, P. C. (1969), Early stages of fertilization *in vitro* of human oocytes matured *in vitro,* Nature, *221*:632.

Elizan, T. S., and Fabiyi, A. (1970), Congenital and neonatal anomalies linked with viral infections in experimental animals, Amer. J. Ob. Gyn., *106*:147.

Ferriera, A. J. (1969), Perinatal Environment, Charles C Thomas Co., Springfield, Ill.

Fialkow, P. J. (1966), Autoimmunity and chromosomal aberrations, Amer. J. Hum. Gen., *18*:93.

Franklin, E. C. (1967), Genetic polymorphism of gamma globulins in man, Amer. J. Med., *43*:1.

German, J. (1969), Chromosomal breakage syndromes, Birth Defects: original article series, Vol. 5, No. 5, p. 117.

Gruenwald, P. (1968), Deprivation of the human fetus: forms, causes, significance, *in* Diagnosis and Treatment of Fetal Disorders, K. Adamsons, Ed., Springer-Verlag, New York.

Harris, H. (1966), Genes and enzymes in man, Cancer Res., *26*:2054.

Harris, H. (1969), Enzyme and protein polymorphism in human populations, Brit. Med. Bul., *25*:5.

Hers, H. G., and Van Hoof, F. (1970), The genetic pathology of lysosomes, *in* Progress in Liver Disease, Vol. III, H. Popper and F. Schaffner, Eds., Grune and Stratton, New York.

Hsia, D. Y. Y. (1967), Clinical variants of galactosemia, Metabol., *16*:419.

Jacobs, P. A. (1969), Structural abnormalities of the sex chromosomes, Brit. Med. Bul., *25*:94.

Jagiello, G. (1967), Streptonigrin: effect on the first meiotic metaphase of the mouse egg, Science, *157*:453.

Kelley, W. N. *et al.* (1969), Hypoxanthine-guanine phosphoribosyl transferase deficiency in gout, Ann. Int. Med., *157*:453.

Kohn, G. *et al.* (1970), Mosaic mongolism, J. Ped., *76*:874.

LaDu, B. N., Jr. (1969), Pharmacogenetics, Med. Clin. N. Amer., *53*:839.

LaDu, B. N., Jr. (1967), Genetic variation in metabolic disorders, *in* Amino Acid Metabolism and Genetic Variation, W. L. Nyhan, Ed., McGraw-Hill, New York.

Lanman, J. T. (1965), Transplantation immunity in mammalian pregnancy; Mechanisms of fetal protection against immunologic rejection, J. Ped., *66*:525.

Lowe, C. U. (1969), Modification of human metabolism, Amer. J. Dis. Child., *118*:817.

Mathai, C. K., and Beutler, E. (1966), Electrophoretic variation of galactose-1-phosphate uridyltransferase, Science, *154*:1179.

Matsumoto, H. Koya, G., and Takeuchi, T. (1965), Fetal Minimata disease, J. Neuropath. Exp. Neurol., *24*:563.

Mellman, W. J., and Kohn, G. (1970), Human cell cultures–their use in the investigation and diagnosis of disease, Med. Clin. N. Amer., *54*:701.

Migeon, B. R. *et al.* (1968), X-linked hypoxanthine-guanine phosphoribosyl transferase deficiency: heterozygote has two clonal populations, Science, *160*:425.

Murayama, M. (1967), Structure of sickle cell hemoglobin and molecular mechanism of the sickling phenomena, Clin. Chem., *13*:578.

Nadler, H. L. (1969), Prenatal detection of genetic defects, J. Ped., *74*:132.

Nichols, W. W. (1966), The role of viruses in the etiology of chromosomal abnormalities, Amer. J. Hum. Gen., *18*:81.

Nowack, E. (1965), The sensitive phase of thalidomide embryopathy, Humangenetik, *1*:516.

Nowell, P. C. (1969), The biological significance of induced human chromosomal abnormalities, Fed. Proc., *28*:1796.

Oski, F. A. *et al.* (1969), Congenital hemolytic anemia with high-sodium, low-potassium red cells, New Eng. J. Med., *280*:909.

Pauling, L. (1964), Molecular evolution and disease, Bull. N.Y. Acad. Sci., *40*:1.

Pinsky, L., and Krooth, R. S. (1967), Studies on the control of pyrimidine biosynthesis in human diploid cell strain, Proc. Natl. Acad. Sci., *47*:925, 1267.

Plotkin, S. A., and Vaheri, A. (1967), Human fibroblasts infected with rubella virus produce a growth inhibitor, Science, *156*:659.

Price, J. (1967), Human polymorphism, J. Med. Gen., *4*:44.

Priest, J. H. (1968), Human cell culture: an important tool for the diagnosis and understanding of disease, J. Ped., *72*:415.

Proceedings of the Seminars on the Lesch-Nyhan Syndrome (1968), Fed. Proc. *27*:1021.

Ranney, H. M. (1960), Clinically important variants of human hemoglobin, New Eng. J. Med., *282*:144.

Redding, A., and Hirschhorn, K. (1968), Guide to Human Chromosome Defects, Birth Defects, Original article series, Vol. IV., No. 4.

Renwick, A. (1969), Progress in mapping human autosomes, Brit. Med. Bul., *25*:65.

Scriver, C. R. (1969a), Treatment of inherited diseases: realized and potential, Med. Clin. N. Amer., *53*:941.

Scriver, C. R. (1969b), The human biochemical genetics of amino acid transport, Ped., *44*:348.

Sever, J., and White, L. R. (1968), Intrauterine viral infections, Ann. Rev. Med., *18*:471.

Smith, L. M., Jr., Huguley, C. M., Jr., Bain, J. A. (1966), Hereditary orotic aciduria, *in* The Metabolic Basis of Inherited Disease, J. B. Stanbury, Ed., Blakiston Co., New York.

Smithberg, M. (1967), Teratogenesis in inbred strains of mice, Adv. Teratol., *2*:258.

Smithells, R. W. (1966), Drugs and human malformations, Adv. Teratol., *1*:251.

Solomon, S., and Friesen, M. G. (1968), Endocrine relations between mother and fetus, Ann. Rev. Med., *19*:399.

Sotelo-Avila, C., and Shanklin, D. R. (1967), Congenital malformations in an autopsy population, Arch. Path., *84*:272.

Stewart, A. L. *et al.* (1969), A chromosome study of unselected live-born children with congenital anomalies, J. Ped., *74*:449.

Stoller, A. (1969), Virus-chromosome interaction as a possible cause of cases of Down's syndrome and other congenital anomalies, Adv. Teratol., *3*:113.

Tschudy, D. P. (1969), Porphyrin metabolism and the porphyrias, *in* Disease of Metabolism, P. K. Bondy, Ed., W. B. Saunders Co., Philadelphia.

Uchida, I. A., Holunga, R., and Lawler, C. (1968), Maternal radiation and chromosome aberrations, Lancet, *II*:1045.

Walzer, S., Breau, G., and Gerald, P. S. (1969), A chromosome survey of 2,400 normal newborn infants, J. Ped., *74*:438.

Warkany, J., and Kalter, H. (1961), Congenital malformations, New Eng. J. Med., *265*:993.

Weatherall, D. J. (1967), The thalassemias, Prog. Med. Gen., *5*:8.

Wyngarden, J. B. (1970), Genetic control of enzyme activity in higher organisms, Biochem. Gen., *4*:105.

INDEX